⌐ on or before
below.

The Nervous System

Its Function and Its Interaction with the World

The Nervous System

Its Function and Its Interaction with the World

Lloyd D. Partridge and L. Donald Partridge

A Bradford Book
The MIT Press
Cambridge, Massachusetts
London, England

This book was set in Times Roman and Helvetica by DEKR Corporation and was printed and bound in the United States of America.

Library of Congress Cataloging-in-Publication Data

Partridge, Lloyd D., 1922–
  The nervous system : its function and its interaction with the
world / Lloyd D. Partridge, L. Donald Partridge.
  p. cm.
  "A Bradford book."
  Includes bibliographical references and index.
  ISBN 0-262-16134-6 (hc). — ISBN 0-262-66079-2 (pbk.)
  1. Neurophysiology.   I. Partridge, L. Donald.   II. Title.
[DNLM: 1. Nervous System—physiology.   WL 102 P275n]
QP355.2.P37   1992
591.1'88—dc20
DNLM/DLC
for Library of Congress   92-6225
                                                            CIP

Contents

Preface

Science and art are arguably the most intrinsic of human activities in which we engage. The English word "science" derives from the Latin word *scire*, meaning to know. A host of other English words concerning knowledge spring from this root: conscious, from sharing knowledge; innocent, from not knowing; and omniscient, from all knowing. Perhaps only in humans, and certainly to the highest degree in humans, do we encounter the native curiosity necessary to acquire knowledge about nature purely for the sake of that knowledge. The directing of this curiosity toward ourselves, and in particular toward the function of our brains, has always held a special place in the quest for knowledge.

Through the ages, the methods by which we obtain knowledge of nature have changed. Much of our approach derives from the philosophy of Sir Francis Bacon, who in 1620 wrote in the *Novum Organum* that "Man, as the minister and interpreter of nature, does and understands as much as his observations on the order of nature, either with regard to things or the mind, permit him, and neither knows nor is capable of more." Although recent studies of dynamic systems are posing a challenge to this method of obtaining knowledge, we still generally adopt Bacon's empirical approach to science.

A book on the science of neurophysiology might be expected to serve as a compendium of refined empirical observations about the function of the nervous system. But there are two serious problems with writing any such compendium. First, the act of writing itself tends to validate what is written. Thus, when published, empirical observations and working hypotheses often solidify to become scientific facts. Second, writing removes the author from any subsequent discourse. The reader lacks recourse for question or discussion. Perhaps this is why Plato favored expressing his ideas as dialogues.

Scientific method is a cycle consisting of empirical observations, hypothesis formation, and hypothesis testing through further observation. We would like, in this book, to interject the reader into this cycle. We will present many empirical observations and some currently accepted hypotheses. We hope to entice the reader to test some of these hypotheses through his or her observations. Sometimes we have suggested demonstrations or experiments that might lead to pro-vocative empirical observations. Sometimes we have suggested that the reader form hypotheses from his or her existing observations. At other times we leave it to the curiosity that derives from a questioning and discerning mind to lead the reader to make observations and to form working hypotheses. The reader should never accept a purely passive position, but rather should be like Luigi Galvani, the premier electrophysiologist, who performed experiments because "I was fired with incredible zeal and desire of having the same experience, and of bringing to light whatever might be concealed in the phenomenon" (*De Viribus Electricitatis in Motu Musculari Commentarius*).

Part of the philosophical legacy that we have inherited from Aristotle is the separation of biological science into function and form. Of this perhaps arbitrary division, he wrote: "Instances of what I mean by functions and affections are Reproduction, Growth, Copulation, Waking, Sleep, Locomotion, and other sim-ilar vital actions. Instances of what I mean by parts are Nose, Eye, Face, and other so-called members or limbs, and also the more elementary parts of which these are made" (*De Partibus Animulium*). Although we might argue against this dichotomy altogether, its application has usually given a primary role to form. Thus, neurophysiology is generally presented as "functional neuroanatomy." Carried to its extreme, the logical extension of this thinking would be that the unique connectivity of each neuron imparts on that neuron a unique function. We are accepting a very different premise in this book, namely that understanding of function can exist in isolation from study of structural localizations. Rather than focus on location, we shall emphasize the classes of information processing that underlie the variety of nervous system functions.

We hope to establish some dialogue with our active readers, to provoke some interaction in the communication of the observations and hypotheses about the function of the nervous system. Perhaps the best place to begin is with the central premise of this book: Do you believe that a significant body of information exists about neural function that can be understood without a consideration of the specific location at which it is accomplished?

Acknowledgments

This writing adventure has been possible because of the skepticism, ideas, and support of many individuals. Our view of the nervous system has grown through hundreds of discussions at scientific meetings, in classrooms, and in university hallways. Two groups have provided especially useful forums for discussion: the group organized by Stan Franklin and others in Memphis, and the neuroscience group in Albuquerque. We appreciate the insight, recommendations, and technical help of Terence Barrett, Donald Cooper, Jim Emerson-Cobb, Evelyn Gladney, Anna Korzeniowska, Joel Neely, Reinhold Penner, Stella Thomas, Gerald Weiss, and Gaynor Wild, and the guidance of the editorial staff at The MIT Press. We express gratitude to our wives and family for tolerance, support, and suggestions. Finally, we would like to thank our students who have asked the provocative questions that led us to undertake this project.

The Nervous System

Its Function and Its Interaction with the World

Chapter 1

Introduction

Rational facilities have been associated with the brain from at least as far into antiquity as Plato. Over the intervening centuries the understanding of the means of this association has changed repeatedly. Our current curiosity about nervous system function has extended the bounds of neuroscience research to topics spanning a spectrum from the function of single molecules to human social interaction.

The nervous system has a special controlling or modifying action over most body functions although its cells depend on the same metabolic processes as do other cells.

The following is a sample of some functions in which the nervous system is involved. The nervous system gives to an individual characteristics that distinguish one personality from another, it controls constriction of the pupil in bright light, it modifies pituitary activity, it coordinates the thousands of muscle units that produce an individual speech phoneme, it reports that a finger is so hot that tissue damage is imminent, it speeds the heart rate during exercise, it holds the urinary sphincter closed for hours, it contracts tiny muscles that increase insulating effectiveness of fur and cause "goose bumps," and it processes information that leads to a scientific discovery or a musical composition. With a moment's reflection, you should be able to add many more items to this list. The neurologist, physical therapist, ophthalmologist, psychologist, electroencephalographer, rehabilitation engineer, neurosurgeon, or psychiatrist has an obvious need to understand nervous system function. Although at times less obviously, nervous system function plays an important role in most other medical and paramedical fields. This is true even without the more subtle consideration that both a patient's complaints and a medical person's responses are products of the function of their respective nervous systems. So, as an example, our current understanding of internal medicine problems such as those resulting from loss of ions with sweating, vomiting, or diarrhea is closely tied to information about cell membranes that was originally acquired in the study of giant nerve fibers of the squid. We will later devote a whole chapter to the interactions between certain ions and large, specialized molecules in cell membranes, interactions that have common characteristics in tissues as diverse as nerve fibers, heart muscle, or kidney tubules.

Usually the investigators who have studied principles of neural function have expected these functions to have survival value, and this bias has affected the design of experiments and the observations of phenomena. There exists a bias in neuroscience toward those phenomena that seem logical in the eyes of the orthodox scientific community. Students can usually take advantage of this superimposed logic as a mnemonic aid in studying neuroscience. One needs to remember, though, that evolution may not have been constrained to the same logic. One must always be cautious to avoid the teleological argument that some function exists specifically to accomplish some particular end. It is always safer to consider some function's *survival value* rather than its *purpose*. Scientific beliefs, as well as beliefs in other areas of human endeavor, grow out of whatever general framework of human knowledge is currently accepted. When part of the general framework changes, as it has in the past and will undoubtedly do in the future, those beliefs previously held to be logical may become absurd. For those who would do useful research in neuroscience, it is necessary to be prepared to change some accepted understandings. Each user of neuroscience must be continually prepared for revision of what he or she understands of specific examples and of general concepts.

Any course of neurophysiology should be considered no more than a foundation on which to build further study of the ever-changing details of our understanding of neuroscience.

We shall not attempt to touch on the many implications of neural function in biomedical fields. Even less can we describe the details of the different functions of the various parts of the nervous system. Yet we shall attempt to bring together a collection of principles from which a working understanding of total neural function can be developed.

The student wishing to pursue particular topics beyond the coverage given here will ordinarily find it advisable to move next to those detailed review articles in which the coverage is more complete than is appropriate for a textbook. Some sources of review articles are the five volumes that make up Section I of the *Handbook of Physiology* entitled "The Nervous System." More specialized topics are found in journals such as *Physiological Reviews, Annual Reviews of Neuroscience,* and *Trends in Neuroscience.* The student should try to find more than one article on the topic of interest since, in spite of careful review and an attempt to be critical, each paper will inevitably emphasize the author's biases.

One journal has an unusual approach that is particularly useful to the person attempting to learn about an unfamiliar area of neuroscience. *Behavioral and Brain Research* publishes a small number of presentations, each dealing with some current subject of controversy. A target paper is written that takes a stand on a particular issue. Then a diverse group of experts in related fields is asked to write commentaries and criticisms of this target paper. The original authors are then given the opportunity to write a rebuttal or comment on these essays. The whole set is published as a single package. This collection can provide a breadth of understanding and recognition of differences that ordinarily would require extended reading through widely scattered publications.

After getting a general feel for the issues and problems in a field, one can read more critically the original research papers and specialized monographs. Those primary sources will, in part, have been identified in the bibliographies of the review papers, but they also can be found by forward and backward searching from them using standard library search methods. Finally, an attempt to duplicate or extend the experimental work described in the literature will give leads to further study that cannot be gained by any amount of unsupported reading.

1.1* Problem: Use one of the papers cited in this book to solve the following problems.

1. Make a single step of *backward search,* that is, list the references cited in the chosen paper. How many sources are cited?

2. What range of publication dates is represented by the citations found?

3. Use a reference publication such as *Science Citation Index* in printed or electronic form to make a single step *forward search.* List titles and references for all papers that you can find that refer to your chosen publication.

*An asterisk following the number of a problem or experiment indicates that further discussion can be found in the Notes section at the end of the book.

4. Are there any overlaps in references found in your forward and backward searches?

5. Why does the use of a combination of a single step of forward and backward search from a single paper leave a gap in the period in which related papers could be found? How can the search be extended to cover this gap?

The nervous system generally has little value in dealing with stationary conditions but provides an animal with the ability to adjust to changing conditions.

The nervous system contributes to the survival of an animal by its action in adjusting responses to varying environmental conditions. In doing this, the nervous system acquires information about those conditions and, after processing this information, generates controlling signals that modify a multitude of individual responses of the animal. These adjustments are important when the conditions change over time and, in fact, the nervous system is especially sensitive to change.

Next to the separation of biochemical processes from the environment by the cell membrane, one of the most critical developments for survival in diverse environments is the ability of a cell or an animal actively to alter its functions in the face of changes in the environment. This ability results from the most basic of nervous system characteristics, *excitability*. Many cells exhibit some excitability, but it is the neurons, receptors (sense organs), and effectors (muscles and glands) of the nervous system that show the property of excitability to the greatest degree. All other actions of the nervous system are dependent on the results of excitation.

Excitation is a process by which a cell changes one of its characteristics, usually an electrical potential, in response to a change in some external factor acting on the cell. There are four important characteristics of this response to a change in the environment: (1) it occurs following a considerably smaller change than would be necessary to damage the cell; (2) it is reversible, allowing the cell to return to the unexcited state on cessation of the environmental change; (3) it is usually graded, being of greater magnitude when the environmental change is of greater magnitude; and (4) it always involves an exchange of energy between the stimulating agent and the excited cell, but the response exceeds the simple passive effects of the stimulus energy.

1.2 Problem

1. Identify a nonbiological process that meets the characteristics of biological excitability.

2. Modify the description of excitability so that it is still biologically accurate but now excludes some functional characteristics of the identified nonbiological case. With this modified definition, return to part (1).

(You may choose to leave this problem before completing it.)

The nervous system contains certain elements that are specialized to move information from a site of origin to more remote points of utilization.

In multicellular animals, most responses to stimuli are accomplished by cells remote from the location of the stimulus. For example, contact of a toe with a tack is likely to produce a response in the thigh muscles. *Conduction* of the effect of excitation is a second function of the nervous system. As Hermann von Helmholtz showed in the midnineteenth century (Helmholtz, 1850), this transmission is at a rate that is slow enough to be measured within only a few centimeters of nerve.

The nerve fiber provides a means of transferring the local excitation to one or more remote effectors with considerable speed and with relative freedom from any distortion by intervening conditions. Phenomena related to the conduction of information along nerve fibers are the subject of chapter 2 and the mechanisms of excitation and conduction in neural structures are the subject of chapters 11, and 12.

1.3* Experiment: Set up a simple experiment to measure "reaction time" to an unpredictable visual stimulus. Use a stopwatch that registers time in 0.01-sec intervals and has separate start and stop buttons. Have someone press the start button without giving any advance clues. The subject must watch for the start of the clock and then press the stop button as quickly as possible.

How long is the response time? What is wrong with the experiment? Do not quit yet; what else is wrong? Use the same equipment but correct these faults and make a better evaluation of response time.

How much does response time vary (1) with repeated trials? (2) between individuals? Is the shortest response time perhaps a more meaningful measure than the mean of a group of trials? Does the best measure of response time depend on the purpose of the measurement?

Note: To describe the variation within a group of measurements of this type, it is usually appropriate to use the *standard deviation.* (Most scientific calculators provide for automatic calculation of the standard deviation.) On the other hand, when evaluating the probable error of the mean or when comparing two means, each determined from several measurements, the *standard error* is used.

1.4* Experimental Design: What is the minimum conduction velocity that could account for the transmission of the effect of visual excitation to a muscle reaction in the response time measurements made above? Identify any deficiencies in this simple estimate of conduction velocity.

Design variations of the experiment to measure response times. Use both different stimuli, such as sound or touch, and different responses, such as foot movement, pupil constriction to light, and blowing into a tube. For these experiments, considerably more ingenuity may be required to make the needed measurements.

Note: Some quadriplegic patients are able to control external devices only by blowing into a tube.

1.5 Problem: For an electric wheel chair traveling at 5 km/hr (3 mph), how many meters (feet) will it travel during one reaction time between visual input and a blowing response?

Information is distinct from the form in which it is represented. Transduction is the process of translating information from one physical form to another.

Transduction, or the changing of information from one form to another, is an important function of the nervous system. *Receptors,* the input elements of the nervous system, change information into nerve signals and *effectors,* the output elements of the nervous system, change these nerve signals into mechanical or chemical responses. Within the nervous system further transductions involve equally great changes, which are generally concealed from casual observation. Transduction of the information from one form of signal to another often is associated with changes of the information itself. The output may differ in magnitude or in time course from the input and often *both* the magnitude and temporal relationships are changed.

Since nerve fibers usually branch, a single stimulus may act on many targeted effectors. Along the different branches the signal is subjected to different delays and transformations, so that a stimulus to a single receptor can have diverse and dispersed effects. In most pathways, signals are transformed in a series of stages between a receptor and an effector. In these ways, the total response to a specific excitation can increase in complexity. Such signal transformations could, on the one hand, be considered as distortion of the signal by the neural elements. They might equally be interpreted as neural computations on the inputs. In any case, the transformations occurring in the nervous system are important in that they give patterns to the output response that do not simply mirror the input stimuli in magnitude or temporal sequence.

The concept of *signals* is central to any discussion of nervous system function. A signal is a representation of time-varying information that passes from one point to another. A signal can remain unaltered even when the physical process carrying it changes. For example, a telephone mouthpiece first transduces sound waves into movement of a diaphragm and then further transduces this movement into a changing voltage. These voltage changes later result in magnetic field changes in an earpiece, movements of another diaphragm, and finally new sound waves. Through this whole sequence, a signal has passed unaltered, and the listener recognizes the information delivered by the speaker. A small time delay has occurred and the form of the information has changed repeatedly as it moved through the system, but the time-varying information—that is, the signal—has passed through the whole system unchanged. If the listener were then to write an interpretation of the message, both a transformation and a further transduction would occur. In this instance, the time-varying signal would be altered.

Not all stimuli are the same, and responses that would be appropriate to one stimulus might be inappropriate to another stimulus. The pattern of excitation resulting from the different stimuli must differ if the responses are to differ. Selective excitability, in which different nervous system elements respond to different stimuli, is accomplished by the selectivity of the different receptor systems. Each receptor has a particular type of external stimulus to which it best responds. Characterization by the nervous system of an individual's environment depends on the pattern of receptors that is responding and the extent to which each responds.

Individual molecules within the membrane of an excitable cell can be selectively altered by particular environmental stimuli. These molecules are the basis for receptor function in higher organisms and initiate simple tropisms in single-cell organisms. The properties of these molecules will be discussed in chapters 11 and 12. In chapter 4 we will discuss ways in which a small number of types of selectively alterable molecules in receptors provides the wide range of sensory sensitivities of a human.

Effectors transduce neural signals into physical responses and contribute significantly to the combination and processing of these signals.

Effectors are, of course, essential for a response to occur. Biological effectors typically contribute critical transformations to the signals as well. The most obvious effectors associated with the nervous system are muscles, which convert neural signals into mechanical effects. A second group of effectors controlled by the nervous system is glands. These provide an adjustment of chemical processes that serves to maintain the internal environment of the individual. Neural signals also have a third target of action that is easily overlooked. This is the modification, by previous neural signals, of the rules by which future neural signals will be handled. Muscle and glandular outputs will be discussed in chapters 7 and 14, and modifications of the internal rules for processing signals will be discussed in chapter 9.

There are three types of muscle, which differ in the way that they are controlled by the nervous system. Mammalian *skeletal muscle* is active only when driven by neural signals and inhibition occurs only by removal of an excitatory signal. *Cardiac muscle* operates independent of neural signals but can be modified in its action by nerves that increase or decrease various aspects of the muscle function. *Smooth muscle* commonly has two different types of innervation. These two types of innervation often, but not always, have opposing effects on the smooth muscle. Smooth muscle can have different responses to a particular neural signal depending on the hormonal status at the time.

Although neural signals regulate the activity of various glands in a variety of ways, the role of neural control of glands can be subdivided into two functional classes. Neural excitation causes some glands to produce a product, such as a digestive enzyme, that has a direct action. Neural excitation of endocrine glands, on the other hand, adjusts the release of hormones that have an indirect action.

The hormone becomes, in effect, the next stage of the information transfer process. The final action is transmitted some distance at a speed roughly the same as that of the slower nerve fibers. The endocrine signal often has a more diffuse action and is generally more persistent in its effect than signals transmitted entirely by way of nerve fibers. Because of its extensive treatment as a separate topic, the endocrine signal transmission system will not be considered in any detail in this book.

Often the only effect that occurs during the lifetime of a particular signal is the alteration of the rules of the system. The changing of rules for processing future signals is what is ordinarily called learning, or plasticity of the nervous system. Although this is not strictly an output, it is a consequence of the neural signal, and it influences future outputs even after the active signal has disappeared.

Neural control requires that there be a prediction of future needs and conditions.

Prediction of future responses is a most important function of the nervous system. The nervous system deals with information about things that are changing in time and, as the information ages, it usually becomes obsolete. Because of the delay inherent in conduction and the lags common to neural circuits, the nervous system is always acting on information about the past to determine future responses. Sometimes the nervous system does, in fact, fail to solve the problem, so that the response is inappropriate. Much of the time, however, predictive mechanisms present in receptors, in the central nervous system, and in effectors produce an adequate response in spite of the delays and lags.

Sometimes, prediction is simple in that the changes in question are so slow that it is sufficient to treat the slightly old information as if it were still current. In other cases the old information can be updated adequately to predict future conditions based on the rate with which the old information was changing. Alternatively, information of a different type may provide a basis for prediction. For instance, when one decides to start a physical exercise, the nervous system initiates circulatory and respiratory changes before there is a need for an increased oxygen supply. Here, predictions about an intended activity initiate a response to a future need before a deficiency exists.

1.6* Experiment: Hang a weight by approximately one meter of string to make a pendulum. While swinging the pendulum, attempt to point to its position by moving your whole forearm in time with the pendulum. Can you track it?

Adjust the string length until the pendulum period is about four times the reaction time from a visual stimulus for a similar forearm movement (see experiment 1.3). You can either calculate the period from the pendulum length or simply time a series of successive cycles to estimate the period of each cycle. The time that it takes the pendulum to move between mid-position and either extreme is now equal to the reaction time. Does your tracking lag behind the pendulum cycle by an amount approximately equivalent to the reaction time? What information would allow your nervous system to predict pendulum position and make appropriate corrections in arm position?

Devise an experiment to compare tracking of an unpredictable target movement with tracking of a predictable target movement. Devise and carry out an experiment to determine reaction time for ankle movement from visual signals. How does this reaction time compare with the walking cycle, at a slow pace or with rapid walking? How might foot adjustments be made when walking over rough ground with and without visual input?

Note: We are asking open-ended questions. You should be able to produce some answers now and better ones as you study more neurophysiology. It is unlikely that we will ever be able to answer completely the many questions raised. Individuals (often including students) who were not satisfied with the best answers available have in the past made some of the most important discoveries about neural function. If we are lucky, dissatisfaction with the answers to some of the questions that we ask will lead some readers to make advances in our knowledge of the nervous system's function.

Probably the most interesting predictions made by the nervous system are the least understood. These complex predictions lead to many decisions in everyday life. You will recognize that we often make important decisions without the benefit of all the desired information about future consequences and yet the frequency of good decisions under these circumstances far surpasses what we might expect from chance. We have a whole vocabulary of words, ranging from intuition to the occult, to cover our ignorance in such cases. Careful experimental investigations point to an ability of nervous systems to identify and use important patterns of clues without conscious recognition of their existence.

Pattern recognition of this type is a major factor in the improvement of judgment that a physician develops with clinical experience. Since the clues involved are not recognized, it is impossible to include them in either diagnostic programs for computers or in syllabi for medical teaching. For the "art of medicine," experience of an alert physician may be the only teacher.

Normal neural function requires the combination of information entering over a period of time and by way of multiple pathways.

Excitation of a single receptor can produce an effective, but stereotypic, response in some invertebrates, but such minimal excitation is seldom adequate in vertebrates. Ordinarily, only the excitation of individual receptors in combination with that of other receptors is sufficient to initiate an effective response. Appropriately, the combination of signals from multiple sources is the most common type of processing within the central nervous system of vertebrates.

Combinations involve signals coming from similar receptors located in different parts of the body, signals coming from different types of receptors located close to each other, or signals originating in the same or different types of receptors at different points in time. These combinations occur in networks of interconnecting neurons and may result in changes in the magnitude, the temporal relationships, or even the nature of the response to one signal as a result of another signal. Signals from the output of a neural pathway can even feed back into the input of that same pathway.

Does the success that humans exhibit in dealing with their environment result from unique previous experiences combined with the accumulated genetic information? We can use some approximations to try to answer this question. One consideration is how many different input conditions might be involved. A reasonable assumption is that a typical receptor can produce distinguishable responses to at least 10 different levels of excitation. In a human nervous system, with at least 10^7 receptors, there would be 10 raised to the 10^7 power possible different input combinations. This number is far larger than the total number of milliseconds of life of all humans who have ever lived! It is reasonable to rule out the possibility that all input combinations of previous experience could have occurred even in the whole species. Since it is also reasonable to rule out exhaustive training of the species or of the individual for all possible environmental contingencies, it is obvious that another explanation must be advanced to explain the high degree of success humans have in adapting to their changing environment. Humans must respond with a range of adequate responses to a wide constellation of similar, but not identical, receptor excitation patterns. Even highly trained responses must maintain this nonstereotypic quality.

The human nervous system is made up of complex networks of interacting neurons and has many more central units than it does input units (10^{12} compared with 10^7). Because of the different delays and lags between receptors and various central neurons, at any moment the neural signals distributed within the nervous system represent a variety of combinations of information from temporally dispersed inputs. Functional effects of signal combinations and processing in a variety of simple nerve networks will be discussed in chapter 16. Some of the most interesting effects of neural networks are those properties that emerge from the operation of the whole network but are not found in any of the parts making up the network.

Nervous systems and computers both deal with information in a pulsatile form, but the organization and processing details are markedly different.

Comparison is frequently made between the nervous system and an electronic computer. Indeed, like a computer, the nervous system has an input of information that it processes in combination with stored information to produce a valuable output. Both also use all-or-none electrical pulses in the transmission of information. In spite of these and perhaps other points of similarity, though, the internal processing is rather different. Analogies between brains and existing computers are often carried so far that they are misleading.

Recent developments in computer research have introduced many different architectures and algorithms resembling properties of the nervous system, but there is still no computing device that incorporates all the known aspects of neural function. The differences are ironically most distinct in those machines usually considered when analogies are made between the brain and computers. These are Turing machines, in which one processor deals with all the data one step at a time in an ordered sequence. Data and program are stored in separate places in a form that is distinctly different from the computing device itself. Ordinary computer programs are defined in advance, although the sequence of steps may be modified, during execution, with conditional branches. In the nervous system each neuron acts as a processor of information, with all neurons acting simultaneously. There is no distinct separation between information and architecture since neurons or their connections are altered during information storage. The partitioning of the system into computer, sensors, and effectors, although easy in technology, is impossible in biological systems. Both the receptors and effectors combine and process information while the central neurons, like the sensors, behave differently under different conditions. One important characteristic of the nervous system is that it continually readjusts its own internal rules. Finally, the nervous system, with 10^{12} neurons each having perhaps 10^3 inputs, is orders of magnitude more complex than any current electronic computer.

Computer modeling of brain function or programming artificial intelligence systems has provided investigators in brain research with one type of important information. It has revealed the nature of the complexity of the formal logical solutions to problems, such as speech recognition, and the human nervous system can do this simultaneously with such other complex activities as the control of walking.

In the following chapters we shall attempt to outline how the nervous system accomplishes tasks of processing information in a way that leads to control of the relationship between an individual and an ever-changing environment. Some faults that occur clinically will be indicated and some internal operations will be expanded to a molecular and ionic level of description. We hope that you will find excitement in examining some parts of the nervous system's function. At least when you finish this study you should feel that function in the nervous system, although complex, is orderly and no more obscure than any other in biology.

Chapter 2

Transmission Phenomena

Coordination of activities in different locations implies communication, whether by neural or other means.

Most biological processes, to be effective, require the coordination of activities at multiple locations. External influences at one site lead to responses at sites remote from the direct influence. Effective responses of individual cells usually require the coordinated response of other cells and larger assemblages of cells require compensation or support from other multicellular structures. This type of interrelated activity represents either the direct communication among the participating units or the common receipt by each unit of related signals from a common controlling structure. A variety of means of communication among separated parts of animals will be discussed in this chapter.

The single-cell organism *Paramecium* can avoid obstacles in its environment by making coordinated responses. To do this, the animal has both an *affector,* or sensory, process and an *effector,* or motor, process within its single cell. Mechanoreceptive calcium channels (to be discussed in chapter 12) in the cell membrane at the front of the animal respond when the animal bumps into something. These channels open and allow the flow of Ca^{2+} ions into the cell. As a result, the electrical potential within the cell becomes more positive, causing the cilia that propel the animal to reverse the direction of their beating. By contrast, the mechanoreceptive potassium channels in the cell membrane at the rear of the animal respond to contact by opening, thereby increasing the flow of potassium ions out of the cell. This causes the electrical potential within the cell to become more negative; as a result the cilia increase their beating in the forward direction. Thus information about the environment is transduced into an electrical potential, which, in turn, is transduced into a functionally useful response of the animal.

How nerve fibers function is one of the most thoroughly understood biological processes. This knowledge has grown through intensive study during the past two centuries. Our knowledge today spans topics from the interaction of individual ions and molecules to the combined activity of nerve fibers in humans. Many details are missing and there is some disagreement about the facts that are known, but the current knowledge of the general principles of the function of neurons is well established. An understanding of these fundamental principles is essential to understanding any other function of the nervous system. Topics related to the operation of individual nerve fibers will be discussed not only in this chapter but in several later chapters. Part of chapter 4 deals with the initiation of nerve impulses in sensory fibers. Chapter 10 discusses electrical excitation of, and recording from, nerve fibers. Chapters 11 and 12 are almost entirely devoted to mechanisms involved in the production and propagation of nerve impulses. Most of the rest of the book addresses, either directly or indirectly, the role of activity in nerve fibers.

Neurons are unique among cells in having long, thin cytoplasmic extensions. These processes are collectively called *neurites*. Long neurites that conduct impulses away from their cell bodies are called *axons* (from the Greek, αξων for axis). The long neurites that conduct impulses from the periphery toward the centrally located cell bodies of sensory nerves have similar anatomical and conducting properties, and there is some debate whether these also should be called axons. To avoid this issue we will use the term *nerve fiber* in the general case and *sensory fiber* when we wish to be more restrictive. The term *dendrite* (from the Greek, δενδροσ, for tree) is used for the short neurites that convey information toward the cell body. We will use the term axon to describe neurites that convey information away from the cell body by means of nerve impulses. (For a further discussion of this topic that carries nomenclature to a consideration of neural development, see the article by P. Sargent (1989) entitled, "What distinguishes axons from dendrites?")

Most of the electrical properties of nerve fibers are directly applicable to skeletal, smooth, and cardiac muscle fibers. It is important to recognize this similarity when dealing with interventions intended to alter impulse function in one of these tissues, since the intervention may have adverse side effects on other tissues that function by similar mechanisms.

Mechanical, chemical, and electrical phenomena by which conditions in one location influence conditions in another location are capable of communicating information.

Although the nerve fiber and its associated impulses are the usual topic of consideration concerning internal communication, many other pathways in an animal also communicate information over a distance. Any mechanical, chemical, or electrical change can act as a means of transmission of information. Often multiple mechanisms are involved in communication between different structures within the individual. Some of these communications operate at energy levels approaching the theoretical limit of detection, and they are often overlooked by any but the most careful investigation.

Our previous example of communication within a single-cell organism might seem of little interest to those studying human biology. Yet evolution has retained, or directly elaborated on, many primitive mechanisms found in organisms of lower phylogenetic development. Study of these more primitive mechanisms has frequently led to insight into the function of higher organisms.

Mechanical actions that communicate information from one location to another may range from mechanical actions on, or in, individual cells to gross skeletal movements.

An ameboid cell, when extending one pseudopod, maintains a constant volume by retracting another part of the cell. A similar hydraulic communication is found in skeletal muscle cells (fibers). When muscle fibers are arranged in complex patterns, lateral pressure communicates information to a fiber about activity of adjacent fibers. This pressure, in the constant-volume muscle cell, results in alterations of the tensile force that the muscle cell can deliver. (This topic will be further considered in chapter 14.) At the other extreme is the mechanical communication that occurs in the coupling of separate joint movements through the linkage of multijoint muscles and the connective tissues that span more than one joint.

2.1* Demonstration: Have someone grasp a 2- to 3-cm diameter rod. Test how firm this grasp is with the wrist extended. Now have the subject maximally flex the wrist and recheck the firmness of the grasp. Why does wrist position effect finger flexion? How might an animal use this type of mechanical communication?

Information about a chemical event occurring at one location is reflected in changes of chemical quantities appearing later at other locations. Chemical communication pathways are a type of communication that is of major importance in both plants and animals. Chemical communication can involve metabolic agents such as glucose that appear in considerable quantity throughout the body, or, in other cases, chemicals such as neurohormones or neurotransmitters, whose effective quantities are very small. Some chemical action is very general, affecting cells throughout the organism, whereas other chemical action is very specific, affecting only discrete locations in an individual cell.

The magnitude and effectiveness of chemical signals depend on the rate of delivery, transportation dynamics, rate of removal, volume of distribution, and quantitative effectiveness of these molecules along different chemical communication pathways. The most basic mechanism of chemical distribution is diffusion. Diffusion of a local quantity of a chemical causes its concentration to fall rapidly as a function of distance from the source. Simple diffusion of a chemical agent in free solution is too slow to provide communication of useful biological information over distances greater than a few millimeters (figure 2.1). Biological systems, however, have many chemical pathways that communicate information about quantitative variations. Communication pathways that are effective over short distances may not be effective over long distances, and those that deal effectively with slowly changing information may not be effective for rapidly changing information. Simple identification of the agents involved and the locations of delivery and action are not an adequate basis for understanding chemical communication without the inclusion of quantitative information about dynamics.

Junctional transmission between cells (discussed in detail in chapter 13) can carry rapidly varying signals. At the well-studied neuromuscular junction, this process involves preformed transmitter molecules, that can be released within less than a millisecond and can be removed at a rate that reduces the quantity by one-half every few milliseconds. The dilution space can be microscopic in size; and transport, although by diffusion, may span distances of only tens of nanometers. In junctional communication, the chemical source and site of action can be both close and sharply localized.

Communication using insulin or thyroxin as chemical messengers involves distribution throughout the body with release and removal processes timed in hours. Blood circulation provides the necessary mixing and transport. Each agent is released at a specific site but the action of each involves most of the tissues of the body. On the time scale of accumulation and removal, transport is essentially instantaneous, since distribution by way of the circulation involves only a few seconds.

The six hormones secreted by the anterior pituitary are under the control of chemical releasing factors that are produced in the region of the brain called the hypothalamus. The anterior pituitary, although located adjacent to the brain, receives no neural input from the brain. Hypothalamic releasing factors are delivered to the circulation in a very localized region and are transported only a

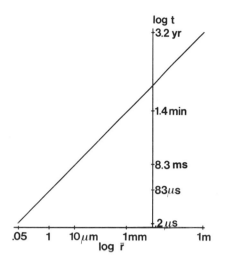

Figure 2.1
Log diffusion time vs. log mean diffusion displacement. Mean diffusion displacement, r, is calculated according to Einstein's 1905 solution to the Fick equation for three-dimensional diffusion. Mean displacement,

$$r = \sqrt{6Dt}$$

an approximate diffusion coefficient for small ions is

$$D \approx 2 \times 10^{-5} \text{ cm}^2/\text{sec}$$

The distances plotted are approximately equal to the following: 0.05 μm, synaptic cleft; 1 μm, small nerve fiber diameter; 10 μm, neuron cell body diameter; 1 mm, internodal length; and 1 m, length of a long nerve fiber.

few millimeters by the circulation from their release site to their point of action in the anterior pituitary. In the process, dilution is into only a small volume of blood. The transport delay is probably only a fraction of a second. Effective removal occurs after the blood passes through the pituitary simply by dilution into the general circulation followed by a slower removal. As a result, these hormones never accumulate in the general circulation to a sufficient level to be effective.

A variety of materials is transported within nerve fibers both toward the cell body and away from the cell body. Transport of different agents occurs at rates from about 1 to about 400 mm/day. This transport of materials differs both in speed and in the direction of transfer. Although much of this transport provides materials for the metabolic maintenance of branches of the cell, evidence is accumulating that this transport also provides a relatively slow communication pathway in parallel with the rapid impulse pathway. As we will discuss in chapter 9, such slow pathways may be particularly important in memory. There is also some indication that some pathological states of the nervous system result from defects in these slow transport systems.

Chemical signals influence ionic movements and thus introduce potential changes and electrical currents in cells. Electrical current, resulting from the flow of ions, is a signal-carrying mechanism distinct from the chemical pathways already considered. Voltage changes further influence chemical processes and the release of chemical signaling agents. Most nervous system functions involve a sequence of alternating electrical, chemical, and often mechanical signaling processes. The chemical signals are typically carried by a variety of chemical species at different points in the system. Differences in the type of signal carriers between different pathways are an important basis for differential sensitivity to drugs, endocrine agents, disease, and the general chemical environment.

2.2* Problem: Write a set of equations to describe the generalized dynamics of a chemical communication system and identify the coefficients needed to describe a specific case. Consider release, dilution, and removal of the agent involved. For a first trial, assume that there is no transportation delay (i.e., dilution volume is thoroughly and immediately mixed). If you are familiar with computer implementation of difference equations, program your equations and solve them with a variety of values for the coefficients until you are comfortable with predicting the effect of any change. Several simple assumptions about types of transport are possible, but the development of a realistic model for a specific case is most likely a difficult research problem.

Currents and voltages (see appendix A) are more than just a by-product of the electrical charges associated with chemical agents moving in the body. Electrical potential differences cause movement of ions through the space in which the potential gradient exists. These ion movements in turn provide information to the surrounding area about changes of the source potential. Electrical fields can influence ion movement around the source much more quickly than can diffusion of uncharged chemical agents.

Biological sources of potential are generally limited to only about 0.1 V. The intensity of electrical fields around a biological source drops abruptly with dis-

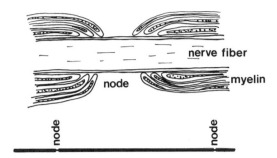

Figure 2.2
Node of Ranvier. The upper schematic drawing shows one periodic interruption in the myelin that wraps a nerve fiber. Nodes expose the nerve cell membrane to the interstitial media. The lower schematic figure shows the approximate scale of internodal length (1–2 mm) to fiber diameter.

tance from the source and generally falls below effective levels within a few millimeters. In some brain regions, even within this small volume, there can be millions of nerve cells. The effect of the external electrical fields of one cell on adjacent cells is difficult to measure and has not been well studied. Local electrical effects are a part of the information processing of sensory receptors, have effects at some junctions between neurons and muscle fibers, and are important in the generation and propagation of the nerve impulse. Some of the local electrical phenomena mentioned here will be discussed in other chapters.

In the 1850s, while attempting to account for problems encountered in sending telegraphic signals over a transoceanic cable, Lord Kelvin developed equations to describe the effect of distance and time on the electrical potential along an insulated conductor submerged in a conducting solution. Later it was recognized that under some conditions these equations could be used to describe the spatial and temporal distribution of potentials along a nerve fiber.

Human nerve fibers are cylindrical structures with diameters from 0.5 to 12 μm and lengths from about 1 to over 1000 mm. All nerve fibers are bounded by a membrane that is about 10^{-8} m thick and are filled with electrolytes, large molecules, and specific subcellular structures. Some nerve fibers are enveloped by a fatty *myelin* covering with periodic interruptions, known as *nodes of Ranvier* (figure 2.2). Leaving aside the complications imposed by myelin, the nerve fiber is thus a conductive core surrounded by an insulating cell membrane, which is, in turn, surrounded by a conductive external medium. The passive electrical properties of this combination cause it to respond to the local application of a constant voltage across the membrane with characteristics of a *cable conductor* so that the voltage falls exponentially with distance from the point of application. The voltage falls thus to about one-third of its initial value within less than a centimeter. In addition, electrical *capacitance* of the membrane results in a lag of voltage change across the membrane at points remote from a driving source. The voltage driving the charging of each successive section of the membrane rises slowly as the voltage in the preceding section charges, thus, at successively more remote sites, the voltage change is progressively slower. The passive electrical influence of local currents on adjacent regions of a neuron is the basis for rapid transmission of information in the nervous system over distances up to a few millimeters. Such *passive spread* is ineffective at distances much greater than a centimeter. Long distance transmission of information requires the repeated renewal of currents that underlie the propagation of nerve impulses.

Specialized properties of the membranes of excitable fibers provide for the renewal of spatially decrementing signals. This allows nondecremental communication at a distance with relative independence from intervening local conditions.

As we will discuss in chapter 12, nerve fibers as well as muscle fibers and certain other excitable cells can respond to small local potential changes by producing rapid, stereotypic changes in their transmembrane potentials known as *impulses* or *action potentials* (figure 2.3) (see appendix B). Whereas the initiating action in a particular part of a membrane can be driven by electrical energy from outside that point, the energy that completes the regenerative local response is derived from locally stored electrochemical gradients across the cell membrane. Consequently, above a certain threshold level, the active response that develops is independent of the stimulus intensity. The threshold level and the active response magnitude are affected primarily by the local ionic distributions and by the presence of chemical agents (e.g., anesthetics) that modify molecular events in the membrane. The nerve impulse response is *all or nothing* and a stimulus can be classified as either *subthreshold* or *suprathreshold* based on the presence or absence of an impulse.

Besides the small, presumably random, fluctuations of threshold for nerve excitation (see appendix C), some rather large variations are known to exist (figure 2.4). Following a nerve impulse, there is a period during which the mem-

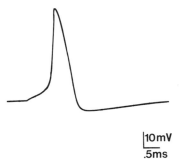

|10mV
|_
.5ms

Figure 2.3
Single action potential. Typical intracellular action potential as recorded from a squid giant axon (see appendix C). This waveform is strikingly similar to that seen in most other excitable cells.

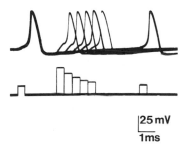

|25 mV
|_
1ms

Figure 2.4
Refractoriness. Recovery of excitability from immediately after the absolute refractory period until the end of the relative refractory period (see appendix C). The six superimposed records show responses to near-threshold stimuli, each following a preliminary conditioning stimulus. The interval between these two stimuli was varied between each record. The lower line shows the preselected, just-minimal stimuli at the different interstimulus intervals.

brane is first unexcitable and then has a depressed excitability. This interval, known as the *refractory period,* is of variable duration among excitable fibers but is characteristic in a particular type of nerve or muscle fiber. Some nerves even exhibit a *supranormal period* during which threshold is below that of resting nerve. Another means by which threshold is altered is in response to a slowly applied stimulus. This process, known as *accommodation,* causes a rapidly rising stimulus voltage to be more effective in initiating a nerve impulse than is a slowly developed stimulus.

2.3* Problem: Design more than one alternate way to either evaluate or minimize the effect of stimulus sequence on the measurement of threshold. If, while generating a graph such as that in figure 2.4, you found that you could draw only an irregular line to separate all the subthreshold from all the suprathreshold measurements, how would you decide whether the irregularities represented underlying complexity in the threshold function or variations in your testing?

In a nerve fiber where the membrane can generate impulses, the current flow from an excited area of membrane causes local current flow that will bring the adjacent areas of excitable membrane toward threshold. The local currents, drawn by excited regions, lead to a wave that progresses along the fiber. This wave includes a sequence of potential changes and refractory periods that move past any point on the fiber. Figures 2.3 and 2.4 show the potential change and subsequent refractory period experienced at one point as the wave moves past.

   The ability to conduct impulses over nerves is common to both primitive and the most highly developed animal nervous systems and similar actions can even occur in some plants (figure 2.5). Coordination of activity in widely separated parts of an organism almost invariably requires impulse transmission. Even in those situations in which the information originates near its site of action, transmission of impulses over long nerve fibers can be involved. Thus muscle fibers are often excited because of signals that start from receptors within the same muscle but then travel over an intervening *reflex arc* in which the impulses are transmitted on nerve fibers to the central nervous system and on other nerve fibers that return impulses to the muscle of origin. Similar pathways come from and return to such organs as the heart and kidney. These long pathways might seem wasteful but they allow the information to be processed and combined with information from other sources before the result is returned to a site near its origin.

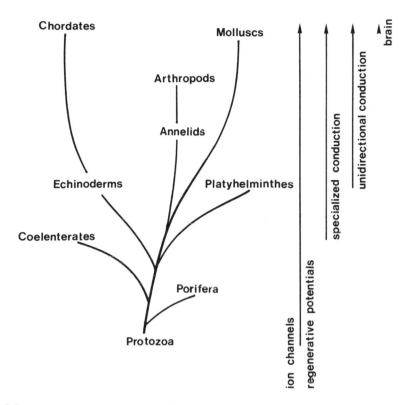

Figure 2.5
Phylogenetic relationship of various electrical conduction properties. Selective ion channels and regenerative potentials are found in cells of all animal (and some plant) phyla, whereas specialized conduction systems are related to the ability of the animal to exhibit coordinated multicellular actions. Both the chordates and the molluscs include animals with complex brains in which regions with specialized functions are interconnected by specialized fiber tracts.

Impulse-conducting nerve fibers make up the principal part of all peripheral nerves (figure 2.6). There are three general classes of peripheral nerve fibers: *primary efferent fibers* that originate in the central nervous system (brainstem or spinal cord) and pass out to terminate on muscles or peripheral ganglia; *postganglionic fibers* that originate in (autonomic) peripheral ganglia and carry signals on to glands, blood vessels, the heart, or other visceral structures; and *afferent fibers* that originate peripherally in sensory receptors and pass in to terminate at various locations within the central nervous system. Many of the neurons of the central nervous system, called *interneurons,* carry internal information between various locations. In the human brain, 99% of the fibers interconnect various brain structures. Peripheral and central nerve fibers can range in length from less than a millimeter to about a meter. If one assumes an average fiber length of 1 cm per neuron, the human nervous system contains more than 10^6 km of nerve fibers! Aggregates of nerve fibers within the central nervous system make up the *white matter* and are often grouped in bundles of related fibers that are called *tracts*.

Once initiated, an impulse will travel the length of a fiber but generally it does not affect activity in other fibers.

Nerve impulses themselves do not cross the junctions between neurons but generally rely on specialized mechanisms at these *synapses*. Since these junctions commonly transmit information in only one direction, and since impulses originate at sensory receptors or central neurons at the end of nerve fibers, nerve fibers usually conduct information in only one direction. An artificial stimulus can, however, produce an impulse that will travel in the opposite (*antidromic*) direction until it encounters the first synapse.

Although communication carried by impulse transmission on nerve fibers overlaps, to some extent, the speed of other forms of communication, it generally provides the fastest nonmechanical communication pathway within an organism. Since the distribution of nerve fibers is often discrete, impulse transmission generally has the most specific locations of action.

Both the velocity of conduction and the size of the impulse are independent of the stimulus, given that the stimulus is suprathreshold. Normally action potentials are considerably larger than the minimum necessary to stimulate adjacent regions of the fiber and this provides a *safety factor* in impulse transmission. Threshold,

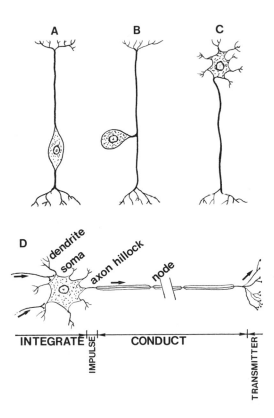

Figure 2.6
Neuron types. Three general morphological types of neurons are classified as (A) bipolar, (B) unipolar, and (C) multipolar according to the number of processes that originate at the cell body. The functional areas of a neuron, as diagrammed in (D), include the postsynaptic regions on the soma and dendrites where *integration* occurs, the axon hillock where frequency encoding occurs by *impulse* initiation, the axon where information is *conducted* to a distant site, and the presynaptic terminals where *transmitter release* occurs.

however, is high enough so that fibers are not stimulated by current from an action potential in an adjacent fiber. Thus an impulse originating in a fiber in a peripheral nerve or in a central fiber tract will have a high probability of reaching the end of that, but only that, fiber.

Under certain conditions, propagation of impulses on peripheral nerves can be artificially influenced. Stimulation of a peripheral nerve either electrically or mechanically, such as hitting your "funny bone," produces impulses that are exactly equivalent to those of more usual origin. Such impulses have the same sensory or motor effects at their terminal as would impulses that were generated normally. On the other hand, transmission of normally originated impulses can be blocked by several means. Local anesthetics act by blocking transmission in peripheral nerves. Local compression or lack of oxygen also can block the transmission of nerve impulses on peripheral nerves. (On recovery, trains of impulses may originate in the recovering region causing the paresthesia, or abnormal sensation, of the limb that has "gone to sleep.") Finally, application of high potassium solution or cooling can temporarily block impulse transmission in peripheral nerves.

The *conduction velocity* of nerve impulses can be fast, although slow enough to be measurable in a length of nerve of only a few centimeters.

Conduction velocities from less than 1 to over 100 m/sec have been recorded in mammalian nerve fibers. (See table 2.1; also see table 10.1 and figure 15.2.) For the same reasons that fiber diameter and membrane electrical properties affect the passive spread of current along a fiber, these parameters determine the speed of impulse propagation.

Shortly after it was proposed that nerve impulses traveled so fast that their velocity could never be measured in the short distances available, Hermann von Helmholtz (1850) showed his mentor, Johannes Müller, to be wrong by measuring the delay of conduction over a measured length of frog nerve. He used a muscle contraction, recorded on a moving smoked surface, to show the response to electrical stimuli applied at two different distances along the nerve. He determined differences in muscle response time with a resolution of 0.0001 sec and combining this information with the known conduction distance, he calculated the conduction velocity of the nerve impulse.

Table 2.1
Conduction Velocities and Times

Process	Velocity (cm/sec)	Time for 10 cm (sec)
Slow axonal transport	1.2×10^{-6}	8.6×10^{6}
Diffusion of K^{+}		8.3×10^{5}
Fast axonal transport	4.6×10^{-4}	2.2×10^{4}
Circulation, small artery	10	1
Circulation, aorta	50	2×10^{-1}
Slow nerve conduction	10^{2}	10^{-1}
Speed limit (65 mph)	2.9×10^{3}	3.5×10^{-3}
Fast nerve conduction	10^{4}	10^{-3}
Sound (air)	3.3×10^{4}	3×10^{-4}
Light (vacuum)	3×10^{-10}	3.3×10^{-10}

The conduction velocity of impulses travelling over nerve fibers is sensitive to temperature with a Q_{10} of about 2.6 (see appendix D). The implication of this temperature coefficient is that physico-chemical processes and not the passive electrical cable properties dominate in the determination of conduction velocity.

Although nerve impulses are the fundamental element in the transmission of information from one location to another, a single nerve impulse on a single nerve fiber is almost meaningless both theoretically and in terms of the usual response of the nervous system to an isolated event. Theoretically, an isolated nerve impulse can carry only one increment of information (one bit) (e.g., only the occurrence of an event), with no ability to convey further information about the magnitude of the event. The information content of a single impulse is only about one-fifth that carried by a single letter of the alphabet—a very limited message.

The pattern of successive impulses on a nerve fiber and the relationship of the activity on different fibers, rather than single nerve impulses, define the information communicated.

A train of impulses, repeated on individual nerve fibers, is the normal basis for signal transmission in nerves. The magnitude of a signal is, in general, represented in the repetition rate of the impulses and a changing signal is usually represented by a corresponding change in the firing rate of impulses.

Figure 2.7A shows two pulse rate representations of a time-varying signal. This *pulse rate code* is one in which the interpulse interval is proportional to the

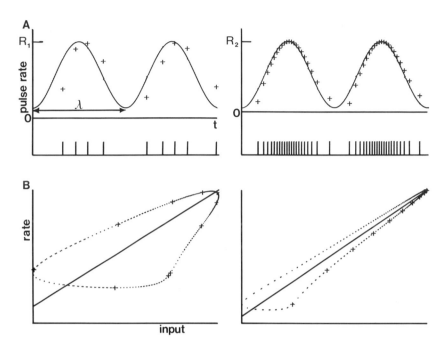

Figure 2.7
Different representations of a sinusoidally varying signal. (A) At the top of each illustration is shown a solid line time graph of two cycles of the input signal. Each impulse is generated at such time that the instantaneous pulse rate is proportional to the average of the input signal in the pulse interval terminated by that impulse. A constant signal equal to or below the line marked 0 produces no impulses. For the graphs on the left the pulse rate interpretation is scaled such that a steady input at the level marked R_1 would produce eight impulses per cycle period, λ, of the sinusoidal signal. On the right, a steady signal of magnitude, R_2, would similarly produce 40 impulses per cyclic period. For each impulse the instantaneous rate represented by the interval it terminates is marked on the input graph as a (+) at the time of that pulse. In (B) the instantaneous rates are graphed against the input signal for enough cycles besides those shown in (A) to generate a total of 300 impulses. The diagonal line on each graph shows the input-output relationship that would occur at various steady input levels. The signal magnitude that just fails to generate impulses is marked by 0 in (A) and by the baseline in (B).

(continued)

Figure 2.7 *(continued)*

Pattern 1		Signal		Pattern 2	
Nerve type	R_1PPS	f(Hz)	λ(sec)	R_2PPS	Nerve type
Visceral	0.8	0.1	10	4	Visceral
	1.6	0.2	5	8	
	4	0.5	2	20	Motor
Motor	8	1	1	40	
	16	2	0.1	80	Sensory
	40	5	0.2	200	
Sensory	80	10	0.1	400	None
	160	20	0.05	800	
None	400	50	0.02	2000	
	800	100	0.01	4000	

This table shows relative signal frequencies and pulse rate encoding ranges that would give patterns of encoding as are shown in the figure. These signal frequencies span the range subject to pulse rate coding in mammalian nervous systems. The encoding of each signal frequency (column 3) or wavelength (column 4) is represented by two patterns. Pattern 1, which is also represented on the left in the figure, occurs with the pulse rates that would represent a steady signal of magnitude R_1 (column 2). Pattern 2, represented on the right in the figure, would represent a steady signal of magnitude R_2 (column 5). The labels visceral, motor, and sensory show the general range of firing rates ordinarily found on the corresponding nerve types.

average of the amount of the input signal that is above threshold during that interval. By rescaling the time axes on the figure, this model can illustrate pulse encodings that represent several types of nerve fibers.

2.4* Problem: Examine the different responses to the same driving signal that are shown in figure 2.7A noting in particular the effect of the two different scale rules on the encoding of the slow and fast parts of the input signal. Select several interpulse intervals in these records and carefully project the time of occurrence of the starting and the ending pulse to intersect with the input signal curve. Estimate the average magnitude of the input signal during that interval. As the pulse code is being generated, when does this information about the input signal become available in the output? In what ways does the pulse code information differ from the input signal that generates it? Although the encoding is based on precise rules, notice that there is variability in the encoded signals with each scale and during different cycles using the same scale. Why might it appear that the encoding by a particular rule was subject to noise when comparing results of repeated tests? Describe a general relationship between the rules and the parts of the input signals that are most accurately encoded. If the nervous system used rules similar to these, what are some probable limitations in its encoding ability?

2.5* Problem: Compare the graph scales in figure 2.3 with those in figure 2.7A and note the difference in appearance of single nerve impulses at these different time scales. Why would it be appropriate to use different scales on different occasions?

In 1846, Weber used a hand-cranked generator and a battery to stimulate the nerve to a muscle. He showed that a steady muscle contraction resulted when the nerve was stimulated in a repetitive fashion and that a steady stimulus was ineffective. In the 1920s and 1930s Adrian finally succeeded in measuring individual nerve impulses and showed that an increased level of sensory or motor excitation was related to an increased number of active nerve fibers and an increased rate of firing in the individual fibers. He describes some of this Nobel prize-winning work in a very readable manner in his book entitled *The Basis of Sensation.*

Nerve impulses are relatively immune to varying conditions but their discontinuous nature limits a nerve's ability to communicate information about continuous processes.

Just as individual impulses travel along a nerve fiber almost without influence from the local conditions, so a train of impulses is usually transmitted the length of a nerve without change. Although there is a temporal delay between the beginning and the end of the fiber, all the impulses are delayed equally so that the rate and pattern of firing are preserved.

In general, muscle increases its response when the rate of nerve impulses being delivered to it is increased. The response is, however, not linearly related to the instantaneous impulse rate. Sensory neurons produce a firing rate that is related, also in a nonlinear manner, to the stimulus magnitude (figure 2.8). The input–output relationships of central neurons are very hard to define. Some increase their response rate to an increasing input level and others decrease their firing rate with increased input. In normal function, the total input to a neuron is difficult to evaluate. Still, all neurons, to a first approximation, use a variable

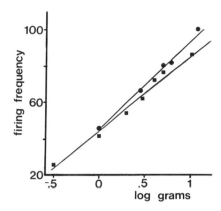

Figure 2.8
Relationship of firing frequency to stimulus intensity. A redrawing of one of the earliest published graphs of the input-output relationship for a receptor. Here, published by B.H.C. Matthews (1931), there is a logarithmic relationship between the load and the firing rate of two different stretch receptors.

impulse repetition rate to encode some magnitude of their input signal (see appendix E).

The smallest interval over which firing rate has meaning is the interval between successive impulses. Thus the pulse rate information about a signal's magnitude is delivered intermittently only with successive pulses (see figure 2.7). The inverse of each interval, or the *instantaneous frequency,* can convey a point value of some magnitude. Certain problems in interpretation are introduced because continually varying signals are sampled only periodically. For instance, when light intensity varies continuously, an optic nerve fiber reports the intensity of the light only intermittently with the arrival of each nerve impulse. This granularity of pulse-coded signals requires the firing rate of the pulses to be higher than any variations in the signal that can be encoded. It is often acceptable to represent a sine wave with a pulse-coded signal in which the average pulse frequency is 10 times higher than the frequency of the sine wave (see appendix E). A 200 pulse/sec nerve signal can define only about a 20-Hz-signal. A light flashing at 50 flashes/sec is ordinarily interpreted as a steady light. (Motion pictures are projected at 48 images/sec and North American fluorescent lights flicker at 120 flashes/sec.) This suggests a limit in the visual system imposed by pulse-coded signals in the optic nerve. Encoding may represent a general limit on the temporal resolution of nervous activity.

Records of physiological activity in a variety of nerve fibers show different types of pulse patterns. Sometimes firing rate changes smoothly over time. In other cases, impulses tend to repeat in closely spaced pairs separated by longer intervals. Often patterns consisting of bursts of closely spaced impulses alternate with silent or nearly silent periods. The significance of these patterns can, to some extent, be surmised by examination of the inputs that initiate them and the responses of the structures to which they are delivered. The nerve fiber delivers these patterns, albeit faithfully, without regard to what they represent.

2.6 Problem: Pulse rate signaling has, of course, no negative values. Physiological signals very commonly take on both positive and negative values. Describe how a pulse rate encoding mechanism could represent both positive and negative values.

2.7* Problem: A pulse rate code is used to encode a sinusoidal input signal. What are the largest and the smallest values for the average magnitude of the part of a sine wave in an interpulse period that includes the wave maximum and spans 1/10 cycle?

It is easy to be misled by diagrams of neural pathways into thinking that these connections involve only a single nerve fiber. In fact, when we look at a peripheral nerve we are looking at a bundle of hundreds to thousands of nerve fibers. The total number of fibers carring information into the spinal cord is around a million and the optic and auditory nerves each carries similar numbers of individual fibers. A similar consideration can be made on the output side where hundreds of thousands of fibers carry signals to muscles, viscera, glands, and other effectors. Within the central nervous system one fiber tract will typically carry hundreds of individual nerve fibers.

2.8* Problem: Although we probably will never know how many nerve impulses enter the human nervous system during any period of normal function, we can hazard some guesses. Individual sensory nerve fibers tend to be active at rates between 5 and 200 pulses (samples)/sec. Use the information provided here or more accurate numbers from other sources to estimate a range for the number of impulses arriving at the central nervous system. How does this number compare with the input to various digital computers when acquiring information from a fast analog-to-digital conversion?

Multiple fibers carrying related information provide a safety factor in case of fiber loss but cannot eliminate some effects introduced by the discontinuous nature of pulses.

Whereas modulation of firing of impulses carried on a single nerve fiber can transmit information about the changing magnitude of some variable, most motor and sensory functions involve modulated activity on many individual fibers. Although many fibers can carry more information than can a single fiber, the individual signals are not fully independent and thus the amount of information delivered does not increase in proportion to the number of active fibers. The overlap of information among fibers provides a redundancy and safety factor against individual fiber failure.

The information carried on a single fiber of a nerve trunk is a scalor, that is, it is unidimensional time-varying information about a single magnitude. Generally these scalors represent the magnitude of separate vector signals. These vector magnitudes are subject to changes as parts of the complex input change that occurs over time. Since there is overlap of the information that determines the magnitude of the vector signal carried on different fibers, a redundancy exists within a group of fibers. Thus, neural information can be preserved through loss of individual fibers even when no two fibers are carrying identical information. How the preserved information is retrieved without distortion is an intriguing research topic.

Since signals on separate nerve fibers within a nerve trunk carry independent information, it is essential that impulses in one fiber do not excite adjacent fibers. When two impulses travel in adjacent fibers, the local currents may slightly alter the excitation time and thus conduction velocity in adjacent fibers, each of which is propagating its own impulses, but this effect is unlikely to be of much importance. The information on adjacent fibers is essentially independent.

There are several factors that lead to parallel organization of neural pathways. Growing nerve fiber tips are sensitive to environmental conditions and this sensitivity modifies the direction and growth rate of that fiber. Similar fibers, developing simultaneously, are thus likely to follow a similar course. Nerve fibers within a peripheral nerve or central tract tend to originate close together and stay together. Fibers that carry similar information tend to travel together in bundles. Since neural processing of related signals is often important, there is a value supporting any tendency for functional organization of nerve fibers.

Because of the functional organization of central neurons and nerve fibers in peripheral nerves and central tracts, pathological changes and localized trauma often produce dramatic and specific functional defects. The background for recognizing such correlations between structure and functional defects is normally covered in neuroanatomy courses. For those unfamiliar with neuroanatomy, a brief examination of figures in F.H. Netter's *The Nervous System* under the classification of lesions will show schematically the type of analysis involved.

Although both digital computers and the nervous system use pulses to communicate, the way that these pulses are used is rather different in these two cases.

Although the arrangement of multiple parallel signal pathways in peripheral nerves and central tracts resembles a signal handling bus in a computer, it does not function in the same manner. Information about signal magnitude is carried in a single nerve fiber. Although large signals often involve activity in more fibers than do small signals, individual details are not encoded in the relationships among a group of fibers as is customary in parallel paths in a computer bus. In nerve trunks, each fiber is dedicated to a particular signal dimension and carries information about the variations in magnitude of that dimension over time. The dimensions represented by different nerve fibers are not strictly independent as are the signals on individual wires in a computer bus. Whereas single pathways in a computer bus carry information about different functions at different times, nerve fibers are generally dedicated to a particular signal dimension. To further depreciate any analogy between these two systems, parallel nerve fibers can conduct at significantly different velocities and be differently affected by existing temperature gradients. Such desynchronizing effects would totally disrupt parallel transmission on a computer bus.

In summary, internal communication in an individual involves multiple types of pathways that are effective over varying distances and that differ in their ability to deal with rapidly changing signals. Generally, conveying information over a distance introduces delays and may modify the details of the signal. Different pathways overlap in function but generally neural fibers provide the most rapid means of information transmission and the most discrete localization of action available to an organism.

Chapter 3

Information Inputs

The nervous system controls processes that adjust both internal operations of the individual and relations between the individual and the external environment.

For the nervous system to make an ideal adjustment of a function within the individual, it would have to be provided with complete information about both the state of the world and the state of the individual. This information would include all the factors that might have an effect on the individual's immediate and future condition. Some classes of information of importance to this function concern potential injury, needed supplies (e.g., food, water, oxygen, heat), internal status (e.g., blood constituents and temperature), and relationships to the immediate and remote environment (e.g., gravity direction, posture, contacts, location, and the nature of surrounding objects). In addition, special emphasis is placed on changes in any of these variables.

3.1. Problem: Make some of your own additions to the above list. (There are important omissions, so you should have no trouble.) For some items in your extended list, define the measurements that you might make with instruments to obtain that information. Do your individual measurements dependably separate each important type of information from all others?

Humans continually experience a vast array of stimuli from the environment. An extensive, but arbitrary, set of classifications and quantitative measures have been developed for use in describing the status of, and changes in, these conditions of the environment.

In any animal, the presence and magnitude of stimuli from the environment are important information. Equally important in determining the appropriate response is the distance and direction of those stimuli. Even within the limited behavioral repertoire of a single-celled organism such as the *paramecium,* responses are based on differentiation among several stimuli. In humans the effectors are usually remote from the sensors of environmental information so that nerve fibers are required to carry the signals. Since each fiber carries only information about the time-varying magnitude of one measure of some part of the stimulus world, there must be at least as many individual fibers as there are independent measures of the world to be reported to the central nervous system (CNS).

The terms that best describe the stimuli to an individual are frequently different from those terms to which we have become accustomed in describing physical measurements. Physical nomenclature often is transferred directly to descriptions of nervous system inputs. In this chapter, we will follow this physics-based nomenclature for most of the discussion. We do not intend to imply that the nervous system has evolved with the ability to differentiate those specific dimensions that we use in our descriptions of physical stimuli, although our *perceptions* of the world have most certainly biased the choice of dimensions that we choose for physical descriptions. Although both visible and infrared light are electromagnetic radiations, we ordinarily deal with them separately. This is because our retinal receptors are distinct from skin "warm" receptors.

The richness of the environmental information available to species as diverse as *paramecia* and humans is comparable, but the amount of this information that is differentiated and used by the human is much greater. Furthermore, the complexity of the human organism adds a great diversity of important information about internal relationships that becomes necessary for coordination of activity among cells, organs, and systems. In contrast, most protozoans require no coordination above the cellular level. Intercellular, organ, and system relationships provide a whole class of information that has sensory value only in more complex organisms.

Besides an external environment that is shared with unicellular animals, most multicellular animals have an internal environment the status of which is of major importance.

Unlike the *paramecium,* the human has an internal environment in which the individual cells are relatively independent of the extremes in the external environment. The maintenance of the internal environment within tolerable limits is, to a large extent, dependent on nervous system actions. Control of the internal environment consumes a considerable part of the total activity of the nervous system. This control depends on information from the inner environment itself sensed by a variety of receptors.

Certain classes of information exist only within higher animals, and, therefore, the importance of this information must have developed during the evolution of these animals. This information relates to things such as the location of various materials, the anticipation of future demands for these materials, and the presence of internal conditions that might cause damage to or modification of function of parts of the system. Internal O_2, CO_2, urea, and glucose concentration and blood osmolarity and pH are important to the control of the conditions within which all the body's cells operate. Concentrations of ions such as K^+, Na^+, Ca^{2+}, and Cl^- are particularly important because of their role in the function of nerve, muscle, and secretory cells as we will see in chapters 11 and 12. Since the levels of various hormonal control agents provide important signals for general body functions, sensing these levels is important to the coordination of overall control. Temperature information is important because of the denaturation of proteins that occurs above about 40°C and because of the destructive effect of cell freezing. In humans, the restrictions on internal temperature are even more severe because coordination of multiple internal functions becomes inadequate at reduced temperatures even considerably above freezing. Because of the large and different temperature coefficients of important enzyme reactions, small temperature changes can cause loss of critical coordinations among different body functions. This disruption of the balance of activities is seen during hypothermia at temperatures not any lower than about 25°C.

The quantities of most substances in the internal environment that are sensed and controlled by the nervous system are subject to accumulation in one or more pools. These quantities are acquired or produced at a limited rate and are then removed by a depletion process that requires a finite time. Three examples of such quantities are heat within the body mass, sodium ions within the extracellular fluid, and blood gasses within the tissue space. As will be discussed in chapter 15, lag-producing processes largely eliminate any rapid changes in these parameters. In discussions of body constituents, this effect is largely a result of *buffering*. Because of buffering, or lag, most of the quantities of the inner environment do not change rapidly, and, thus, frequent measurement or fast reporting is not necessary to represent adequately their dynamic status for control.

Not only does the internal environment of higher animals raise the need for controlling a new set of variables, but the controlling systems themselves introduce additional requirements for stabilization in order to operate consistently. *Controllers require controlled conditions.* This interdependence poses some interesting questions about evolution. Maintenance of body temperature probably requires a posture that holds the body off the ground, but such a posture on flexible limbs requires a controller that operates consistently at a nearly constant temperature.

Objects and conditions that make direct contact with the surface of an animal have an immediate effect on the future of that animal.

The internal conditions of the body provide the immediate environment of the cells; these conditions directly influence cell function. The mechanical, chemical, and thermal conditions at the surface of the body are not only spatially remote from most of the individual cells, but the effects of these surface conditions are often temporally remote from the individual cells. The important physical properties of these external influences usually involve their qualitative character, magnitudes, locations of application, spatial distribution, and time course. Chemical agents and thermal processes at the body surface act on internal cells only after the appreciable time required for chemical diffusion or heat transfer. Forces acting at the surface of the body govern accelerations that develop velocities and displacements; the effect of these displacements on the internal cells is often complex. Generally, information about surface conditions concerns actions that will influence the internal environment of the future. Often it is desirable to change external relationships so that these future changes are either enhanced or avoided before their effects on the inner environment accumulate.

Frequently, the contents of the gastrointestinal tract, the urinary bladder, and the respiratory tract are included as part of the external, albeit immediate, environment of the individual. For the current discussion, such an inclusion is appropriate. For these hollow organs, however, the important mechanical information is structured somewhat differently from the important information at the external surface of the body. On the body surface, localization of forces is available in considerable detail, and information about the three-dimensional direction of these forces can be critical. In contrast, for the enclosed surfaces, localization detail does not need to be precise; information about force is in the form of pressure and is independent of direction.

Important quantitative information must be obtained regarding objects that contact the body surface. Besides object identification this information is necessary to predict how the contact will change on its interaction with the surface.

There are two kinds of information of importance about surface interactions at a specific external locus: (1) information defining a modality and its magnitude such as force, temperature, or concentration, and (2) information describing related properties of the source of the contact stimulus such as its stiffness, viscosity, inertia, thermal conductivity, thermal capacity, or chemical quantity. This latter type of information is especially useful in answering important qualitative questions. Is the object easily moved? Does it provide a solid support? Would fast movement through it be particularly difficult? Will the concentration of the substance change rapidly by local exchange? Will the object readily absorb body heat? Will the substance cause chemical damage to the skin?

3.2.* Questions: Do you, in everyday activity, properly distinguish among temperature, thermal capacity, and thermal conductivity? For example, do you make such a distinction when first anticipating, and then placing your hand on either a car body or blanket when both are at the same subfreezing temperature? How does your experience of this thermal difference relate to the usual information that would be obtained from an ideal thermometer? What is the importance to the individual with respect to the potential of a burn of (1) temperature, (2) thermal capacity, and (3) thermal conductivity of contacting objects?

3.3.* Questions: Do you consider the compliance of a contacting object when applying a force? Is an anticipation of an object's inertia important in predicting the effect of an applied force? Consider a few examples.

Chemical composition is especially important at the point of entry into the respiratory or gastrointestinal tracts, where it provides an important basis for selection between those agents that are toxic and those that are essential. Within the hollow organs, chemicals take on importance if they require special treatment or if they approach the point of causing tissue damage. For example, information about the concentration or the presence of some chemical agents can be a valuable influence on both the secretory and motor activity of the gastrointestinal system. On the body surface, distinguishing between chemical agents is usually of little importance. Thus information about any external agent takes on particular importance only when its characteristics approach the point at which they might have an action of sufficient intensity to threaten tissue damage. The threat of tissue damage, even without specific information about the physical basis of that damage, is usually sufficient to justify some immediate avoidance response.

The relationship between geometry of an external object and its pattern of contact with the surface is dependent, in part, on the configuration of the part of the animal making the contact.

To interpret information about the geometry of objects making surface contact or to organize mechanical responses in an effective way, it is necessary to consider the configuration of the body at the time. This information is represented by joint angles, torques, and velocities; muscle lengths; tendon loads; body rotational and linear velocities and accelerations; as well as a variety of soft tissue configurations. If properly combined, such information can provide a reference geometry and inertial frame of reference from which other geometric information can be derived. This mechanical or geometric information is largely internal to the individual but is essential in controlling and interpreting external relationships.

Most joint movements are rotational with from one degree of freedom (in hinge joints such as the elbow) to three degrees of freedom (in the intervertebral and hip joints). There are also sliding movements (as in the jaw) and rotational movements in which the center of rotation slides (as in the knee). The number of degrees of freedom becomes uncertain when separate movements are not independent (like the individual joints of a finger, or the separate vertebral-rib joints). Sensory configuration-of-self information includes both information about joint positions and about individual muscles and parts of muscles. Most joints have several muscles acting on them and usually the number of muscles considerably exceeds that needed to control all the degrees of freedom of the joint. Although there is considerable overlap between the information that can be acquired from individual muscles and from the related joints, there is never a complete redundancy. For example, when antagonist muscles are active simultaneously, they can each produce internal force without causing any net joint torque. Furthermore, mechanical compliance of a joint is important, but it may be best represented by information about muscle status. A full representation of muscle status would require several measures from each muscle fiber.

Information about changes at a remote location (e.g., sound, light, and airborne chemical substances) provides a basis for predicting possible future direct interactions.

Beyond the range of direct contact are a variety of things that are important to an individual because of the possibility that, in the future, they may result in contact. Information about these objects and events is often available at the location of the individual as patterns of light, sound, or airborne chemical substances. In some vertebrates, both magnetic fields and electrical fields provide added information about remote objects. In many ways, information about remote objects differs from that available by direct contact, and thus requires different processing to be of use. It does not carry the direct information about interaction that is available in contacting stimuli. Variability is inevitably introduced when the source of the information is remote either in space or in time. Finally, the energy that delivers the information is often small when compared with the energy exchanged between a contacting object and the individual.

The nature of the information delivered from a remote object by light or chemicals or sound depends very much upon which of these carriers of information is involved. It is thus convenient to separate the different carriers of information in most of the following discussion.

Characteristics of the light source are usually of less importance in light-transmitted information than are those modifications that result from intervening reflecting and transmitting media.

Although light always originates in a luminous source (figure 3.1), most of the information delivered to the visual receptors involves light that has been altered by being reflected from, or transmitted through, remote objects in a way that is characteristic of those particular objects. The important information content is about these remote objects rather than about the light carrying the information. There are several aspects of light that can be modified to carry information: wavelength, intensity, spatial distribution, polarization, and temporal variation. The possibility of different combinations of these properties makes light a powerful agent for information transmission.

One limitation in the analysis of light-transmitted information is the frequent absence of independent information about the light source. Since transmitted or

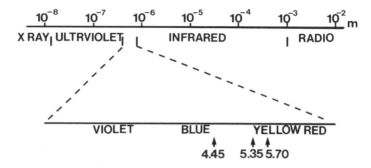

Figure 3.1
Electromagnetic spectrum. The visible spectrum encompasses only a short segment in the center of the whole electromagnetic spectrum. The colors that we perceive are distributed across this spectrum. In mammalian retinas colors are distinguished by the differential absorbance of only three classes of receptors (cones) that have absorbance peaks at 4.45, 5.35, and 5.70×10^{-7} m.

reflected light must first originate in a luminous source, the light information from a particular object is not ordinarily constant, but depends on the distribution of light that reaches the object at a particular moment. Ideally, the light transmitted, reflected, or emitted by an object gives all the necessary information to make a spectrographic analysis of the chemical composition of the object. This potentially valuable information would require determining the ratio of the wavelength-dependent intensity of the transmitted, reflected, or emitted light to the wavelength-dependent intensity of the source light. Without this complete information, the visual system usually operates based on relative information.

3.4.* Experiment: Obtain a set of colored objects such as a set of painter's color chips, a photographer's color card, or an artist's color wheel. Observe these objects under different lighting conditions such as a sodium vapor light, a mercury vapor light, a neon light, a tanning light, or a heat light. Record your perception of a representative set of color samples under the different lighting conditions. Now examine them again under sunlight and under household (incandescent) illumination. Presumably the physical samples of color are not changing. Which colors appear the darkest and the lightest under each light? Can you properly identify all the colors under the different lights?

Characteristics imparted by the sound source are usually of more importance in sound-transmitted information than are those modifications that result from intervening reflecting and transmitting media.

Sounds provide necessary information for the identification and localization of objects. Sounds also function in the very important role of symbols for communication between individuals. Sound information, like light information, is carried in several properties, including frequency, phase, intensity, and spatial and temporal differences. Because of the many simultaneous combinations and temporal changes in these properties, sound provides a rich channel for carrying information from one point to another.

Sounds, in general, originate in the objects that they identify. Both bats and dolphins, however, emit sounds and localize objects by the reflection of these sounds. Humans, too, especially the blind, sense sound reflection as a source of information about the location of large objects. Selective transmission of different sound frequencies, comparable to optical color filtration, is probably not a source of added information for humans.

3.5.* Question: Can you identify a practical situation in which selective absorption of particular sound frequencies provides useful information about some remote or intervening object?

The basic unit of relative sound power is the Bel, named in honor of Alexander Graham Bell. This unit is generally too large for convenience, so sound intensities are usually described in decibels (dB). (The dB used to describe sound is the same unit used to describe deviations from uniformity in the response of amplifiers, earphones, and loudspeakers and to specify hearing loss.) One dB = 0.1 Bel and is about the smallest change in sound intensity that is noticeable. The Bel and the dB are not direct measures of sound intensity but are units used to compare two intensities. One Bel (10 dB) describes the ratio of two sound powers when the power being described is 10 times as great as the sound used for a reference. To deal with ratios easily and to span a range of *powers* of more than $1:10^{12}$ (a pressure range of $1:10^6$), the numbers used are logarithms of the magnitudes. To describe a sound intensity in decibels, it is necessary first to identify the reference level being used. The reference level can be chosen arbitrarily, but for certain purposes specific levels have become conventional. In hearing measurement there is an internationally agreed standard that is the power delivered by a sound pressure of 20 micropascals (μPa) (0.0002 dyn/cm^2) (figure 3.2). When this standard is used, it is indicated by the abbreviation *SPL* (*sound pressure level*). This reference is approximately the lowest human threshold for sound detection under ideal conditions.

For technical reasons, the threshold value is stated in sound pressure, whereas the ratios involved in dB comparisons are determined in sound power. The ratio of a particular sound *power*, P_1, to a reference sound power, P_r, is proportional to the square of the sound *pressure* ratio, F_1/F_r, of the two sounds, that is

$$\frac{P_1}{P_r} \propto \left(\frac{F_1}{F_r}\right)^2$$

This ratio can be expressed in decibels as 10 times the log of the ratio of measured power to reference power:

$$dB = 10 \times \log\left(\frac{P_1}{P_r}\right) = 10 \times \log\left(\frac{F_1}{F_r}\right)^2 = 20 \times \log\left(\frac{F_1}{F_r}\right)$$

3.6. Questions: The range of hearing is approximately 120 dB, ranging from the threshold of hearing to sounds so loud that they are painful. (Note: 1 dB = 20 $\log(F_1/F_r)$ where F_1 is a particular pressure and F_r is a reference pressure.) What is the ratio of sound pressures encompassed in this range? What is the range of sound powers that this represents? (You might want to refer to the log graph given in figure 11.3.)

The specifications of two computer printers state that the ink jet model produces 53 dB SPL and that the impact printer produces 65 dB SPL. Is this difference (1) just noticeable, (2) large enough to be recognizable under office conditions, or (3) the difference between tolerable and painful?

Biologically important distinctions of sounds commonly involve time-variant patterns of changing intensities over multiple frequencies.

Rarely in normal activity, and regularly in some hearing tests, we are exposed to sounds of a single, constant pitch (frequency) and loudness (amplitude). Otherwise, most sounds are composed of mixtures of components that change in

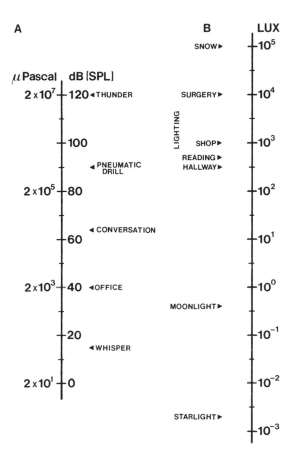

Figure 3.2
Log intensity scales.(A) Decibel scale. The SPL (sound pressure level) decibel scale is referenced to 20 μPa or 0.0002 dyn/cm². The audible range encompasses 6 orders of magnitude of sound pressures. (B) Lux scale. The range of light intensities to which the human eye is sensitive covers almost 8 orders of magnitude from about 10^{-3} to about 10^5 lux.

amplitude and frequency over time. In the normal sound environment, interfering sounds (background noise) are often as loud as the sounds of interest.

The lowest notes on pipe organs may be as low as 16 Hz, a pitch that is felt as much as heard. The bottom of the range of many bass singers is the F below the bass clef (87 Hz). An audible hum of either 60 or 120 Hz is emitted by many electrical appliances. One of the highest written notes in the soprano repertoire is the F above the treble clef (1396 Hz) in Mozart's *Magic Flute*. (Interestingly, in the accepted pitch of Mozart's time, this note would have been sung at about 1318 Hz.) Figure 3.3 relates several notes on the musical scale to their corresponding frequencies. For adequate understanding of conversations, telephone bandpass for voice lines is only 300–3000 Hz.

Overtones that give sounds their individual characteristics are at frequencies above those of the primary pitch. The narrow range of primary pitches listed above is somewhat misleading in that it does not include these important overtones. The differences in timbre of a flute, a trumpet, and an oboe each playing the same note arise entirely from the combination of, and the relative strengths of, the frequencies making up the sound. Similar differences in frequency combinations exist between voiced vowel sounds of *a, e, i, o,* and *u* when sung at the same pitch (figure 3.4). Differences in frequency combinations often identify the remote source of the sound and communicate other information about the nature of the source.

Besides specific frequency combinations, temporal changes of both amplitude and frequency are important features in identifying sounds such as a note from a bell, a violin, an organ, or a human voice (see figure 3.5). These changes in frequencies and amplitudes are generally slow when compared with the changes of sound pressure that are responsible for the instantaneous sound. As the information carried in the individual notes or speech sounds (phonemes) is combined into chords or words and then further combined into musical phrases or sentences, there is a progressive increase in the information content of the sequence. The meaning of a sequence of sound variations may not be apparent until the completion of the whole sequence many seconds later. For many sound objects, the distribution in time has an importance for identification that is comparable to the spatial distribution of other types of objects.

3.7.* Demonstration: Consider the spoken sentence: "It is that which we do know which is the great hindrance to our learning that which we do not know" (Claude Bernard, 1865). At the time you recognized the meaning of the whole sentence

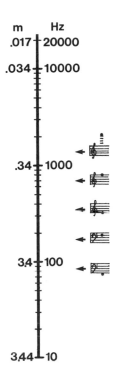

Figure 3.3
Auditory frequency range. The usually quoted ranges for human audition are about 20–20000 Hz. The numbers to the left show the wavelength of these sound pressure waves in air at 20°C (speed of sound = 344 m/sec). Several notes over the range of the normal human singing range are shown.

were you still using information from the first part of the sentence? What was the interval between reading the first part of the sentence and using that information?

3.8.* Experiment: Examine some properties of sound by using a microphone and an oscilloscope. Use an internal trigger and rapid sweep to compare the waveforms of several sustained speech sounds spoken at the same and at different pitches. Compare the same sounds spoken at the same pitch by different individuals. Do the sounds perceived as similar have the same waveform in the different trials? Compare the waveforms generated by different musical instruments playing the same note. Use a slower sweep to examine the amplitude modulation in

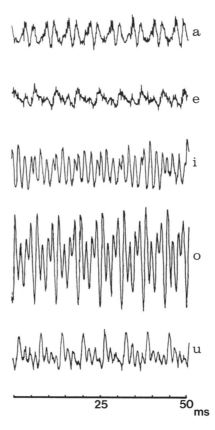

Figure 3.4
Vowel waveforms. Each of the vowels a, e, i, o, and u were sung into a microphone and the resultant outputs displayed as a function of time. See whether you can determine the pitch at which each was sung. How do these records differ from what you would expect if a whistle was played at each of these pitches?

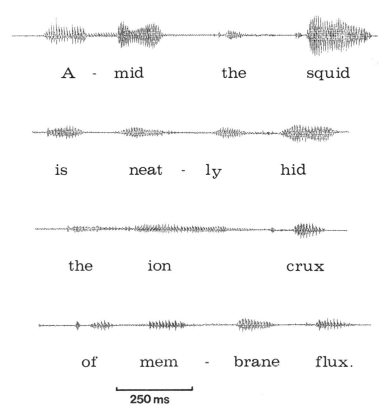

A - mid   the   squid

is   neat - ly   hid

the   ion   crux

of   mem - brane   flux.

250 ms

Figure 3.5
Speech sound pressure waves. Oscillographic record of about 4.5 sec of speech with pronounced syllables placed approximately under the appropriate pressure waves. What information must the ear extract for these pressure waves to be recognizable as speech?

a spoken sentence. Produce a series of sounds at increasing intensities to learn the subjective experience of the loudness of sounds that differ by various measured decibel steps (e.g., 1, 2, 5, 10, 20, and 50 dB). (If available, use a sound meter such as that used for acoustic balancing of stereo equipment.) Depending on the particular type of microphone used, the voltage output may not be proportional to the sound intensity over the whole range. It will generally be more linear than if you used calibrated input steps to produce test outputs from a loudspeaker. For accurate calibration, microphones can be tested against a calibrated sound meter at an audiometric facility or at a recording studio.

Information from specific, remote sources can be modified in transmission through intervening media and mixed with information from extraneous sources (noise).

Information from remote sources is available to an individual only when it actually reaches sensory receptors and, as a result, the intervening medium can easily influence remote information. Information from remote sources is also subject to masking by extraneous signals added by other sources in the environment.

Under the most simple conditions, the intensity of signals from a remote point source decreases with the square of the distance with a negligible time delay for light, a noticeable time delay for sound, and a large time delay for chemical agents. Simple intensity information with respect to sound, light, or chemical substances does not unequivocally define the distance of the source, because both the intensity at the source, and the transmission losses are usually unknown. As a further complication, with each of these carriers of information, the information arriving at any point in space is a mixture of that coming from all sources, attenuated and altered by effects in the intervening space. Information about the location of the sources in space does exist in the small differences in these mixed signals as they arrive at different points.

While the spectral distribution of light reflected from, or transmitted through, a substance is dependent on the optical properties of that substance, it can contain no spectral components that were absent from the original light source. Incident light reflected from or transmitted through a nonluminous object does not have a characteristic spectral pattern, but it does have a characteristic ratio of alterations of its spectrum. In fact, the action of a transmitting or reflecting object is to transmit or reflect characteristic fractions of each spectral component in the light source. Further alterations of the light may occur because of fractional attenuation by the media between the object and the sensory receptor.

3.9.* Question: Photographers are familiar with the greenish color of faces in color slides of people taken when a major part of the light reaching the face was first reflected from grass. (In prints, this effect may be minimized by color correction.) The color difference is most obvious in a side-by-side comparison of a slide taken in direct sunlight and another made in reflected light. What factors can you identify that might account for why side-by-side, or rapidly sequential, comparison of color slides accentuates a difference in color balance more than does successive viewings over a long period?

Since sound is reflected or absorbed by various surfaces and its intensity is attenuated with distance, sound intensity and pattern can be significantly altered by the environment. In a normal room, from 50% to 90% of the sound received from a source arrives after reflection from one or more surfaces. Reflection from complex surfaces can introduce canceling interference between adjacent waves with the effect that incident sounds are absorbed. Further, the reflection of sound from a solid object, such as the human head, leaves a sound shadow behind it, an effect that is most obvious at frequencies above about 1000 Hz. The complexity in the acoustics of a concert hall results from the sounds arriving at different points in space after undergoing different attenuation, reflection, and absorption.

Not only is sound intensity decreased as the square of distance, but it is absorbed as it passes through air. Absorption increases with distance and varies with temperature and humidity. Air absorption amounts to about a 1 dB loss for each 2 m at 16 kHz and increases to twice that amount at 40 kHz.

3.10.* Question: What possible biological significance does sound absorption have?

Reflection of sound is intentionally enhanced in the design of halls intended for musical performances. Lecture halls, by contrast, are designed to control carefully the amount of sound reflection. Before the days of electronic amplification of sound, it was difficult to combine these two uses into a single room. A partial solution was found in the use of chanting in large cathedrals whose acoustical properties better fit the organ than speech.

When sound passes from one medium to another (e.g., from air to water), the ratio of sound reflected at the surface to sound transmitted depends on the closeness of the match in sound transmission properties of the two media. This poses a physiological problem, because sound waves in air need to reach the receptors of the inner ear, which are immersed in fluid. Solutions to this problem will be discussed in chapter 5.

3.11.* Experiment: At a swimming pool, have someone tap two stones together, both in the air above the water and below the surface of the water. Observe these sounds while your head is above the water and while you are completely submerged. Is the attenuation of sound dependent more on the distance or on the presence of an air-water interface? Does the direction of the interface affect the result? What are the complicating factors in interpreting the results of this experiment?

At a sound velocity of 0.33 km/sec, the wavelength of a 2-kHz sound wave (on the musical scale, approximately the C three octaves above middle C) will be about equal to the distance between a human's ears. As a result, for sounds up to moderately high pitches, the instantaneous difference in sound phase at the two ears is related to the direction of the source.

3.12.* Problem: What are two types of information in sound that might be used by a human to localize the sound source? What are the advantages and limitations of these two as a source of sound localization information?

3.13.* Experiment: Use a small source of constant sound (e.g., an audio oscillator-driven earphone) and one or two small microphones attached to an oscilloscope to demonstrate some points discussed in this section. Observe the effect of interposing your head between the source and one microphone. How does this effect depend on the sound frequency and the locations of the source and the microphone with respect to your head? Use either a source-synchronized sweep or two microphones to examine the effects of (1) the distance from the source, (2) the differences between rough and smooth surfaces in sound reflection, and (3) the effect of background sounds.

3.14.* Problem: Individuals with moderate hearing loss often have difficulty in understanding conversation in an environment with background noise. By contrast, individuals with normal hearing use high-frequency components of the conversation to localize the source and thereby attain a 20- to 30-dB improvement. With these facts in mind, design a better hearing aid. That is, with two or more microphones, design a system that would select sound from one location over that from sources in other locations.

Although the whole preceding discussion of physical information has been organized in terms of the site of origin of sound information, it is entirely conceivable that this information could be organized to a different end. For example, information about the internal need of glucose, glucose level in the blood, glucose available in the gastrointestinal system, and external sources of glucose are all important pieces of related information. A neural system that brought these facts together probably would be more useful than one that organized this information based on only the site of origin of the information about glucose. Careful consideration of neural function will reveal many cases in which diverse types of information are combined to produce a specific response.

All the sensory receptors together provide a characteristic response to only a small fraction of the information from internal and external sources.

The total amount of information reaching a human body from internal and external sources is great. There are no reliable numbers for comparing this with the total sensory nerve array that must carry all neural information from its point of detection to where it is used by the central nervous system. Making the reasonable assumption that each sensory fiber carries information about a given sensory dimension, the sensory nerves could not report even 1% of the total input information at any instant of time. We will support this statement by comparing some approximations of the dimensions of sensory input with estimates of the number of sensory fibers serving these sensations.

   The mechanical inputs of force, pressure, acceleration, velocity, position, or distention describe interactions at one instant, whereas inertial, viscous, elastic, or frictional compliance represent important properties of interacting objects. At any point on the body, each of these variables might be directed in any solid angle and pairs of forces might affect rotation in any possible plane. The total effective interaction can be described as the vector sum of three rectangular plus three rotational directions, each of which is an independent dimension. Additional

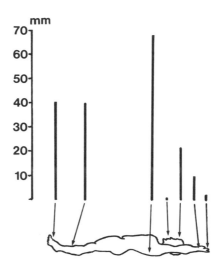

Figure 3.6
Two-point discrimination. The distance between two just-distinguishable points is shown for various selected locations of the body by the length of the solid bars over these sites. What does this figure imply about the density of "touch" receptors? What does the density of these receptors imply about the touch perception of the world?

information about temperature, thermal capacity, and thermal conductivity of all interacting objects increases the total information present.

The skin surface of the adult human body is at least 1 m^2 (10^6 mm^2). If there were as few as 100 dimensions of independent mechanoreceptive input at each point on a 1 mm grid this would account for 10^8 total dimensions of input to the skin (figure 3.6). This estimate is three orders of magnitude greater than the number of sensory neurons serving the skin, although less than the total number of central neurons that might be involved in storing and processing information about these inputs. The total area of enclosed surfaces of the lungs and gastrointestinal tract is roughly 100 m^2. Both the dimensions of independent mechanoreceptive input and the density of sensory neurons are considerably reduced over these surfaces.

Points of independent input within the body are harder to estimate because, to a certain extent, conditions tend to be less independent from one interior point to another. Information about joint and muscle action is an exception. All the joints of the human body account for a few hundred degrees of freedom. Even in the extreme assumption that useful information is developed in each independently controlled group of muscle fibers (a motor unit), the number of independent inputs from muscles is about 10^5. Thus the degrees of freedom in body mechanics give an input of information with about as many dimensions as there are sensory nerves serving the skin. This number is certainly smaller than the error in the previous estimate of the number of independent input dimensions to the skin, and thus does not alter the previous estimate of the total physical input of information.

Adjacent points on the surface, or within the body, are provided with separate nerve fibers that add to the capacity to carry information centrally. Any information that is duplicated spatially can be delivered to the nervous system through the cooperative action of nerves from these different points. On the other hand, some information arriving at the different points is independent and thus adds to the total input load. Mechanical input to points differing by only a millimeter (e.g., on the tongue) is different enough that humans can sense and use these differences.

A further explosion in dimensions of information occurs when we include those dimensions needed to describe incident light. At any point, the solid angles of incidence can be described as the sum of three orthogonal vectors. The plane angles of polarization can be described as the vector sum of two-dimensional components. Since different wavelengths of light can be present simultaneously, any complete description of light as a vector sum introduces as many dimensions as there are wavelengths in the continuous spectrum. Sound information further increases the dimensions of the sensory stimulus. The auditory system extracts pitch and amplitude information from complex sound pressure waveform signals. In addition, this auditory signal is used for very accurate timing information.

An interesting contrast of sensory dimensions arises when we compare the information processing of the auditory and visual systems. Both sound and light signals contain wavelength, intensity, and location information, but our sensory perceptions of these two forms of signal differ considerably. Both systems resolve differences in intensity well but are each impoverished in one of the other two dimensions. Wavelength (pitch) is maintained as distinct information in the auditory system and as a result we can clearly distinguish each simultaneous note of a chord. On the other hand, we can determine only one apparent wavelength (color) from any location in the visual system and Newton showed that we cannot determine the component wavelengths of a mixed color signal. Our localization ability for auditory signals is only rudimentary, and allows for considerable mixing and ambiguity. The visual system, by contrast, very accurately resolves locations and preserves this information through most of its subsequent processing.

Although it requires meticulous counting, determination of the number of afferent fibers in the auditory and visual systems is unambiguous since these fibers are restricted to two pairs of symmetrical specific nerve trunks. The best measurements give about 6×10^4 total auditory fibers and 2×10^6 visual fibers.

The number of independent dimensions required to define the interacting chemical agents is even larger than the number of dimensions of thermal and mechanical inputs. Although there is no exact description of the dimensions of chemical sensation, this could be as large as the number of different chemical agents encountered by the organism. There are 2×10^4 compounds well enough known to be tabulated in the *Handbook of Chemistry and Physics,* and it would be naive to assume that this list is by any means complete.

Besides external chemical information, another important source of chemical information is the composition of fluids in the tissues. Here the number of independent points could be directly related to the vast surface area of the capillaries or to the number of cell surface receptors, and at each point several chemical entities are probably important. We do not know how to make even a rough estimate of how much added information exists in this form.

In spite of the inaccuracies in our estimates, we can still confidently conclude that there are not enough sensory nerves to provide the nervous system with all the information that impinges on, or originates within, the body. We are fortunate that our ancestors did not evolve enough nerve fibers to do that job, because that would have given us a bulk of nerve fibers greater than our present body mass. If, as in computers, the processing of information increases in complexity exponentially with the amount of information to be interrelated, if all this information was delivered to the CNS, it probably could not be analyzed anyway.

The information reaching the body from many sources is both redundant and too extensive to be processed and stored by any finite system. The amount of information required to represent changing conditions increases as the required temporal resolution of detail increases.

The nervous system is limited in its ability to deal with all the dimensions of input that act on and in the body. For the information sensed in any interval of time to be delivered to the CNS without loss, the transmitting fibers must have an adequate temporal transmission capacity.

The rate of delivery of information in a single dimension depends on the product of the amount of information at one instant and the frequency with which that information takes on new, independent values. The amount of information in an input depends on how *unpredictable* that input is. The uncertainty about an expected input is related to the number of possible values it might have. The information content of a signal increases both as the possible range of its values increases and as the resolution of detail within that range increases.

Information in the form of total light flux, concentration of a particular chemical agent in arterial blood, internal body temperature, and mechanical pressure has been chosen here to represent the variety of physical inputs that might act at a point. You might find it interesting and instructive to add some examples from your knowledge.

The smallest increment in light input is the addition of one photon. The maximum natural value of light flux probably is that from direct sunlight at high altitude, which is roughly 10^{16} photons per second on 1 mm^2 of surface. It is possible to have exceedingly rapid changes within this range. In well-mixed, buffered arterial blood the concentration of a chemical agent, such as H^+ (pH), at one point will be essentially the same as it is at any other point. Thus, the amount of independent information is not much more than the information in the value sensed at any one point. The temperature at any deep body location cannot change rapidly under any survivable conditions because of the buffering effect of the heat capacity of the body. Again, the number of independent values per time is small. The information about mechanical pressure at a location can account for a very high information delivery rate. Maximal meaningful pressures are those that approach disruption of the skin. Minimal values that could be separated from "noise" are probably not much larger than the pressure fluctuations due to random molecular collisions of the air. Pressure changes occur from as slowly as hours (atmospheric pressure) to as rapidly as tens of thousands of cycles per second (sound).

3.15.* Questions: Would you expect the pressure fluctuation resulting from random molecular collisions, averaged over a surface, to be influenced by the area of the surface? (Would this be important in the design of small microphones for hearing aids?) The time course of even a short sample of a random collision pattern can be approximated by a combination of sinusoidal signals. Would the magnitude of the part of a random signal that is fitted by a sine wave of a particular frequency be expected to become larger or smaller as the number of cycles sampled is increased? Explain your answer.

3.16.* Problem: Set up the equations necessary to make an estimate of the pressure variation on a 1 mm^2 surface due to random bombardment of air molecules under normal conditions. What assumptions have you made? Extend these equations to predict the probability distribution of this noise over different frequencies. Find the necessary quantitative values and solve your equations. How would you modify the calculations to distinguish light intensity differences as a function of total light flux? In what way do the results of these calculations suggest a type of threshold for audition and vision?

3.17.* Problem: From your knowledge of physical systems, prepare a table of the range of frequencies at which each type of biologically important physical signal is known to change. Compare this table with what you know about the limits of information transmission on nerve fibers.

It is not only impossible with our nervous system but probably also counterproductive for any nervous system to have the ability to acquire all the information that is available to the individual at any moment. The nature of pulsatile signals and the reporting ranges available over single nerve fibers dictate that even among those dimensions that are sensed, there are some for which the actual information input cannot be reported on a single nerve fiber. The next two chapters will examine how particular dimensions are selected by receptors. They also will survey selections and compromises in receptor systems that provide the nervous system with information that, although incomplete, is statistically good enough to allow the individual to survive in the environment. The sensory system that actually evolved reflects chance, the importance of specific information, and the cost of its acquisition. You will recognize some instances in which missing information seems to introduce no problems and other instances in which the incomplete information results in misinterpretation of the relevant facts.

Chapter 4

Receptor Selectivity

Isaac Newton wrote, "We no other way know the extension of bodies than by our senses" (*Principles*, Book III, rule III). This chapter will deal with the ways that we use our senses to know the extension of bodies and to determine a multitude of other dimensions of the world.

Common to all information-handling systems is the requirement that information enter the system. This usually entails a change of the form in which that information is found.

In this age of home computers, the word input has become a household word. Computers have become so "user friendly" that we can seemingly talk with them in English. The internal language of the information system, however, is different from the language of the world in which the information originated. The input process thus often involves a translation. The process that transforms one form of information into another form is called *transduction*. Not only do computer terminals transduce input information, but transduction is the essential function of all sensory receptors. We have considered transduction to be the modification of the form of information. It is important to recognize that transduction requires that there be an exchange of energy between the stimulus source and the receptor.

Sensory receptor systems differentiate between different sources of energy.

Just as a *paramecium* responds differently to different stimuli, it is important that humans differentiate among diverse stimuli. A receptor system that simply summed the total energy incident on the body might be useful in some situations but it is generally more useful to distinguish between various types of energy and to delineate details about each specific energy source and sink. Humans have evolved some marvelously sophisticated means to transduce those specific forms of environmental energy that evolution has found to be especially important.

Sensory receptors have been categorized by several classification systems. An especially useful one was established near the turn of the century by Sir Charles Sherrington. This classification system is based on the source of the information that is transduced. *Interoceptors* transduce information from within the organism. *Proprioceptors,* literally "self-receptors," transduce information regarding the location of the body parts with respect to each other. *Exteroceptors* transduce information from outside the organism. The category of exteroceptors can be further subdivided into *teloceptors* that transduce information from remote sources and *somatoceptors* that transduce information presented at the body surface.

Encoding with pattern codes and transmission over labeled lines are two means by which distinct types of sensory information are internally differentiated.

At least two means have evolved by which the brain is told which type of sensory information is being received. Over the years, these two have alternately gone into and out of favor as a basis to explain sensory differentiation; probably the nervous system uses both means. In the first system, often called a *pattern code,* a unique neural firing code exists for each specific type of sensory information. Such a system allows for the transmission of multiple forms of sensory information over common "party lines." Pain may, in part, use such a system, sharing neuronal transmission lines with other forms of mechanoreceptive information. The second system is one in which *labeled lines,* or specific nerve fibers, are committed to specific forms of sensory information. In this case, any information received by the brain over a specific nerve is always interpreted as representing that particular stimulus. The visual system is one good example of a system with labeled lines to sensory areas of the brain. As a result, any stimulus that is capable of exciting peripheral visual neurons (even a blow to the eye) is perceived as light.

4.1.* Experiment: You can demonstrate this effect without the risks of stepping into a boxing ring. Turn your eyes as far as possible to the left. Now the retina of your right eye is in a position directly inside the right hand corner of the right eyelid. Close your eyes and gently tap the right corner of the eyelids of the right eye. This produces a pressure stimulus to the right eye that is seen as a purple spot surrounded by a yellow ring. Where does this spot appear in your visual field? Why would you expect it to be in that location?

The idea of labeled lines in sensory physiology is associated with the nineteenth-century physiologist Johannes Müller. His observation is given special import by being called "Müller's law of specific nerve energies."

Julius Bernstein wrote in 1876, "If, under accidental circumstances, the auditory nerve had been attached to the eye, and the optic nerve to the ear, then every ray of light would produce a sound, and every sound in our ear would produce an appearance of light in our imagination; we should then see a symphony, and hear a picture." Less poetically, everything that we know about the world enters our nervous system as changing spatiotemporal distributions of nerve impulses. These nerve impulses are determined by the independent actions of our sensory receptors.

This chapter will deal with some selective capabilities of individual receptors. The next chapter will describe specialized accessory structures that further diversify and enhance the selectivity of various receptors. Both of these means of selectivity include mechanisms that suppress the effects of unwanted forms of energy and enhance the response to the forms of energy that constitute the adequate stimulus.

The various modalities of sensation represent the dimensions of sensory space.

The specific form of energy to which a receptor best responds defines the *modality* of that receptor. We live in a world whose dimensions are determined by the modalities of the specific sensory receptors that we possess. The dimensions of "sensory space" are thus ultimately a result of the fine tuning of specific receptors to limited parts of the total energy exchange. Loss of sensory dimensions is encountered in various pathological situations in medical practice. In these cases, because of the sudden removal of the dimension, or the lack of built-in compensations, the individual is handicapped by the lack of that particular dimensional information. Trauma (or surgery) can result in the loss of either receptors or the sensory nerves between the receptor and the central nervous system. Partial or total blindness results from damage to the retina or optic tract and deafness from similar insults to the auditory system. In addition, age, loud music, and certain drugs can all lead to the loss of specific auditory receptor cells. Olfactory nerve fibers are sometimes disrupted in head trauma. The senses of touch, temperature, and even pain are lost following trauma to peripheral nerves. Genetic deficits result in the loss of specific sensory dimensions spanning the spectrum from loss of one color component to complete loss of pain. The importance of pain sensation is dramatically shown by the frequency of trauma in parts of the body that have become anesthetic. For instance, smokers who have lost the sense of pain in their fingers often have many cigarette burns there.

Mechanoreceptors provide sensitive responses to a wealth of different mechanical stimuli.

Many different receptors respond to direct mechanical deformation. These include muscle spindles, Pacinian corpuscles, Golgi tendon organs, stretch receptors, joint receptors, and various skin receptors. In addition, nociceptors respond to high levels of mechanical stimulation. Other mechanoreceptors that respond to second-order mechanical stimuli are the hair cells of the vestibular and auditory systems. These receptors have cilia that when mechanically displaced cause a response in the sensory receptor.

We will see in chapter 11 that potential changes in neurons result from the opening or closing of ion channels in the cell membrane. Sensory transduction in some way, then, must incorporate mechanisms that affect membrane channels. For mechanoreceptors, physical distortion of the membrane in some way causes specific ion channels in the membrane to open. Stretch-activated channels have been observed that open for distortions that cause less than 2% change of membrane area.

The mechanoreceptors in the auditory system are specialized and respond to a unique type of mechanical stimulus. To encode sound information, individual auditory hair cells must respond to a specific narrow range of frequencies of sound pressure waves. A part of the determination of this specific frequency results from secondary structures that will be discussed in chapter 5. In addition, at least in lower vertebrates, the membranes of auditory hair cells are electrically tuned to specific frequencies (figure 4.1). The frequency of electrical resonance corresponds to the specific frequency of sound pressure wave to which the cell responds best.

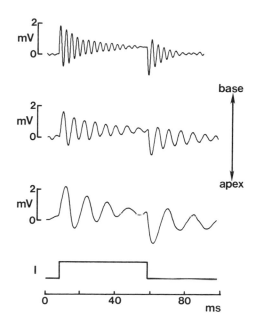

Figure 4.1

Auditory receptor response. The primary auditory receptor, called a hair cell, gives the largest response at a sound frequency (pitch) that is specific to that cell. As we will see in chapter 5, accessory structures to the receptor allow a specific receptor cell to receive a maximal mechanical stimulus at a specific frequency. This figure shows the electrical tuning of three auditory receptor cells. When these cells are stimulated electrically with a brief pulse of current (lower record), the membrane potential oscillates with a damped oscillation at the frequency to which the cell normally responds. These records are arranged according to the location of the cells from the base to the apex of the cochlea. (Data from Art and Fettiplace, 1987.) The mechanism of electrical tuning of lower vertebrate auditory hair cells has been studied extensively in recent years. These cells contain excitatory calcium channels and inhibitory calcium-dependent potassium channels. (Membrane ion-selective channels will be discussed in chapter 11.) Bending of the hairs on these cells produces an excitatory potential that opens the calcium channels, which leads to the continued excitation of the cell. The calcium flowing in through these calcium channels eventually causes Ca^{2+}-dependent potassium channels to open. These potassium channels then terminate the excitation. The interaction of these two processes, one causing excitation and the other terminating excitation, causes the cell to be electrically tuned to a specific frequency of sound pressure. The number and kinetics of the calcium and potassium channels vary from cell to cell in a graded manner so that there is a progression of tuning frequencies along the auditory receptor structure.

Chemoreceptors respond when specific classes of chemical agents contact the receptor cell.

One group of chemically sensitive receptors will be apparent to all readers. These are the cells of the olfactory mucosa and the taste buds. There are, however, a second and a third category of chemical sensitive cells that needs to be considered. The second category includes a group of interoceptors that responds to chemical concentrations in the internal environment. In this category are endings in the gastrointestinal mucosa, carotid body and aortic arch receptors, and various neurons in the brain. The third all-encompassing category is cells that respond to the specific neurotransmitters and hormones that are released at many sites within the body.

The human olfactory sense can distinguish qualitative and quantitative differences among airborne substances ranging in molecular weight from 15 to 300 and with concentrations as low as 10^{-12} M (ethyl mercaptan). There are striking similarities in olfactory recognition and immunological recognition. Both systems are capable of recognizing and responding appropriately and quickly to a vast number of molecules. The olfactory system is capable of making many of the self vs. nonself determinations in the external environment that the immune system makes in the internal environment. There are important similarities in the mechanisms of operation of these two chemosensitive systems. Olfactory cells have excitatory membrane channels that are activated by intracellular second messengers. (Second messengers will be discussed in chapter 13.) These second messengers are released within the cell by molecular receptors in the cell's membrane that are, in turn, sensitive to specific extracellular molecules. An olfactory cell can, like a cell of the immune system, respond to any one of a vast number of molecules by simply creating or modifying existing molecular receptors (figure 4.2). This process can occur with impressive rapidity partially because neither the second messenger nor the ion channel needs to be modified.

While all neurons are affected by temperature, certain neurons respond principally as temperature receptors.

"Cold" and "warm" receptors have maximal responses at different temperatures. In each case, the response decreases when the temperature is either higher or lower than the characteristic temperature. After a long (i.e., 30-min) exposure to

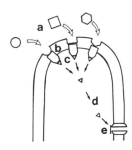

Figure 4.2
Olfactory transduction. The olfactory system can give a specific response to a wide range of different odorant molecules. Individual olfactory receptor cells probably have a select palate of odorant receptor molecules in their membranes. These membrane receptors, however, produce a cellular response through a common second messenger system. When any one of a group of odorant molecules (a) binds with their membrane receptors (b), a common second messenger (c) is released from each. These second messengers convey the message intracellularly (d) to ion channels (e) that determine the receptor cell's electrical response.

heat, cold receptors begin to respond with a "paradoxical discharge," firing at a rate that depends on temperature within the new range. On the other end of the range, cold receptors having been exposed to a low temperature for an extended period stop firing at a uniform rate and begin to fire in bursts. In this mode of firing, the burst pattern is more characteristic of the temperature than is the average firing rate. The details of these mechanisms remain obscure. Incidentally, the response of a cold receptor is driven by an external energy sink rather than by a source.

Mammalian photoreceptors respond to light signals relative to the dimensions of intensity, wavelength, and spatial coordinates.

Each type of receptor cell of the retina (the rods and three classes of cones) responds maximally within a specific range of wavelengths (color) of light. Since the cones operate primarily in bright light and the rods primarily in dim light, the spectrum of wavelengths is reduced to three unidimensional sensory variables in bright light and to a single dimension of graded brightness in dim light. There is a small intermediate range of intensities in which both receptor types are activated.

The details of the visual transduction process have been extensively studied and are known in considerable detail. The photosensitive protein molecules in mammalian retinas are made up of two parts. One part of the molecule, vitamin A aldehyde, is actually sensitive to light. The other, larger portion of the molecule determines the part of the visual spectrum to which the molecule is sensitive. The visual transduction process begins when a single photon strikes this molecule and changes the angle of a specific covalent bond. This begins a cascade of events that ultimately closes membrane channels and results in a change in potential in the photoreceptor cell. In the dark adapted eye, one photon causes about a 3% change in the electrical current flowing in a receptor cell. The human retina is a quantum detector in that it is sensitive to the smallest unit of information in the electromagnetic spectrum, the photon.

Light signals acting on retinal receptor systems include the dimensions of local intensity and wavelength, and the three coordinates of position in space. From these dimensions are derived the characteristics of visual perception, form, color, spatial information, and object recognition. The rod system transduces light signals over a narrow band of wavelengths with high sensitivity, but with lower spatial resolution than the cones. There are three subsets of receptors within the cone system that transduce light signals at three different, but broad, wavelength bands (figure 4.3). This wavelength information is integrated in one neural processing system to produce the sensation of color. Two other neural systems work in parallel to process other parts of the information transduced by the cones. These two systems are relatively color blind. The first of these extracts high resolution information about form of stationary objects; the second extracts information concerning movement and stereoscopic depth.

Artificial color representations such as color TV, color photography, color printing, artist pigment mixing, stage lighting, and color figures on computers all take advantage of the loss of information that occurs in transduction in the human retina. It is necessary to provide only the three dimensions of the wavelength information that is transduced by the retina to produce the whole spectrum of color sensation. Thus red-green-blue, tint-hue-contrast, magenta-cyan-yellow, or hue-saturation-luminosity are each three dimensional, but not equivalent ways of representing what is interpreted by the brain to be a full range of colors.

Color blindness is the result of genetic variations that cause deficiencies of one or more of the color receptor types. Individuals with this condition have a reduced number of light dimensions that they can identify. The result of this loss of dimensions is an ambiguity in distinguishing between certain regions of intensity and the continuous color spectrum.

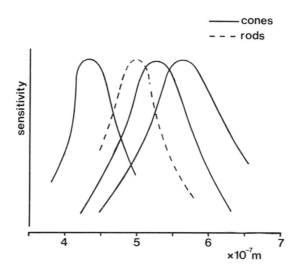

Figure 4.3
Rod and cone sensitivity. Relative sensitivity of the rods (dashed line) and three types of primate cones (solid lines) is plotted against wavelength of incident light. The single rod peak exactly overlaps the absorption of the visual transduction molecule, rhodopsin. There are three distinct groups of cones that are distinguished by their visual pigment and hence the spectral location of their absorption peak. Color determination by the cone system results from the fact that any wavelength of light will produce a characteristic response by the three groups of cones. (What type of ambiguity would arise in a color blind person with only two cone systems?) Differences between sensitivity graphs, as shown in this figure, and threshold graphs are considered in appendix F.

4.2.* Experiment: Take a series of strongly colored paint chips ranging from red to blue to a location that is so dimly lighted that you cannot identify the colors. Arrange the chips in order of a gray scale as you see them. Now turn on bright room lights and inspect the results. Relate these results to the differences between rod and cone sensitivity.

Sensitivity to electric currents and fields, although common in many neurons, is not a well-developed sensory system in humans.

Since neurons operate with electrical signals, it is to be expected that they can be stimulated with electrical currents. In the human, however, there are no known receptors whose primary adequate stimulus is external electrical current. There are many occasions when one cell is stimulated by electrical current from another cell. The high conductance current paths between certain cells are called *electrical synapses*. These occur between certain neurons and between many muscle cells. The low threshold *axon hillock* region of a neuron, where the axon joins the cell body, also might be considered an electroreceptor. This part of a neuron is sensitive to currents flowing between regions of the same cell. The primary specialization of the parts of cells that are sensitive to electrical current is a low resistance pathway from the source of the current. The lack of electroreceptors in the periphery in humans does not reflect the lack of a biological mechanism by which they could operate.

Extreme conditions are likely to damage any cell and as a result will affect the behavior of any neuron. Certain neurons, however, are especially responsive to conditions that are likely to lead to damage.

We have seen that receptor systems usually sense fewer dimensions than are delivered by the external and internal world. For high levels of stimulus strength, many receptors will respond outside their normally most sensitive dimension. In addition, there are a group of receptors called *nociceptors* that respond across a wide range of physical dimensions but only to stimulus levels approaching that sufficient for tissue damage.

Most nociceptors appear to be free nerve endings. This observation is supported by the evidence that the cornea, to which most stimuli are painful, has only free nerve endings. The dimensions of nociception vary. In the gut, chemical stimuli and stretch dominate; on the skin, cut, burn, and tear dominate; in the tooth pulp thermal, mechanical and electrical stimuli dominate.

The exchange of more than a certain minimum amount of energy must occur before a sensory receptor will respond.

The minimum energy necessary to elicit a response from a receptor is called the *threshold*. The threshold is characteristic of a specific receptor and related to the particular form of energy being sensed. In many dimensions, the threshold is difficult to measure because it approaches the theoretical limit for detecting that form of energy. The best available instruments either will not measure such small amounts of energy or absorb too much of the energy to make accurate measurement. Thus, indirect means are used to estimate absolute thresholds.

A single photon can produce a response in a retinal rod. It probably takes about six photons striking the cornea from a particular direction for one to reach a retinal rod. The human auditory threshold is only about 20–30 dB above the level of thermal noise in air. Olfactory thresholds are near the minimum resolution of gas chromatographic instruments. The human threshold for ethyl mercaptan is 10^{-12} M, while it has been estimated that moths respond to single molecules of sex pheromones.

4.3.* Problem: Calculate the number of *molecules* of ethyl mercaptan in a liter at a concentration of 10^{-12} M. How many of these molecules would be in the human nasal cavity with a volume of about 10 ml? What factors might be involved in determining how many of these molecules make contact with olfactory receptors?

Human gustatory thresholds to saccharine and quinine are about 10^{-5} M. A comparison of this value with those given above for olfaction is consistent with much of the sensitivity (and the diversity) of gustatory sense being a result of olfaction.

Our perceptions of the world are limited by the sensitivities of those sensory receptors with which we have been endowed by evolution.

Information handling, be it electronic or biological, is a costly process. A very large amount of information reaches an individual at any one time and it would be exceedingly unprofitable for the nervous system to attempt to deal with all this information. In the interest of energy conservation, sensory systems must continually reject information, preserving only the most important.

We perceive a world whose dimensions are determined by the modalities of the specific sensory transducers that we possess. Although we are continually immersed in electromagnetic field gradients, we are not aware of them. This, though, is a limitation of our receptors rather than anything absolute about sensory dimensions (Withers 1992). Electric fish have receptors for electric fields (with thresholds as low as 1 μV/m) and can perceive the world in terms of electric field gradients. Our visual spectrum runs from red to blue but does not include infrared or ultraviolet. Bees, on the other hand, have ultraviolet receptors, so their visual world also includes the ultraviolet reflections from certain flowers. One could extend this list to include various other dimensions of information concerning our environment. It is important to keep in mind that our seemingly absolute division of the world into various senses is but one of many such arbitrary divisions.

The evolutionary development of a sensory dimension depends on the chance "invention" of a receptor system, on the further chance that there will be a test of its cost-effectiveness, and finally on the new system passing this test of cost-effectiveness. The gaps that exist in human sensations suggest that there has also been an active process to reject certain sensory dimensions. The gaps in our sensory world may have evolved almost as much as did the inputs that are sensed. On the other hand, there is no guarantee that receptors would have evolved for all dimensions of useful information. Unsolved problems exist in our sensory perception. These may represent problems whose solutions were tried and proven not worth the cost or ones that have not yet been tried.

The history of human civilization is too short a period to have allowed for significant further evolutionary changes in humans. Although there might be other forms of environmental information that would be useful to a modern civilized person, our sensory perceptions are those that were important to a hunter-gatherer animal.

Information arriving at the body, especially that from remote sources, often has considerable redundancy.

Evolution seems to have taken advantage of the redundancy of sensory information by providing only enough receptors to *sample* the inputs. As long as these samples are appropriately chosen the remaining redundant information is unnecessary. Differences in sound or light arriving at only two points contain most of the important information about the nature and location of the source. The development of two eyes and two ears and perhaps two nostrils may be based on an optimal compromise about information input.

Often the information that is actually sensed allows partial or complete determination of other information that was not sensed. So, for instance, although position, velocity, and acceleration are independent parameters, sensing but one

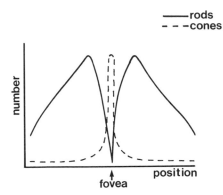

Figure 4.4
Distribution of rods and cones. This graph shows the relative number of receptors at locations along a line drawn across the retina. (This line is assumed not to go through the blind spot where the optic nerve exits the retina.) It is apparent that the cones are concentrated in the central region of the retina called the fovea. Since there is considerable convergence from rods to more central neurons, this system has generally high sensitivity but low resolution. The cone system exhibits little convergence and has high resolution, color sensitivity, but a high threshold. From your everyday experiences with vision, what can you deduce about the unconscious function of the system that includes the muscles that move the eye and thereby determines the direction of gaze?

of these parameters allows a determination of the other two if one is measured continuously over time. Information about movement within an inertial reference frame is acquired only for the head (by the vestibular apparatus). This information might be extrapolated to the rest of the body once further information about body configuration has been determined. This configuration information is obtained by the proprioceptors of the body. Central nervous system calculations can replace the need for sensing additional dimensions.

Another very important economy of sensation is obtained by providing high-resolution spatial information for only a part of the input space with the remainder having only limited resolution. For example, tactile discrimination is high on the tongue and very low on the buttocks. Similarly, visual discrimination is high within a small solid angle around the center of the visual field (the *fovea*) and much lower in the remaining majority of the visual field (figure 4.4). In spite of this great economy of numbers of sensory dimensions, the importance of the loss is minimized by the ability to move the high resolution area to cover the region of greatest interest.

4.4.* Experiment: Obtain a clinical burn chart or other estimate of skin area. Locate an area of your skin where you have the best ability to distinguish between one and two contacting points. Using the same methods, find the skin area with the poorest resolution. Assume that spatial resolution is a direct measure of receptor density. Now calculate the saving in number of receptors accomplished by not having the same high resolution over the whole body surface. What are the functional implications of the locations where the highest resolution contact information is provided?

Sensory receptors limit the response range of the input information.

We have been considering savings in receptors and information input because of limited spatial distributions. Another important economy occurs because of limited response range.

For a sensation such as temperature, a receptor's range is much smaller than the possible range of stimuli. In fact, the temperature range of skin receptors is appreciably less than what is tolerable even over considerable time periods. This range limitation results in a considerable reduction in the information load in this dimension. The response range of light receptors is considerable—about $1:10^{12}$. There are, however, many light sources including the sun, a welding arc, or even sunlight reflected from snow at high altitude that exceed the range of the receptors and can, in fact, damage them. The range of intensities involved in normal human hearing goes from 20 µPa to about 2×10^7 µPa. This range is exceeded occasionally by natural sounds and frequently by technological sounds.

Sensation occurs within specific sensory coordinate systems.

The most primitive receptor imaginable would be an excitable cell that responds indiscriminately to all kinds of incident energy. There are probably no such pure energy receptors. Individual receptor cells, by virtue of their location, membrane composition, or other properties are appreciably more sensitive to one form of energy than others. Although receptors have higher sensitivity to one form of energy, all receptors will respond outside their primary dimension. We name receptors, though, for their greatest known sensitivity or their suspected function and we generally take the names from physical dimensions.

The same information can often be represented equally well in a variety of coordinate systems. There is no a priori reason to expect evolution to have provided receptors that use the same coordinate systems that we have arbitrarily chosen for physical measurements. No known receptor duplicates exactly, in range, dimension, and scaling, a technological measurement definition (figure 4.5). Although it is convenient to refer to our receptors in terms of the dimensions of physical science, we must remember that these dimensions were selected arbitrarily to be convenient for certain manipulations. Because sight and hearing are easily isolated, it is natural that the dimensions of light and sound were selected for use in physics. Selections of other dimensions would be expected to match those of our more concealed receptors only by chance. They, in fact, do not match at all well.

Temperature is one dimension that is invariably added to a receptor's dimensions. All living cells are sensitive to temperature and, at least in the periphery, body temperature can vary by several degrees. Temperature receptors have specific, well-defined responses to changes in temperature but since neuron firing is dependent on temperature, all nervous signaling must in some way account for a ubiquitous temperature sensitivity.

Within muscles there are well-studied receptors, called *stretch receptors,* that respond to muscle stretch. Under carefully controlled conditions one finds that the firing rate of these receptors increases monotonically with the amount of stretch. (As figure 2.8 shows, the relationship between firing rate and stretch is close to a logarithmic function.) From firing rate the central nervous system could ascertain approximately the amount of stretch (length) on the receptor. As early as 1931 B.H.C. Matthews showed that stretch receptor output is additionally dependent on the rate of stretch. This additional dimension influencing the output information from a stretch receptor means that the central system cannot unambiguously determine either length or velocity from firing rate of a single receptor. With further study, it became apparent that there were two types of stretch receptors in a single muscle. Both types respond to length and rate of change of length, but the response of the two receptor types differs in its relative dependence on these two dimensions (figure 4.6). The central nervous system, receiving both inputs, could use these two inputs to make an unambiguous determination of both length and velocity. There is, however, no reason to suspect that the central nervous system makes this conversion to the dimensions of length and velocity instead of using the information while still in the sensory dimensions.

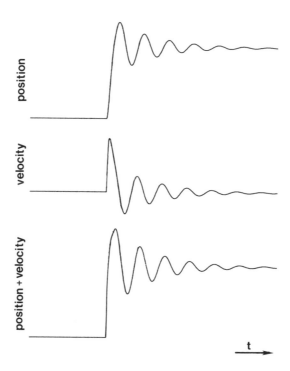

Figure 4.5
Coordinate exchange. A rapid finger movement such as suddenly pointing from one target to another looks, in position vs. time coordinates, like the upper graph. The information received by the nervous system concerning that finger will depend on the type of response of the proprioceptors related to that finger. If those were velocity receptors rather than position receptors, the velocity vs. time graph would determine the neural representation of that finger movement. Actually, the proprioceptors measure a combination of position and velocity. The information that the nervous system receives about the movement is thus like that in the lower graph. Is there information contained in any of these coordinate systems that is lacking in another?

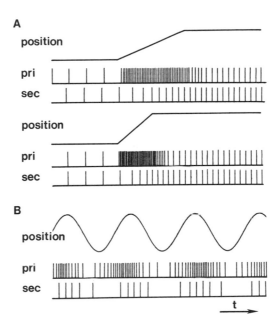

Figure 4.6
Primary and secondary spindle responses. This figure is a simulation of the response of a primary muscle spindle receptor (pri) that senses position and velocity, and of a secondary muscle spindle receptor (sec) that senses mostly position. (A) The responses to a smooth movement between two positions at two different velocities. (B) The responses to a sinusoidal movement. The primary spindle receptor that is simulated here has two noticeable characteristics: its velocity response continues beyond the actual time of movement and it simply adds the velocity and the position components. Would you expect either of these characteristics to be valid for an actual primary muscle spindle receptor?

When receptors respond to more than two dimensions of physical input, the response of a single receptor is necessarily ambiguous in those individual dimensions.

This is equivalent to the case in algebra where there are fewer independent equations in a system of equations than there are unknowns. The requirement for solving algebraic equations is paralleled by the sensory requirement for there being as many types of receptors as there are independent dimensions to be sensed. It is important to remember, though, that the dimensions of sensory receptors need not be transformed into the arbitrary dimensions used in experimental or clinical studies before the unique solution can be achieved. Although terms such as light touch, touch, vibration, and deep pressure are useful for quantifying sensation, they should not be considered to show either specific receptor type or receptor location.

In any instance in which there are fewer independent inputs to a group of receptors than there are members of that group, there is redundancy between receptors. This redundancy provides a safety factor so that the loss of a single receptor does not result in the loss of a particular sensory dimension. Conversely, where there are fewer receptors in a group than there are inputs acting on that group, different combinations of inputs can produce indistinguishable sensory responses. This is the neurophysiological basis for various types of sensory illusions.

Many bilateral receptor systems, although providing redundancy of overlap, extract valuable information from the nonredundant information arriving at the two displaced receptor systems. The bilateral semicircular canals of the vestibular system are an interesting case. Because the canals are rigidly linked by the skull, they receive identical rotational inputs. Pairs of canals, however, are arranged to produce opposite outputs from a given rotational input.

Sensory encoding recurs at multiple steps as sensory information is conveyed centrally. Specific sensory information is selected in this encoding process.

Receptors generally produce graded potentials called *receptor potentials.* As was mentioned in chapter 2, such graded potentials fall off precipitously at even small distances away from their site of origin. In a small organism, such as a *paramecium,* in which the receptor and effector functions reside within a single small cell, this is of little consequence. In larger organisms, where the receptors and effectors are separated by considerable distances, a receptor potential will have no *direct* effect on the effector. Here transmission of information is effected by encoding the receptor information into a pulse code that can be carried reliably over long distances on nerve fibers.

The evolution of large, complex organisms has made necessary the physical separation of receptive functions from central sensory integration and further from effector processes. It is necessary that some form of transmission of sensory information is effected. Seldom do sensory systems function by transmitting a point-by-point representation of the environment to the central nervous system. Just as environmental information is modified by the nature and location of receptors, so it is modified during encoding and transmission.

If the visual system simply consisted of a television camera for the eye and a monitor screen for the visual cortex, we would need to have another television camera to watch the visual cortex monitor. Nothing would have been accomplished in the process toward understanding the incoming information. Actually, signals reaching the visual cortex are distorted in a way that is useful to the organism. Some qualities of the information are lost and others are emphasized and, at every step along the way, some interpretation has occurred. Neurons have been identified that respond to a multitude of specific aspects of visual input patterns. However, no one has found a neuron that provides the equivalent of recognition of "grandmother" from a visual image.

Stimulus amplitude is typically encoded in a nonlinear manner.

Psychophysics has two "laws" that relate stimuli to perception. The *Weber-Fechner law* (proposed by E. Weber in 1846 and modified by G. Fechner in 1860) says that there is a logarithmic relationship between a stimulus and the *perceived* sensation. The *Stevens law* (proposed by S.S. Stevens in 1953), on the other hand, states that it is a power relationship. Both are applicable in approximating psychophysical measurements, depending on the system and the range being tested. Both, though, have three things in common: (1) they predict a nonlinear input-output relationship, (2) they predict a relatively greater sensitivity for small inputs, and (3) they allow for a broad dynamic range of responses by compressing the representation of large inputs.

4.5.* Problem: The Weber-Fechner law says that

$$R = k \log \left(\frac{S}{S_0} \right)$$

where R is the response, k is a proportionality constant, S is the stimulus amplitude ($S \geq S_0$), and S_0 is the stimulus threshold level. What is the necessary increment of the stimulus above an initial stimulus of 10 (arbitrary units) to produce the same increase in response as that found in a stimulus increase from 0.03 to 0.1 units?

Stimulus-response relationships for the whole animal are often close to log or power functions. At which step in the sensory process does this nonlinearity occur? Measuring the response of sensory receptors to various stimulus levels is an experiment that has been repeated for many sensory modalities. (For example, see figure 2.8.) The relationship is usually nonlinear, and it is often a logarithmic relationship over some range of stimulus amplitude and a power relationship over more extended ranges.

Certain other nonlinearities exist in sensory systems, but the original trans-duction step can often explain how the whole animal responds to sensory inputs. Much of the psychophysical input-output relationship may reside at the initial step. The implication of this statement is, of course, that any successive encoding of sensory information is nearly linear. Such a linear encoding relationship is common, at least in encoding a graded receptor potential into a pulse frequency code for transmission.

Spatial and temporal boundaries are emphasized in sensory encoding.

Many sensory neurons send lateral branches that inhibit adjacent neurons to produce *lateral inhibition*. This is a simple and rather universal means of modi-fying sensory information as it is relayed toward the central nervous system. The amount of this inhibition typically depends on the level of excitation of the neuron doing the inhibiting. The result of this process is that the spatial boundaries of stimuli are accentuated.

A horseshoe crab in the murky intertidal water or a hunter-gatherer human ancestor wandering in a dark forest is much more concerned with the outline of an approaching predatory animal than with the details within that outline. Such a distortion of sensory information has obvious survival value.

In a manner similar to the emphasis of spatial boundaries by lateral inhibition, temporal boundaries are also emphasized. *Adaptation* occurs when a constant stimulus causes an initial large response that dies away to a lower maintained response. The process of adaptation is common in receptors and will be the topic of an extensive discussion in chapter 15.

There are many mechanisms by which adaptation is produced; two of these are mechanical and electrical. Sometimes, as we will see in chapter 5, structures associated with a receptor cause the actual signal reaching that receptor to diminish with time. Many neurons use electrical means to produce an adapting response. In these receptors, the electrical response to a maintained stimulus has an adapting component to it that results from a slow change in electrical conductance of the cell membrane. The photoreceptive cells of many animals, for instance, exhibit this property.

The word "phasic" comes from the Greek word φασισ, meaning an appearance or more specifically a transient appearance. The term is used in sensory neurophysiology to delineate the transient aspect of a stimulus or response. The word "tonic," on the other hand, derives from the Latin word *tonus*, meaning stretching or, in particular, a maintained stretch. In sensory physiology, tonic is used in reference to the maintained aspect of a stimulus or response. Adaptation serves to accentuate the phasic aspect of a stimulus at the expense of some of the tonic information that also might constitute the stimulus. Partially adapting receptors represent an intermediate in a continuum ranging from purely phasic receptors to purely tonic receptors.

4.6.* Questions: Which of the modalities of sensory information would be most important to be transduced by phasic receptors and which by tonic receptors? Consider this question in terms of both conscious and unconscious sensory input to the nervous system.

Individual photoreceptors in the retina are rather phasic. What mechanism might the eye use to produce a maintained visual input?

To return to a previous example, the horseshoe crab or hunter-gatherer human ancestor is also more concerned with the time of entry of a predator into its visual field than with its maintained presence. A predatory cat, on the other hand, approaches its prey with quick advances interspersed with extended periods of motionless crouching. During much of the time the cat minimizes both the temporal and spatial boundaries of its presence.

Figure 4.7 shows the similarity of adaptation in the temporal domain to lateral inhibition in the spatial domain. In either case boundaries are accentuated at the expense of static information about the stimulus.

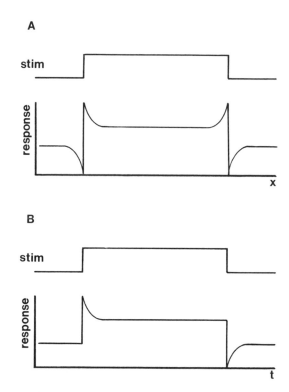

Figure 4.7
Boundary enhancement. (A) The results of lateral inhibition produce an accentuated spatial boundary to a stimulus that begins and ends abruptly in space. (B) Adaptation produces a similar accentuation of the temporal boundary of a stimulus that begins and ends abruptly in time.

Our familiar sensations result from information in many physical dimensions that originates from a multitude of sensory receptors.

There are major discrepancies among the perceived information, the specific receptors that respond, and the physical description of the stimulus. It is important to distinguish which is being described. The table in appendix G provides a partial listing of the terminology used in these categories.

Chapter 5

Accessory Structures to Sensory Receptors

Receptor properties determine the response to the energy that reaches a receptor; other structures selectively affect what part of the energy from the environment reaches each receptor.

In chapter 4 we considered the ability of various sensory receptors to transduce specific forms of energy. That discussion emphasized differences in the properties of the receptors themselves. Further differences in receptor responses are determined by accessory structures that selectively affect the energy before it reaches the receptive cells. Accessory structures, such as the optics of the eye and the mechanics of the middle ear, attenuate, amplify, or in other ways modify selected parts of the energy before it reaches a specific receptor. This process is often the first step in determining the *modality* of a sensory system. This chapter will be concerned with these accessory structures (figure 5.1).

The ultimate step in every receptive process is the opening or closing of the ion channels through which specific ions cross the membrane. The penultimate step, in which the energy is actually absorbed, is often not very specific. Thus the receptors themselves may lack not only the ability to localize energy sources or extract detailed information about the energy but also the ability to even distinguish among various forms of energy.

Differential selectivity, because of accessory structures, can impart unique response patterns to a set of nearly identical receptors.

Nonspecific, but important attenuators of mechanical energy are the soft tissue, the bones, and the fluids that surround particular receptors. The body is then the most general absorber of energy from sources that are extraneous to a receptor. The orientation of the body is extremely important in separating energies that arrive from different sources and directions.

Since many sensory receptors are located in the head, the skull serves an important function in shielding sensory receptors from the mechanical stimuli to

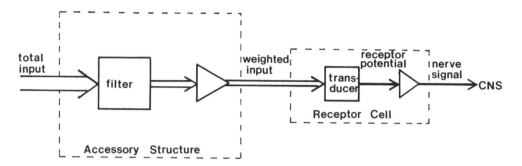

Figure 5.1
Sensory accessory structures. Most sensory systems depend on accessory structures to help define a specific sensory modality. These structures generally act first as a filter reducing some types of energy that is transmitted to the receptor cells. Often accessory structures serve the additional function of amplifying the specific form of energy to which that particular sensory system is most sensitive. As we have seen in chapter 4, receptor cells transduce and amplify the energy delivered to them.

which all receptors are intrinsically sensitive. Thus the skull is an attenuating accessory structure to auditory, visual, vestibular, and olfactory receptors. This accessory function is especially important for the auditory and vestibular systems since these receptors specifically transduce mechanical energy. Because of the attenuation of other forms of mechanical energy, vestibular receptors respond fairly specifically to gravity along with other linear acceleration and head movement whereas the similar auditory receptors respond to sound pressure waves. The vestibular attenuation function goes even further and excludes responses to actions that have no component in a specific linear direction or plane of rotation.

Further isolation of receptors is accomplished by fluid supporting actions. The receptors in the retina, and vestibuloauditory complex, in particular, are contained within fluid-filled cavities. Without the fluid support, these mechanically sensitive receptors would be stimulated to saturation by the gravity-oriented acceleration forces on the receptors.

5.1.* Demonstration: To show the effectiveness of hydraulic support place an intact raw egg in a wide-mouth jar, fill the jar with water, and cover it tightly. Now shake the jar in different directions increasing the acceleration as you become more confident in the effectiveness of the hydraulic support. If you can spare the egg, remove the water and repeat the experiment. Relate these results to the theories proposed by Pascal and by Archimedes.

5.2.* Problem: Patients who have had some cerebrospinal fluid (CSF) replaced by air for certain X-ray studies find it very unpleasant to make any movements until the CSF has been renewed. Where might the receptors reside that are responsible for these sensations? Why are head movements not usually a basis for unpleasant sensations?

One of the simplest examples of attenuation by an accessory structure associated with a receptor is that produced by the capsule of the *Pacinian corpuscle*. Pacinian corpuscles are mechanically sensitive receptors found in the skin, joints, and periosteum that are formed by a mechanoreceptive nerve ending surrounded by a fluid core covered by layers of connective tissue. A rapid compression of the corpuscle distorts the receptor fiber thereby stimulating it to produce a local current flow that triggers nerve impulses. The viscoelastic properties of the onion-like bulbous structure covering the nerve ending dissipate the distorting effect of compression over time. The Pacinian corpuscle produces an adapting response to a maintained compression; however, the adaptation is eliminated if the connective tissue is removed and the compression is applied directly to the mechanoreceptive nerve ending (figure 5.2). The accessory structure here serves to isolate the phasic aspect of a mechanical stimulus that would have produced an essentially tonic response in the underlying nerve ending.

Accessory structures protect the individual mechanically sensitive hair cells of the auditory system from stimuli other than a specific range of airborne vibration.

The auditory system accomplishes another important selection of energy by means of accessory structures (figure 5.3). Here the structures of the middle ear shield the receptors from slow pressure changes that can be as much as 10^5 times as large as the pressures encountered during the normal transduction process of the receptors. The ambient atmospheric pressure on the ear drum is normally balanced, because of the Eustachian tube, by the pressure in the middle ear.

Normally the auditory system encounters only slow changes in ambient pressure. Atmospheric pressure changes are generally no more than 10% and take days or at least hours to occur. The rate at which pressure changes as the result of a change of altitude depends on the means by which the altitude change is occurring. Going from sea level to the top of Mount Everest represents a 70% decrease in atmospheric pressure, but this change in altitude would take weeks

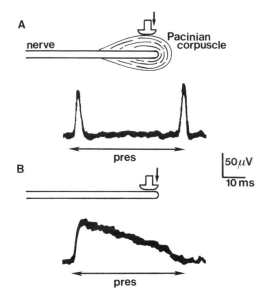

Figure 5.2
Pacinian corpuscle. (A) The Pacinian corpuscle, with its viscoelastic sheath, produces an adapting response to a maintained pressure. When the sheath is removed (B), the response to a maintained stimulus has very little adapting component. (Data from Loewenstein and Mendelson, 1965.)

to accomplish on foot. A similar change in pressure is minimized by pressurization in the cabin of commercial aircraft when similar altitude changes occur in a matter of minutes although the remaining changes in cabin pressure are greater than those ordinarily experienced on the ground. Rapid ambient pressure changes are produced by simply turning the head while standing in a strong wind. Such a change is too rapid to be compensated by the eustachian tube. Pressure changes in diving can be large and fast. A 10 m dive can result in almost a 100% increase in pressure; if this is not compensated by voluntary action it will cause considerable pain and even rupture of the eardrum.

5.3. Demonstration: Close your nose, mouth, and glottis and attempt to exhale forcibly. The resultant increase in pressure in the middle ear via the eustachian tube can be felt (and heard) as a displacement of the ear drum. This experiment is called *Valsalva's maneuver* after Antonio Valsalva (1666–1723). The Valsalva

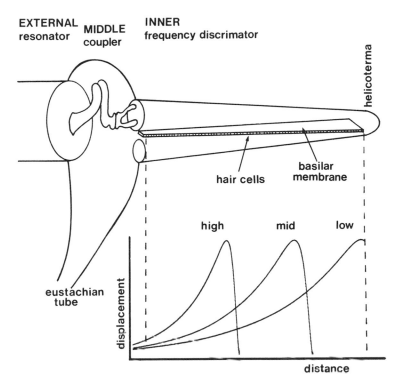

EXTERNAL **MIDDLE** **INNER**
resonator coupler frequency discrimator

helicoterma

hair cells

basilar membrane

high   mid   low

displacement

distance

eustachian tube

Figure 5.3
Auditory accessory structures. Each of the three anatomical divisions of the ear, the external, middle, and inner ear, has specific effects on sound pressure waves. The external ear, because it is a closed tube, acts as a resonator. This resonator improves responsiveness by 5–12 dB at frequencies between 2000 and 5500 Hz. The middle ear is an effective mechanical coupler because of two characteristics. First, the area of the ear drum (tympanic membrane) between the external and middle ear is about 16 times larger than that of the oval window, which separates the middle and inner ears. Second, the ossicles that connect the ear drum to the oval window act as a lever with a mechanical advantage of about 1.3. This makes the mechanical coupling between air and the inner ear about 25 dB more efficient. The inner ear, or cochlea—shown here as if it were uncoiled—contains the actual receptor cells and acts as a frequency discriminator. This property will be discussed in figure 5.7.

maneuver is used to equilibrate middle ear pressure in diving and is useful for adjusting to pressure changes in a commercial airplane cabin.

The ear drum, however, transmits rapid pressure changes that occur only on the external side. Within the middle ear, air pressures are balanced between the round window and oval window of the cochlea. Any maintained differences in pressure, which would be capable of producing a steady displacement of the basilar membrane, are dissipated through the helicotrema. The rapidly changing components of pressure that are related to sounds, though, can be transduced because they are mechanically transmitted to only one window. In addition, the external and middle ear select the direction, frequency, and magnitude of air pressure fluctuations that act on the actual receptors in the inner ear. This selection results from enhancement of some parts of the sound and reduction of other parts.

Although movement of the external ear is only minimally effective for sound localization in humans, most of us have observed that some dogs and cats are very adept at moving their external ears (pinna) to localize sound sources. In humans, the shadow provided by the head is important in producing the sound differential between the ears that is useful for sound localization. In addition, rotation of the head is an important technique that is used to localize the source of a continuous sound.

Enhanced responsiveness to a particular stimulus energy can be produced by structures that either increase the energy converging on the receptor or increase the effectiveness of coupling of a particular type of energy to the receptor.

The abrupt change in mechanical compliance between soft tissue and bone introduces large distortions on those receptors that lie near this interface. This mechanical linkage causes some deep mechanoreceptors to be more sensitive to surface mechanical inputs than other mechanoreceptors nearer the surface.

The vestibular organs, located within the middle ear, include the fluid-filled *semicircular canals,* one in each Cartesian plane (figure 5.4). Each canal is partially blocked by a gelatinous structure in which the hairs of the vestibular hair cells are embedded. The dynamics of the canal system are such that the inertia of the fluid within the semicircular canals makes the fluid tend to remain stationary when the head starts to rotate. For short rotations, the stationary fluid causes a shearing force on the hairs of the receptor cells in a direction opposite to the

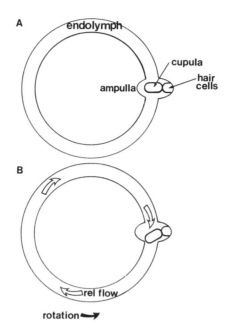

Figure 5.4
Semicircular canals. Part of the vestibular apparatus consists of fluid-filled canals in each Cartesian plane. (A) The canals are blocked at an enlargement, the ampulla, with a gelatinous structure, the cupula. Hairs of the receptor cells (hair cells) are embedded in the cupula so when the cupula is moved the hairs are bent and the hair cells excited. (B) When the body is rotated in the plane of one of the canals (counterclockwise in this instance) the inertia of the endolymph causes it to move relatively in the other direction. This movement is an effective stimulus to cause the cupula to bend. With continued rotation the endolymph will begin to move with the canal and the cupula will return to its resting position. What effect will the termination of rotation have?

rotation. The receptors are directionally sensitive and their output firing increases or decreases depending on the direction and magnitude of deflection. We will discuss the dimensions of the output of the vestibular apparatus in chapter 15.

Energy is inevitably attenuated during transmission and many accessory structures operate to compensate for this attenuation by making the receptor more effective in responding to the energy that does arrive. Since the enhancement mechanism is usually effective only for one form of energy, this is another means by which modalities are distinguished. Mechanical stimuli, for example, are selected and matched to their receptors through direct mechanical linkages. Besides simply transmitting mechanical energy to the receptor, these linkages serve to match the transfer of energy from its source to the receptor. Such linkages are especially effective in the auditory system.

Impedance is a measurement of the resistance seen by time-varying signals. Signal sources have an output impedance and the recipient device, or load, also has an input impedance. Efficient transfer of energy between the source and the load occurs only when the source and load impedances are approximately equal. *Impedance matching* is the means by which such a condition is attained. A small force that can act through a considerable distance can deliver as much energy as a larger force acting over a short distance. A simple mechanical lever exchanges force for distance and thus can match impedances of an energy source and a particular load. A very simple case of such matching is accomplished between air movement and the deformation of mechanoreceptors found at the base of hairs in the skin.

Another important impedance matching operation is accomplished in the outer and middle ears. This compensates for the approximately 30-dB loss of energy at a simple air-to-fluid interface as would occur at the oval window of the cochlea were it not compensated. Liquids, having a greater inertia than gases, require a greater force to cause them to move. The impedance matching problem of the ear is one of transferring large-amplitude, low-force movements of air on a large surface to lower amplitude movements with the force necessary to move the fluid behind the small window into the cochlea.

The first auditory accessory structure to have an impedance matching effect is the external auditory canal—a closed tube with a resonant frequency of about 3 kHz. Within a range around this resonant frequency, sound pressure waves are amplified by about 12 dB. There are two further mechanical mechanisms in the middle ear that produce frequency-dependent impedance matching. The first results because the tympanic membrane has an area of about 70 mm^2 and the oval window has an area of only 3.2 mm^2. The second results because the ossicle chain between the tympanic membrane and the oval window acts as a lever with a mechanical advantage of 1.3. These two mechanisms produce a total mechanical gain of about 25 dB in effectiveness of energy transfer from air to the cochlear fluid. There is thus a frequency-dependent compensation for the impedance mismatch between sound pressure waves in air and pressure waves in the fluid surrounding the actual receptors. The overall best transmission occurs at a frequency of about 1500 Hz.

The modifications of sound by the external ear, middle ear, and cochlea are complex and have been studied in considerable detail. For an introduction to the physical detail, chapters 14 and 15 of volume III of the Neurophysiology Section of the *Handbook of Physiology* are convenient. These chapters suggest many areas in which understanding is still inadequate and also list several hundred references for further study.

The iris and lens of the eye, like the similar components of a camera, are exceedingly well adapted to produce a sharp, albeit inverted, image of the world on the photoreceptive retina at the back of the eye. The iris, by controlling the size of the pupil, modulates the intensity of the light falling on the retina. The powerful but fixed focal length cornea and the less powerful but variable focal length lens operate together to focus objects from various distances on the retina, which is always at the same distance behind the cornea.

A *lens diagram* shows one problem encountered by a fixed focal distance optical system such as the eye. In a camera one can vary the distance between the lens and the film to produce a sharp image of objects at any distance. In contrast, the distance from the cornea to the retina in the eye is fixed, so the eye must use a different strategy to maintain the information from the visual world in focus on the retina. The basic problem is that as objects move closer to any lens, the in-focus image moves further back behind the lens. Without the ability to focus the eye, the in-focus image would move to a position *behind* the retina. To rectify this situation, the eye *accommodates,* muscles attached to the lens contract, the lens thickens, and its focal length shortens.

5.4.* Problem: Draw a lens diagram such as the one in figure 5.5 and convince yourself that without shortening the focal length a near object will be in focus behind the retina.

By the middle of the nineteenth century, Hermann von Helmholtz (1821–1894) had discovered much of what we know of the optics of the eye. In 1856 he

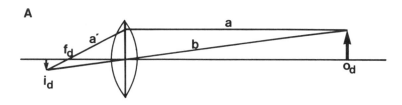

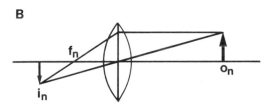

Figure 5.5
Thin lens diagram. The location of an image projected behind a lens can be determined by constructing a lens diagram. First a line (a) is drawn parallel to the center line of the lens from a point on the object to the center of the lens. A second line (a′) is then drawn from this point through the focal point of the lens. A third line (b) is drawn from the same point on the object through the center of the lens. The point where lines b and a′ intersect demarks the corresponding point on the inverted image. (A) A distant object, o_d, in a normal eye with focal length f_d produces an in-focus image, i_d, on the retina. (B) For the eye to also produce an in-focus image, i_n, of a near object, o_n, the focal length, f_n, must be shortened. The eye does this by using muscles to change the radius of curvature of the lens.

published the *Handbook of Physiological Optics* which continues to be a readable and comprehensive discourse on the subject. Much of modern optometric practice is based on the observations of Helmholtz. Technical advances since Helmholtz have, however, made modern optometry a highly quantitative field. Physiological optics are covered in many modern sources. A brief, readable account can be found in the second edition of Kandel and Schwartz, *Principles of Neural Science* (Appendix IIA).

In the eye light coming from a small solid angle that falls over the area of the pupil is collected and most of it is redistributed onto a much smaller area of the retina (perhaps a single photoreceptor). In the center of the retina, the area taken by an individual receptor is about 5×10^{-6} mm^2. The collecting area of the pupil varies between $\pi \times (8/2)^2$ mm^2 and $\pi \times (1/2)^2$ mm^2. Thus the available light for a single receptor can be increased by a factor of 1.6×10^5 to 1×10^7.

The specific location of action and source of energy that causes a particular sensory neuron to respond is the *receptive field* for that cell.

The modalities of sensation are at least partially determined by specific receptors that are more or less specialized to transduce the information carried by one form of energy. Within each *form* of energy certain *sources* of energy, or dimensions of the signal, are especially effective in producing a response within a specific receptor cell. A useful term in describing the spatial distribution of the adequate stimulus to an element of a sensory system is the *receptive field*. The receptive field defines, for a specific receptor cell, the dimension or source of energy, out of all the incident energy on the body, that causes that receptor to respond.

To record the response of a single pressure receptive nerve fiber from the skin, one could probe the skin with a pin and delimit a specific area that caused this receptor to respond. This area would be the receptive field of that receptor. Here the receptive field also could be determined by tracing out the area of skin innervated by the terminal branches of that fiber. The situation is somewhat less obvious with other modalities. In laboratories where the visual system is being investigated, a spot of light is moved on a screen placed in front of the eye of an experimental animal. As the spot is moved around, it will be found to cause one particular neuron in the visual system to respond only in some restricted region on the screen. This region on the screen is then the receptive field of that cell.

5.5. Problem: What is the receptive field of an auditory receptor neuron that lies along the basilar membrane in the cochlea? What is the receptive field of an olfactory neuron in the olfactory mucosa?

Because of the transduction process the information reported by a single receptor is reduced to a single dimension. This reduction occurs regardless of how many dimensions are required to define all the variations of the energy that are delivered to, and absorbed by, that receptor.

Although most objects and events involve characteristics that span multiple dimensions, individual receptors transduce their inputs into a single-dimensional output signal. A single receptor seldom produces a signal that uniquely defines the source of its stimulus. The usual biological solution to this problem is to divide the stimulus dimensions among a series of receptors, each of which then senses the magnitude in only one dimension. For instance, sound is characterized by the dimensions of frequency (pitch) and amplitude (loudness). The auditory accessory structures separate the frequency dimension over a series of separate receptors and each receptor responds to intensity within a narrow range of frequencies. A narrow frequency range is thus the receptive field for each auditory hair cell.

Identification of the receptive fields of cutaneous receptors provides an example of the partitioning of the dimensions of mechanical stimuli. Receptors distributed over the skin respond only to the intensity and location of a mechanical stimulus of a particular type. Many cutaneous mechanoreceptors will respond to low-frequency movements with a signal that follows the temporal pattern of intensity of the stimulus. These receptors, however, are unable to distinguish between higher frequency oscillations and a steady stimulus. The Pacinian corpuscle, on the other hand, transduces only fast changes producing a single pulse per cycle up to signal frequencies of roughly 200 Hz. Thus the skin's mechanoreceptors form a limited set of submodalities that further delimit cutaneous receptive fields (figure 5.6).

Light signals include the dimensions of intensity, wavelength, and the three coordinates of position. Resolution of spatial dimensions ultimately depends on the location of receptors within the retina and the optical accessory structures of the eye. Within the low-intensity rod system and again within the high-intensity cone system, light intensity transduction depends on the number of photons striking a given receptor. The dimension of wavelength is partially preserved in the transduction process because the rods and three categories of cones have specific wavelength peaks in their sensitivity. The wavelength sensitivity of rods and cones was graphed in figure 4.3.

The oscillating pressure waves of sound lie mostly above the frequency that can be carried directly by the pulse code of a single neuron. The pattern of vibration, however, that reaches the cochlea results in a response that is spatially distributed along the basilar membrane. Individual receptor cells respond to amplitude at a specific frequency. The dynamic range of amplitude information is further extended because there are receptor cells with different thresholds at any one location on the basilar membrane.

The problem solved by the auditory system in analyzing complex sound waves is essentially the problem solved by a *Fourier transformation*. Baron Jean-Baptiste-Joseph Fourier, in 1807, devised a method for solving the equations for heat

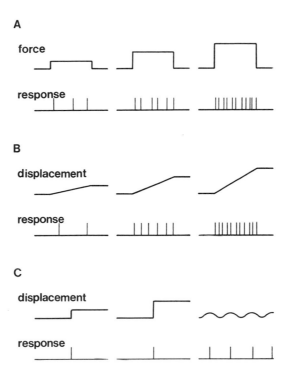

Figure 5.6
Schematic representation of the response characteristics of mechanical receptors. Many morphologically distinct mechanoreceptors exist in the skin. Although their responses extend through a continuum, they are often grouped into three categories based on their ability to produce a maintained response. (A) One group (e.g., Merkel's disks) can produce a sustained response to a maintained stimulus (force) with a greater response to a greater force. These are classified as *pressure receptors* or *intensity detectors*. (B) A second group (e.g., Meissner corpuscles) will eventually stop responding to a maintained stimulus (displacement). These receptors are classified as *touch receptors* or *velocity detectors*. (C) A third group (e.g., Pacinian corpuscles) stops responding almost immediately when the stimulus (displacement) is maintained. These receptors are classified as *vibration receptors* or *acceleration detectors*.

conduction in solid bodies. His technique has since been extensively applied to many other functions that vary in time. Fourier analysis, done either mathematically or electronically, takes a complex waveform and breaks it down to determine how much energy there is within each frequency component of that wave. The inner ear is an active mechanical Fourier analyzer that takes complex pressure waves in air and sends information to the brain regarding how much sound energy there is in each frequency component (pitch) of that wave (figure 5.7). The observation that the ear is a Fourier analyzer goes back at least as far as Helmholtz, who wrote in 1877 (*The Sensation of Tone,* p. 35), "that this analysis (Fourier) has a meaning in nature independently of theory, is rendered probable by the fact that the ear really effects the same analysis."

Single receptive cells provide some information about the location of a stimulus simply because of the location of their receptive fields. Further information is obtained in the difference between the signals that arrive at two spatially separated receptors from a single source. Binaural directional information about sound location is somewhat ambiguous but it does establish one dimension of the direction of the sound source. Two eyes can provide depth information, or *stereopsis,* for distances to about 5 m because of the binocular disparity of the images from a single object (figure 5.8).

5.6.* Problem: What additional mechanisms might provide for depth perception at distances greater than 5 m? Why is the sense of depth not entirely lost when one eye is closed?

Efferent neural signals often effect alterations in the relationship between an individual receptor's response and the conditions in the environment to which the receptor responds.

Some receptors are so located that they are influenced by neurally driven (efferent) actions. These receptors have a special relationship to information processing because they can combine external information with information from other sources. Neural influence on receptors can include direct modification of the receptor itself, action on accessory structures that modify the signals reaching the receptor, and modification by muscular action of the receptor input because of changes in the situation of the receptor. Information sent to the central nervous system by these receptors does not have a constant relationship to the environ-

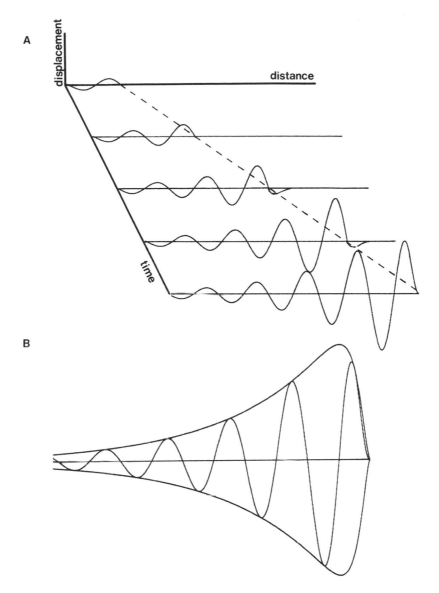

Figure 5.7
Frequency discrimination by the basilar membrane. (A) As sound pressure waves travel along the basilar membrane their amplitude varies with distance along the membrane. The basilar membrane is narrow and stiff at its base near the oval window and wide and flexible at its apex. As sound pressure waves travel along this membrane they displace it most at a location that depends on the frequency of the wave. High-frequency waves displace the membrane most near the base and low-frequency waves have their maximum displacement near the apex. Since the receptor cells (hair cells) respond to displacement of the basilar membrane, they are differentially stimulated dependent upon the frequency of the sound. (B) The envelope of the traveling wave shows how the basilar membrane is displaced along its length. It is the top half of this envelope that was plotted in figure 5.3.

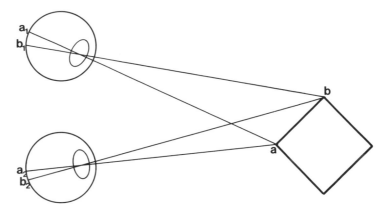

Figure 5.8
Stereopsis. Information concerning depth can be derived from several sources. The two eyes must converge for a given point on an object (*a*) to fall in the center of the two retinas (a$_1$ and a$_2$). Since the *distance* to the object can be calculated with simple trigonometry if the distance between the eyes and the angle of convergence is known, the information from sensory and motor signals can be used to judge distance. The *depth* of the object will cause two points (*a* and *b*) to be represented by different distances (a$_1$ b$_1$ vs. a$_2$ b$_2$) on the two retinas. The nervous system can use this information first to give the perception of only the distance *a b*, and second to derive information about the depth by which *b* lies behind *a*. Why does a perception of depth remain if you close one eye? How good is this perception when applied to unfamiliar objects?

ment but rather results from an integration of external information with the effects of efferent neural action.

Muscle *stretch receptors* are one example of receptors that are directly influenced by neuron action. These receptors lie on special muscle fibers called *intrafusal fibers*. These fibers are, as are all skeletal muscle fibers, innervated from the central nervous system by motor neurons. These motoneurons are called *fusimotor neurons* or sometimes *gamma efferent neurons* because many of them fall into this fiber diameter category. Thus, although the stretch receptors respond to muscle stretch, they are also directly influenced by the activity of the fusimotor nerves. Stretch receptor output, which includes information regarding length, velocity, and fusimotor activity, represents the magnitude of a complex vector function. These receptors provide a complex computation in which mechanical inputs are combined with efferent fusimotor activity. The result of this computation is afferent proprioceptive information that is, under some circumstances, a function of error of position.

Two muscles, the *tensor tympani* and the *stapedius,* are attached to the ossicles of the middle ear. These muscles are under unconscious control by the central nervous system. Their contraction allows adjustment of the impedance match and energy transfer in the middle ear. Their major function is probably one of reducing the possibly harmful effects of sustained loud sounds. Besides the efferent control to the middle ear, there are about 500 efferent fibers in the cochlear nerve that travel to the inner ear. These fibers make synaptic contact with certain auditory hair cells and can presumably influence the receptor properties of these cells. Their actual functional significance is unknown.

We have already mentioned the effect of muscular action in adjusting the focal length of the lens in the eye. Additional muscles control the diameter of the pupil and thereby regulate total light flux to the retina. A third group of muscles, the extraocular muscles, allows voluntary and involuntary movement of the eye. In each of these three cases, muscles provide control, by the central nervous system, of the energy transduced by the receptors. Visual relationships depend on integrating information about the position of images on the retina, eye position, head position, and body position. An abrupt movement of the eyes to locate an object is often followed by a head movement in the same direction coordinated with the return of the eyes to their original position in the head. The net result of these complex movements is that the image is maintained in a nearly constant location on the retina.

The action of sniffing converts a steady olfactory stimulus into an oscillatory signal. Varying chemical concentrations, at frequencies to about 5 Hz, are more effective than constant ones in producing an olfactory response. Thus transient, but more rapid, air flow establishes better conditions for olfactory receptor response.

Motor control is an essential aspect of tactile sense. Tactile sense is largely determined by the interaction of mechanoreceptive input with motor activity in exploratory examination. Defects in the neural control of muscle impede exploratory testing of external objects. Would you expect that cerebral palsy patients, with complex involuntary movement, might have disturbed tactile sense?

5.7. Experiment: Try a standard neurological examination procedure on yourself. Have someone place a small familiar object (neurologists typically use a coin, a safety pin, or a key) in your hand without your knowing what the object is. First attempt to determine what the object is without any manipulation of it. Now manipulate the object. Why can you make a better determination when you manipulate the object? What processing is necessary to use the manipulation information?

Although prolonged changes in accessory structures can alter the response of sensory receptors, sometimes the central processing of signals from those receptors is altered in a compensatory manner.

Sometimes we can readjust our interpretation of sensory information to account for changes that occur before the information reaches the sensory accessory structures. Thus an individual wearing inverting prisms can soon interpret the world to be the right way up rather than being inverted. Often, if the defect is in the accessory structure itself, we have no means of making effective compensation.

Defects in the optics of the eye produce many well-known problems as is obvious from the number of people who wear corrective lenses. Common optic defects include myopia, hyperopia, presbyopia, astigmatism, and cataract.

5.8.* Problem: Use a lens diagram, such as the one in figure 5.5, to understand the following optical problems. *Myopia* results when the focal length of the eye is too short for the length of the eyeball and objects are focused in front of the retina. Myopic persons can, however, see close objects. Why is this so? *Hyperopia* is the opposite condition; the object is focused behind the retina. Why would accommodation help in this condition? Given that there is only a certain amount of accommodation available, why can these people not see close objects? *Presbyopia* is a condition of the elderly in which the lens becomes less elastic. What would you expect to be the limitations of vision under these conditions? *Astigmatism* results when the refraction along different meridians of the eye is different. How would this affect the ability of the eye to produce an in-focus image on the retina? A *cataract* is a condition in which the lens becomes opaque. Treatment for a cataract often entails surgical removal of the lens. What impairment would you expect in a person following this surgery? (Be sure to consider what has already been stated about the relative powers of the cornea and the lens.)

About 9% of the population suffers from hearing loss. This, perhaps more than any other sensory loss, leads to profound social isolation. Deafness results in an increase in the threshold level of sound with no change in the upper limit or pain threshold. As a result, there is a compression of the auditory range. In addition, high frequencies are often the most impaired and since high frequencies are very important for sound localization, deaf people are handicapped in their ability to localize sounds.

Otosclerosis is a condition in which additional bone formations limit conduction through the middle ear. Perforation of the eardrum results in loss of the mechanical amplification of the middle ear. In each of these cases, defective accessory structures greatly reduce the ability of the sensory receptors to function. Traditionally, hearing aids have simply amplified the sound in the external auditory canal. More recently, direct cochlear stimulator implants have been developed. Technology has limited these devices to stimulating only a few points along the cochlea. Surprisingly though, in some cases, a single channel stimulator is effective in restoring a useful degree of hearing to deaf persons. The mechanism by which such stimulation works is not understood.

Different species, having evolved in different environments, have sensory systems that respond to stimuli that are important in those environments. Often one species will respond to conditions that are not sensed by another species.

As the result of the determination of modalities and submodalities by the characteristics of receptors and by their accessory structures, the nervous system has distinct information about a variety of internal and external environmental conditions. Certain forms of energy are not sensed and, in addition, all sensory systems have limited amplitude ranges, thresholds, and dimensional limitations. These vast gaps in the information that is sensed mean that there are significant deficiencies in our direct knowledge of the world. These sensory limitations are probably explicable because of evolutionary demands rather than because of any innate inability to sense specific forms of energy. Because of the added bulk of additional receptors, and the additional central processing needed in dealing with extra information, an input is profitable only when it contributes to (significantly) useful interactions of the organism with its environment.

Visual information reaches an individual from all solid angles of a sphere, has spatial resolution to the microscopic level, and contains information over a wide span of wavelengths, intensities, fluctuation frequencies, and polarization angles. Out of this wide range of information, humans sense light from approximately a hemisphere of solid angles with a spatial resolution of about 1 minute of angle at the eye. Sensed light is within a spectrum from violet to red, has an intensity range of $1:10^{15}$, fluctuates more slowly than about 50 Hz, and lacks information about polarization angle.

5.9. Problem: Use a variable-frequency strobe light to determine the maximum frequency at which you can move your hand. Does this value offer any suggestion about the evolutionary pressure for the range of fluctuation frequencies sensed by the visual system? Can you provide any other examples to justify some of the aforementioned visual system information limitations?

Auditory information arrives from a sphere of solid angles, covers a wide range of intensities, and extends to those very high frequencies used by echo location in bats. The human auditory system restricts input, however, to two poorly defined cones, to an amplitude range of 20 to 2×10^7 μPa, and to a frequency range of 20 to 20,000 Hz.

Out of the vast range of chemicals that exist, the human olfactory sense is capable of identifying only about 90. The human olfactory sense has a threshold of sensitivity of about 10^{-12} M. By comparison, dogs have an olfactory sensitivity about 100 times as great, possibly because they have an olfactory mucosa with about 100 times the area.

In the two previous chapters we have considered the transduction of information by the sensory systems. The sensory systems of humans are both impressive for their extreme sensitivity to some energy forms and notorious for their complete lack of sensitivity to other energy forms. We tend to think of the world in terms of the specific sensory dimensions that we superimpose on our most common sensory systems. Such a superimposition may restrict our understanding of the function of sensory systems that operate within their own sensory dimensional coordinates. Of importance, along with the sensitivity and dimensions of those forms of energy that we sense, are those areas that are not sensed. Information processing restrictions are probably an important factor in the limitations placed on the forms of energy that are sensed.

Chapter 6

Convergence

Information is usually carried in the nervous system by multiple nerve impulses that can be distributed over time on individual fibers and over multiple fibers in the same time period.

Although information is conveyed over appreciable distances in the nervous system by means of nerve impulses, a single nerve impulse, on a single nerve fiber, has little significance in neural function. Information must exist in combinations of impulses and the nervous system must deal with these combinations. The afferent information that is extracted by individual receptors affects most efferent neural control in a way that responses are not directly driven by the action of a single receptor but rather by combinations of information from many receptors. Without the combination of information from different nerves, the nervous system would be very limited in its actions. The simple combinations of the effects of individual nerve impulses will be the topic of this chapter. More complex, but less well-understood, combinations will be discussed in chapter 8 and the details of the local process of combination will be discussed in chapters 12 and 13 and the effects of these combinations, in simple networks, will be discussed in chapter 16.

Important background reading for anyone who wishes to understand our current knowledge of combinations of signals in the nervous system is Charles Scott Sherrington's Silliman Lecture, published in the monograph *The Integrative Action of the Nervous System*. Here he summarized results of his first decade of published research on reflex function. Other publications, spanning the whole first half of the twentieth century, earned him both the Nobel Prize in 1932 and the appellation "Father of Neurophysiology." His terminology still dominates functional discussions in neurology and will be used in this chapter. Thus the word *integration,* in the context of nervous system research, is still more likely to refer to his usage, meaning a general bringing together of parts, rather than to the formal mathematical process that is now used in many analyses of neural data.

Junctional regions between different nerve cells are usually the site of computation and signal modification.

Neural pathways, which include junctions between different neurons, exhibit a variety of properties not found in individual nerve fibers. Usually the output in these pathways is not the simple, time-delayed duplication of the input that would be expected from a continuous fiber pathway. It is these junctions that allow the interaction of inputs, including those that originate at different times on the same fibers and those that originate on different fibers at either the same or different times. Such combination is possible because junctional activity, unlike nerve fiber activity, is not all or nothing.

The graded activity in junctional regions is sensitive to a variety of conditions. Many drugs act through modification of junctional transmission and certain pathological conditions are the result of modifications of the effects at junctions. The graded activity at junctions is also influenced by the input history of that junction, a property that is the basis for learning and memory.

Multiple, separate nerve pathways generally converge on each neuron in the central nervous system.

Central nervous system neuron cell bodies and dendrites are usually covered profusely with the terminations of axons originating with many different central neurons or receptors. This anatomical arrangement provides the morphological basis for the combination of actions of different nerve fibers. Estimates of the number of inputs that converge on some central neurons range up to 10^6, although a commonly used figure for the typical number of inputs converging on a single perikaryon and its dendrites is 10^4. The morphological evidence of convergence of neural pathways is consistent with functional demonstrations of signal combination. The often quoted statement about function—that all neurons are connected to all other neurons—is a considerable exaggeration of morphology. The richest connectivity observed for a neuron's synapses is many orders of magnitude less than that needed for such an all-encompassing network. There can be, however, a high degree of connectivity within the central nervous system as suggested by the extensive dendritic branching of neurons such as the cerebellar Purkinje cell shown in figure 6.1.

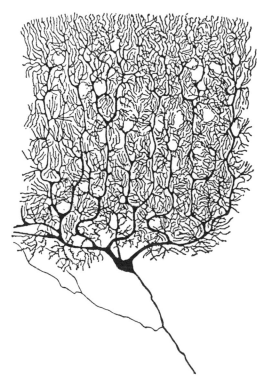

Figure 6.1
Dendritic arborization. The intricate arborization of dendrites of a cerebellar Purkinje cell is shown in this often copied figure of Cajal.

Many methods have been used over the years for testing the effects of convergence of neural signals. A century ago it was known that certain gross motor responses occurred reflexly when any one of several appropriate stimuli was delivered. Sherrington defined a *final common pathway* as a single neural output that, on separate trials, could be excited by different inputs. Sherrington's research, using quantitative recordings of reflex timing and amplitudes, is the basis for much of our understanding of these multijunctional combined effects. The monosynaptic pathway between sensory inputs and discrete motor responses was soon recognized and exploited to study relationships involving a single junctional action. Study of electrical activity in muscle permitted the isolation of the outputs of individual motor units, while the physical isolation of single fibers later extended this resolution of details to single fiber pathways. Recordings of electrotonically spread potentials on spinal roots showed relationships between local potentials in neurons and impulse generation in their axons. Gesell in 1940 recognized that the summation of local electrical processes was the necessary drive for impulse generation. Several years later, the development of intracellular microelectrodes by Ling and Girard (1949) allowed the measurement of events in individual nerve cell bodies and led to the general recognition that local potentials sum to drive impulse generation in individual neurons.

Limitations of methodology and instrumentation at the time of the early studies of the combination of neural signals led to rather holistic studies in relatively intact animals with observation of gross responses. Soviet neuroscience, following the lead of the great Russian physiologist I.P. Pavlov (И. П. Павлов), has continued to place emphasis on the study of the significance of reflexes in the whole animal. It is easy to read into the results of this work various considerations of the practical advantage to the animal of the observed signal combinations. As we have just described, research progress in western countries has generally taken a different, more reductionist path. When the function of a system is not understood, some fraction of the system is then studied more intensely to determine the underlying principles. Both approaches have their strengths and weaknesses in elucidating the process of signal combination by the system.

Today one can stimulate single peripheral nerve fibers and use microelectrodes to record the effect of *temporal summation* from those fibers on the electrical activity of a single central neuron. *Spatial summation* can be studied by applying isolated stimuli to two single fibers that act on the same neuron. The addition of more inputs considerably compounds the difficulty in interpretation. As a result little attempt has been made to study the convergent action of large numbers of independent inputs onto a single vertebrate neuron. Most of our current information has been extrapolated from simpler experiments such as those using synchronous volley inputs on multiple fibers. In a few invertebrate ganglia, the inputs to single cells have been extensively mapped and rather complete control of their inputs seems almost possible.

With the formalization of various tools used by engineers to study interactions among dynamic subsystems, a synthetic approach to the study of biological systems has become possible. From a beginning at around the middle of this century, growth of this approach has accelerated with the ready availability of small computers. Presently this synthetic approach is giving a new direction to much of western neurophysiology. Faults, found in synthetic predictions of the behavior of neural systems, have demonstrated important deficiencies in our understanding of these neural systems. Recognition of these faults has allowed errors in this understanding to be corrected. One possible outcome of this synthetic approach is the possibility of consolidating many isolated observations into more general principles. Synthesis from known details sometimes shows that what often appear to be entirely different details of behavior can be simply the result of small variations in the internal parameters.

Successive nerve impulses, when delivered to a neuron in the central nervous system over a short period, usually lead to a nonliner cumulative result.

During normal function, nerve fibers carry trains of impulses with interpulse intervals typically well less than 1 sec. Cumulative response effects are observed when nerve impulses are generated by electrically stimulating nerve fibers at these natural rates. This *temporal summation* of effect has been shown in many neural pathways using a variety of test methods.

6.1. Experiment: Conduct an experiment on a friendly pet dog. Lightly scratch the skin over the lower rib cage area to elicit the dog's scratch reflex. Over successive trials, record the duration of both the interval between the beginning of the stimulus and the beginning of the response, and the interval between the end of the stimulus and the end of the response. Observe any quantitative changes in the reflex response over a series of trials.

Many experimental paradigms include the stimulation of afferent fibers and the measurement of the consequent efferent response. An *afterdischarge* is a response that continues after the termination of a stimulus. The afterdischarge can last for many seconds in mass reflexes of paraplegic and quadriplegic patients. The heightened spinal reflexes in these patients cause even a brief afferent input to trigger prolonged and complex reflex responses (mass reflexes), including such diverse components as limb movements, micturition, and defecation.

The nature of junctional activity introduces several forms of variability into the combination of input signals. This variability has important consequences in reflexes including the scratch reflex in dogs and various mass reflexes in humans. Besides being variable, these responses show considerably longer periods of summation and afterdischarge than would be expected from the simple summation of junctional potentials in individual mammalian neurons.

The receptive field of a neuron in the central nervous system includes all types and locations of stimulation that directly or indirectly produce an identifiable alteration of the response of that neuron.

Even a casual comparison of the information that receptors deliver and the important nervous system outputs makes it clear that most outputs from the nervous system represent combined effects originating from multiple receptors. Stimulation of two separate inputs, whether nerve trunks, nerve fibers, sensory receptors, or various combinations of these, can result in a response on an output pathway that differs appreciably from that following any input alone. Such combined responses show *convergence* of the input signals. When the combination results in a response that is greater than any input alone it is spoken of as showing *spatial summation*. Sometimes spatial summation produces a response when any of the inputs, if delivered alone, would have been subthreshold.

Spatial summation involves not only signals from different sensory receptors but also signals originating within the nervous system. The central neurons producing these signals are driven by the summation of signals from still other neurons. Frequently, such combinations cause the output of that neuron to eventually determine part of the input to that same neuron, thus forming a *feedback pathway*.

Although most sensory neurons branch and supply a multitude of central neurons, most of the neurons in a human nervous system do not receive any direct input from sensory nerves. On the other hand, many neurons without direct sensory connections do have an identifiable response to a specific sensory input. In chapter 5, we defined a receptive field in terms of the dimension of the adequate stimulus to a receptor. This definition can be extended to all inputs that are effective in modifying the activity of a neuron. The receptive field defines the limits of information available to a neuron.

It is easy to misinterpret the function of those neurons in which more than one type of converging input acts separately to modify their activity. The first experimental stimulus that produces a response can be easily interpreted as the only adequate stimulus although other equally effective but untested inputs were overlooked. In one such example, seven hair cell receptors in a species of fly were studied in several different laboratories. The combined results of these studies would imply that the seven receptors were stimulated uniquely by more than seven specific stimuli.

Some cutaneous receptive fields are simple and receive inputs from receptors of only one particular type, located in a small area of the skin. The value of convergence of information from these receptive fields is easy to imagine. More complex combinations of signals from different types of receptors also have apparent functional significance, e.g., rods and cones that report local brightness within their respective ranges converge onto a single cortical map of the visual world. Unexpected convergences have also been shown in which neither local nor similar information converges onto a single neuron, e.g., skin and gallbladder inputs converge onto individual spinal interneurons. Many neural responses are not understood and may require combinations that look to us to be unusual.

Just as a mechanoreceptor responds to a mechanical input by generating a local current flow that is a function of the input, a central neuron generates a local current flow that is a function of its local environmental conditions and synaptic inputs. Local currents excite the low threshold, initial part of the neuron's output fiber in a manner that is dependent on the cumulative effects of these local currents. The temporal pattern of the local currents is represented in the time course of the impulses generated. One might look on central neurons as a special class of receptor characterized by being especially responsive to convergent synaptic inputs. The effect is, in either case, a summation of the local potentials on the target neuron. Impulses arriving at different synaptic junctions may not all be equal in their effectiveness, but inputs arriving by different pathways or successively on one pathway will generally interact. D.P.C. Lloyd (1946) gave a convincing demonstration of the interaction of afferent inputs onto spinal motoneurons. His results, showing a facilitating interaction of synergistic inputs that lasts more than 10 msec, are a classic example of the interaction of inputs through synaptic junctions (figure 6.2).

Several important terms are used by neurophysiologists to describe summation of signals. A *neuron pool* is a group of neurons that act in common on a particular target. Most commonly, a *motoneuron pool* is a group of motoneurons that innervate motor units within a particular muscle. The term *volley* is used to define nerve impulses that arrive at a neuron or in a neuron pool nearly synchronously. They may originate by electrical stimuli to many fibers in a peripheral nerve

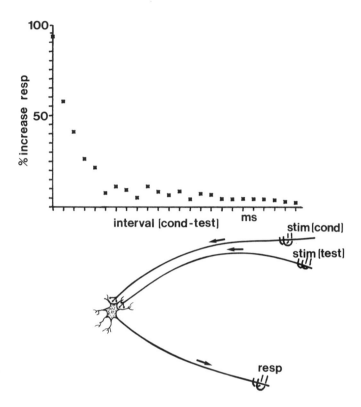

Figure 6.2
Facilitating synaptic interactions. This figure schematically summarizes the results of D.P.C. Lloyd's classic experiment. This experiment dealt with a stimulus to two afferent fibers both of which synapsed on a single efferent fiber. (Actually he stimulated and recorded bundles of fibers but conceptually the results are identical.) With a stimulus to the *test* fiber alone, a response of a specific amplitude was observed. With a stimulus to the *conditioning* fiber and the *test* fiber simultaneously (condition − test interval = 0) there was a dramatic increase in the response. The effect of the conditioning stimulus on the test stimulus decayed with time. The facilitating interaction of these synergistic inputs lasted more than 10 msec.

trunk or they may follow a stimulus such as a sudden tendon tap that stretches a muscle and simultaneously activates many muscle stretch receptors. These atypical stimuli are clinically and experimentally useful because they can be made to elicit specific responses. The tendon tap stimulates only selected fibers—those from stretch receptors. A similar selection of electrically stimulated fibers can be obtained by careful adjustment of the stimulus form and conditions.

Both the facilitory effectiveness and the time course of the action of an impulse delivered to a neuron are subject to variation depending on where it arrives on the neuron.

An important aspect of the interaction of impulses is termed *facilitation*. Facilitation always indicates that the total effect of the combined inputs is greater than that of either input alone. Sometimes facilitation is used to mean only that the responsiveness to the second (facilitated) input is increased by the first (facilitating) input. Here the facilitating input may not actually produce a response by itself. In any case, the term facilitation is used to suggest simply that the output is in some way increased whether this is additive, multiplicative, or enabling. In single neurons, facilitation always causes larger summed junctional potentials and a subsequent increase of impulse rate of the output fiber. In a neuron pool, facilitation also leads to *recruitment* of additional units for which the individual inputs are subthreshold.

Many of the studies of convergence with facilitating effects have involved inputs by way of the *somatoceptive* pathways. The term *somatic* derives from the Greek word σῶμα, for body, and somatoceptive information is sensory information about the body and its contacts with the environment. Receptive fields on the skin for different sensory fibers often overlap in area. Facilitating convergence onto second-order neurons may blur the localization represented by the output of these second-order neurons.

Spatially converging inputs can have rather varied sites of action on the target cell. This spatial distribution of inputs can be important in determining the details of function. In an extensive theoretical study, W. Rall (1967) showed that the combination of separate input signals can be much more complex than would be expected by simple summation. Experimental studies of spatial convergence have often shown facilitating effects. These effects have many similarities to the cumulative effects of temporal convergence.

Inhibition is at least as important as excitation in the action of nerve signals arriving at a neuron in the central nervous system.

The combination of inputs from two pathways sometimes causes an increase in the output. Often, however, the addition of a second input reduces the response from the first input. *Inhibition* within the central nervous system is at least as important to orderly activity as is excitation. An important point is that the decrease of firing of a nerve fiber due to an inhibitory input is just as much a signal as is the increase of firing due to an excitatory input.

Inhibition is manifest in many ways in the nervous system. A direct inhibitory junctional effect (see discussion of IPSPs in chapter 13) is perhaps the most obvious. Inhibitory action also can include a reduced output pulse rate and a reduced effect of excitation on membrane potential. An additional inhibitory effect, the reduction of neuron firing when the inhibition has actually occurred at some "upstream" site, is called *defacilitation*. Defacilitation is common in motor responses since inhibition of skeletal muscle is always due to a decrease of motoneuron activity and not to a peripheral inhibitory signal.

We have discussed junctional effects in this chapter with the implication that two neurons are involved, one before (*presynaptic* to) and a second after (*postsynaptic* to) the junction. Another important inhibitory effect occurs when three neurons and two junctions are involved. The mechanism of this *presynaptic inhibition* will be considered in chapter 13 (see figure 13.10). In presynaptic inhibition, the primary junction is an excitatory one in which the prejunctional neuron produces a fairly constant postjunctional excitation. The presynaptic inhibitory neuron, when active, reduces the size of the excitatory junctional effect. It can be thought of as multiplying the prejunctional neuron's effectiveness by a number that is less than one.

Both the facilitory and the inhibitory actions of nerve impulses act over a period of time that is appreciably longer than the initiating action potential.

Both excitatory and inhibitory actions sum and decay over time and thereby introduce dynamic properties that are not present in single nerve impulses. Further, the dynamic properties of different pathways can differ appreciably at any one time. These dynamic differences not only affect the timing of individual

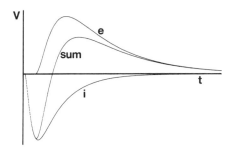

Figure 6.3
Combination dynamics. Excitatory (e) and inhibitory (i) potential changes in a neuron usually have different time courses and can occur with any conceivable timing. As shown in this schematic example, dynamic interaction of inputs can produce complex (biphasic) sums.

events but can be important in determining the results of responses to a combination of signals. Often the time course of the excitatory action on a neuron is appreciably different from that of the inhibitory action on the same neuron (figure 6.3). Most of these dynamic effects are lost in the representationally convenient models of neural function that treat neural response as simply on or off.

The dynamics and sign of an action depend on stimulus rate because of the different time courses of temporal summation (figure 6.4). For example, at one stimulus rate, an action that decays slowly will dominate, whereas at another rate one giving the largest response to each impulse will dominate. The effects of combination dynamics are especially important in the actions of networks and will be discussed and illustrated in that context in chapter 16. Some of the largest differences in dynamics of pathways were found in classic experiments in which the dynamic functions were not investigated at the single neuron level. In many of these cases, multiple stages of action are involved with the resultant dynamic time constants partly dependent on network effects.

A reflex is usually a somewhat stereotypic motor response to one of a restricted range of stimulus variations.

We have been using the term *reflex* without being very specific about its meaning. Part of this is intentional since the word is difficult to define exactly. One convenient approach is to list four characteristics of reflexes without attempting a

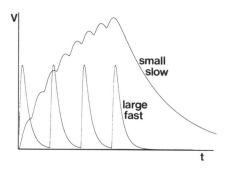

Figure 6.4
Stimulus rate. Comparison of small, slow responses with large, fast responses. At a high rate, summation of the more slowly decaying response can cause it eventually to exceed an initially larger rapidly decaying response.

specific definition. Reflexes involve the response to a stimulus where (1) the response is often rather stereotypic, (2) the stimulus activates specific receptors, (3) some form of integration occurs within the central nervous system, and (4) peripheral effectors produce an output.

A single impulse, arriving at a single synapse, can produce a small excitatory or inhibitory junctional potential in the postsynaptic neuron. Stimuli that have been used to study reflex outputs are usually repetitive impulses on many converging fibers and the studies of reflex response include the intrinsic spatial and temporal combination of individual nerve impulses. Although these older studies did not attempt to discriminate internal mechanisms, they generally produced results that were clearly related to function. These same reflexes are often still used in clinical testing, are altered by pathological change, and account for effects observable in normal day-to-day activity.

Before the work of Sherrington at the end of the nineteenth century (1898), it was generally believed that only efferent fibers connected muscles with the CNS. Sherrington and his co-workers later showed that afferent information left muscles and that this information was used in reflex maintenance of muscle tone (Sherrington and Liddell, 1925). Both simple and complex pathways are now known to join the sensory inputs to motor outputs. A *monosynaptic reflex* is one involving only an afferent and an efferent neuron, topologically the shortest possible pathway. The prime example of a monosynaptic reflex is the reflex using afferent information from stretch receptors in a muscle the output of which acts, through a single synapse, on the motoneurons that excite the same muscle. This reflex causes contraction of the muscle fibers in response to stretch of the stretch receptors of that muscle. The stretch can be induced by various maneuvers and is called the *stretch reflex,* or *myotatic reflex,* or *tendon reflex,* or *tendon jerk.* Figure 15.1 represents the neural circuit that underlies this reflex.

The monosynaptic connection describes the simplest pathway for any reflex, but even this reflex is subject to descending bias and sensitivity adjustment. Spinal cord transection is followed first by *spinal shock* when reflexes below the transection are depressed and later by *hyperreflexia* when some of these reflexes are accentuated. Both of these modulations of reflex activity show that the monosynaptic reflex is not isolated from influences of higher centers.

Most of the early reflex studies were in *polysynaptic pathways,* although they were often not identified as such. Polysynaptic pathways introduce the possibility of considerable complexity of signal combination in reflex action. So, for example, plantar contact alters the stretch reflex in a manner that increases extensor activity—in effect, a reflex multiplication. The reflex response to a noxious stimulus to the same plantar surface of the foot instead results in flexor withdrawal and demonstrates an override of the extensor response. The postural extensor reflex is further altered by signals from the vestibular system that represent head movement.

6.2. Problem: This problem illustrates how a valuable function of two signals can be derived without an independent determination of the two signals. Use this approximation:

$$\Delta L_{(t+\Delta t)} \approx F(R_1, R_2) = \Delta L_{(t)} + \Delta t \times V_{(t)}$$

where ΔL is the deviation of muscle length from its resting length, t and Δt are a point in time and an increment in time, V is the velocity of length change, and R_1 and R_2 are firing rates of two receptors that respond differently to length and velocity.

Assume that the responses of the two receptors to the same stretch at time t are

$$R_1 = 9\Delta L + 3V = 33 \text{ pps}$$

and

$$R_2 = 5\Delta L + 5V = 35 \text{ pps}$$

Set up an approximation for L at some future time, $t + \Delta t$, by combining present values of R_1 and R_2 with appropriate scaling factors. Then solve that equation for ΔL at $t + \Delta t$ where $\Delta t = 0.01$, 0.03, and 0.1 sec. How could these predicted values be of use to a motor response that involved three different reflexes that relate to the same input and output? In what ways do the assumptions of this problem deviate from what would be expected in combinations of actual neural signals? In spite of these deviations, what reasonable conclusions can you make from this model about the combinations of neural signals?

A pair of motoneuron pools that innervate muscles with antagonistic actions is frequently reciprocally innervated.

An important aspect of reflex function, which was thoroughly explored in the early part of the twentieth century, is the phenomenon of *reciprocal innervation*. This is inhibition of ongoing activity in one muscle at the time when an opposing muscle is excited. For example, excitation of flexor motoneurons serving one joint is accompanied by inhibition of motoneurons driving extensor muscles at the same joint. In many activities, such reciprocal action has obvious functional value.

Respiration is driven by a variety of inputs that increase both inspiratory and expiratory response in an alternating manner. Here there is a reciprocal effect in which the stimulus increases one phase and inhibits the opposing phase of respiration followed by reversal of these actions. Clearly those neuron pools involved in one activity receive not only information about the total stimulus that drives both phases but also information about the status of those neurons that drive the other half of the total activity. Alternating limb movements, as in walking, are subject to similar dual drives. The reciprocally related motoneuron pools that cooperate in producing alternating activity have been called *half centers* (Graham-Brown, 1912; Gesell et al., 1947; Gesell, 1951; Shik et al., 1968).

Although the overall reflex response may be stereotypic, the response detail may vary depending on the "local sign" of the stimulus.

Some stimuli simply trigger a response that is characteristic of a range of stimuli but is independent of variations of the stimulus within that range. An example is the eye blink reflex in response to sudden mechanical or visual inputs. On the other hand, many kinds of reflexes can be excited by a variety of similar, but not identical, stimuli with results that differ in a way that is dependent on the value of some variable of that stimulus. Thus a stimulus at one point on the skin can initiate a response that is related to that particular point, whereas a similar stimulus to an adjacent point will produce a slightly different response directed at the different target. Although a dog scratches in a stereotypic manner, these scratches are not indiscriminate but are directed at the location of a flea. For these reflex responses, stimuli are not simply a trigger but provide additional information used in deciding the detail of intensity of firing and selection of active units making up the response. A response that varies with the specific location of the stimulus is said to carry a *local sign*.

Selective drive has been shown even in a dog with a transected spinal cord by means of two "electrical fleas." (This experiment will be further discussed in chapter 8.) These inputs converge to produce a coordinated motor output in the spinal cord but a decision is made to scratch either one site, the other site, or the two sites alternatively. The reflex response is never, however, to scratch midway between the two stimuli. The spinal cord has the capability to make simple decisions.

The nonlinear properties of reflex pathways often lead to interactions among different inputs such that the responsiveness to one input varies with the magnitude of other inputs.

To this point, most of our discussion of combinations of signals on neurons could be interpreted simply as additive combinations (including those with a negative sign). Combinations are generally neither so simple nor so limited in their computational power. The output of a neuron can reflect a true combination of incoming signals rather than the simple superposition of signals. The presence of one signal can increase or decrease how effectively another signal changes the output. In the extreme, this can be a switch action where one signal can prevent another from affecting the output. In other cases, this can be a multiplying action where one modifies the effectiveness of another to produce an output that resembles a product of the two input signals. Figure 6.5 gives examples of such a multiplicitive effect and an additive (*biasing*) effect on the input-output relationship of a reflex pathway. Such differing combinations are the basis for generating a variety of functions that are useful in evaluating the stimulus world.

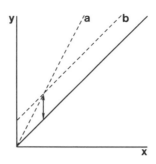

Figure 6.5
Input-output relationships. An input-output relationship between the X input and Y output, shown here as a solid line, can be modified by changing its slope (a), a multiplicative combination of input A with input X, or by changing its intercepts (b), an additive or biasing combination of input B with input X. A single measure of the change in value of Y would define both A and B inputs as facilitating response to input X, but would not distinguish between the types of action and at one point would even show the same quantitative action.

An important means by which one neural signal modifies another is through the release of chemical agents called *neurotransmitters*. Such chemical signals can have spatially diffuse or relatively local actions but in either instance tend to act at specific cells and synapses. Since there are perhaps 100 different types of membrane receptors for chemical agents, this provides a multitude of specific types of neuron sensitivity to *modulation*. Chemical modulation introduces another level of interneuronal connectivity that is not found in electrical transmission, obligatory synaptic transmission, or axonal propagation over fiber pathways. There is considerable current research involved in investigating how these levels of communication interact in the output of neuronal firing.

The response to converging inputs, like the response to successive inputs, is nonlinear. Signals falling below threshold or rising above saturation are, in effect, turned off to the transmission of information. Inputs to a system that exhibits a sigmoidal input-output relationship, such as in figure 6.6, combine linearly only over a very small range. Ordinarily combinations in such a system lead to either an increase or a decrease in the responsiveness to one signal when it occurs in the presence of the other signal. These changes of responsiveness in the nervous system have been called *facilitation* and *occlusion*.

The size of the efferent reflex discharge to a given afferent stimulus reflects the number of motoneurons activated and the intensity of that activation. D.P.C. Lloyd (1946) made extensive studies of the effect of stimulating different afferent

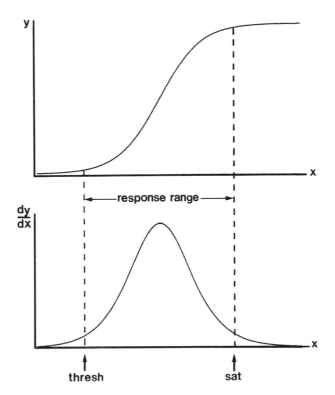

Figure 6.6
Nonlinear input-output relationships. Typical input-output relationships are sigmoidal, being limited at the lower end by threshold and at the upper end by saturation. The derivative of the output vs. input graph (dy/dx) represents the sensitivity of the relationship. A sigmoidal input-output relationship will have a peak of sensitivity near the midpoint of the response range.

fibers on the reflex response. Neurons that are always fired by a given input are said to be in that input's *discharge zone,* whereas those brought closer to, but still not exceeding, their threshold are said to be in that input's *subliminal fringe.* In the original analysis, it was assumed that facilitation occurs only when the subliminal fringe of two inputs overlap, causing the output to exceed the size that would result from simple summation. When the responses to two inputs were less than the sum of the responses to two inputs delivered separately, this was called *occlusion.* Occlusion was interpreted to result from the overlap of discharge zones made up of all-or-none responses of neurons. With the recognition of graded excitation within individual neurons by Gesell, it became apparent that the nonlinearity behind facilitation and occlusion could reside in individual neurons as well as in pools of neurons.

Feedback pathways are common in the nervous system in which the response of a neuron acts directly or indirectly as part of its own input.

A general pattern of signal combination found throughout the nervous system is that in which a feedback signal is combined with an input from another source. Anatomical evidence for feedback pathways is available sometimes where distances are small and only one or two neurons are involved. Over longer distances, or with multiple neurons, identification of specific fiber pathways is difficult to obtain. Vital staining techniques have greatly improved the resolution of our knowledge of the exact connections in such pathways. Less complete functional evidence shows feedback action to be widespread in local circuits, among separate neuron pools, and even in pathways that include effectors that activate sensory pathways producing signals that subsequently return to the originating neurons.

6.3.* Demonstration (Pupillary Light Reflex): Use a willing subject and observe the diameter of his or her pupil. Determine how this diameter changes with distance from a single point light source. Calculate the relative light intensity and the resultant area of the pupil at various distances from the light source. What factors, other than source intensity and distance, influence your results? Try to reduce the influence of these factors. When you have refined your measurements to a reasonable degree of confidence, use them to determine how pupillary feedback affects light intensity at the retina.

Very different types of stimuli often produce responses that interact to generate specific neural responses.

When pressure on one area of skin produces a response and addition of pressure over adjacent areas of skin produces a greater response, the response can be described as one that is dependent on the total force in that region. It is considerably more difficult to give a name to the combination of a visual and an auditory stimulus that leads to turning of the head. Tissue-damaging input and vibration input combine in an opposing manner in determining pain experience (Melzack and Wall, 1965). Similar interactions of stimuli are seen in the combinations of lights of different wavelengths that give a single color experience or in the head rotation and ankle flexion that drive excitation of a single muscle (Kim and Partridge, 1969). Unlike the simpler combinations discussed up to this point, these more interesting and complex combinations are difficult to represent in computer or mechanical models. Before discussing these multimodal combinations in more detail in chapter 8, we will look, in chapter 7, at some control problems that are dealt with by effectors.

An important multimodal combination is found in the vestibular input to the extraocular muscles that is known as the *vestibulo-ocular reflex*. This reflex normally operates to maintain a stable retinal image during head movement. For many years it was thought that this showed a fixed connectivity between vestibular input and specific extraocular muscles. A dramatic demonstration of the plasticity of this combination, however, is obtained from experiments using prisms that laterally reverse the visual field. Not only do subjects learn to deal with the altered visual field, but the vestibulo-ocular reflex appropriately reverses direction. You may have experienced a similar reflex plasticity in adjusting to the change of angular relations introduced by corrective glasses. What additional physical complications are introduced with bifocal glasses?

Interactions in the relationships between sensory input and motor responses also can lead to activity patterns that emerge from the system rather than from any individual part.

Although some central neurons receive input directly from sensory receptors, most central neurons receive extensive input from other central neurons. Among these interconnections are extensive reentry pathways by which the output of individual neurons ultimately contributes to the input of those same neurons. These second and higher order neurons are not simple relay sites for sensory signals but act as convergence points that produce outputs that are complex functions of combinations of the sensory signals. Such closed pathways tend to introduce output patterns that emerge from the network itself and are not generated by either the individual components themselves or combinations of the original sensory input patterns. We will return to these *emergent responses* in chapter 16 but will suggest here a formal symbolic approach to representing combinations of neural signals. The reader should realize that one encounters some difficulties when attempting to fit a more formal description to actual function. The advantage, though, of a formal description is that it highlights theoretical limitations.

For those readers who are comfortable with the concepts of linear algebra, it will be natural to interpret the following paragraphs in terms of vectors and matrices and their operations. The time-varying signals of individual central neurons can be represented as time-varying vectors with dimensions of the stimulus world. At no place in the nervous system is this resolved into a set of orthogonal vectors. Both vector redundancy for some external information and complete loss of other information are common. The real world is at the same time overdetermined (with inconsistencies) and underdetermined in the signals in the nervous system. It is important to bear in mind that to be realistic, linear analysis must be modified to deal with the fact that actual neural systems are quite nonlinear. It is possible that important aspects of neural function lie within these nonlinearities. Effective representation of neural systems in a formal way is a legitimate, although rather difficult, research topic today.

We have seen that the response of individual receptors is ordinarily related to the magnitude of more than one physical variable in the environment. A receptor's response varies in a dimension that is often different from the dimensions measured by physical instruments. The dimensions sensed by different receptors are different, if only because they sample conditions at different locations. Our sensory representation of the world is the result of the response of all of our sensory receptors. This world information is expressed in a sensory coordinate system that is defined by the properties of these receptors and their accessory organs. Each object in the world is represented by a variation of excitations distributed in space and time over an array of sensory receptors rather than by activation of some object-specific receptor. When the responses of different receptors are combined in the response of second-order neurons, the external object acquires a new distributed representation with a relative weighting of external details that is dependent, not only on the receptors themselves, but also on the effectiveness of those different input neurons onto the target neurons. With each successive redistribution of input information by convergent and divergent signals, the objects are represented in a coordinate system that is characteristic of that level of neuronal abstraction. Neural function can be represented as a complex series of coordinate changes that depend on the rules that are built into the existing connections. Additional complication arises when the effectiveness of the connections changes in a manner that is dependent on the past use of the system.

Recall that by combining algebraic equations we can extract information about variables in those equations that cannot be extracted from any one of the equations alone. Similarly, by combining neural information, the nervous system can potentially extract information that is not identifiable in any individual receptor signal. No amount of central processing can derive information that did not originally exist in the total sensory input. It does not follow that central processing is organized in such a manner as to extract the arbitrary dimensions used in physics and engineering for measuring the stimulus world. The signal from Golgi tendon organs, which are often described as force receptors, actually contains mixed information including force, rate of change of force, temperature, and so on. There is no reason that pure force information must be extracted at any point in a central pathway.

6.4.* Problem: There have been many attempts to derive an algebra by which combinations of neural signals can extract specific subsets from the set of information that makes up the total sensory input. One way to understand this research is to attempt to develop a simple example for yourself. The specific logic derived is not as important as is the development of the underlying thought process. This problem, although simple, should provide an opportunity to explore such thinking.

As we have discussed, sensory receptors respond to several types of signals, albeit with different levels of effectiveness. A single receptor's response can be given by its inputs scaled by their relative effectiveness (see figure 6.7A). Second-order neurons are typically driven by signals from more than one sensory neuron. The effectiveness of these interactions varies and the interactions can be excitatory or inhibitory. Write algebraic equations for these interactions. Assign arbitrary values to the signal magnitudes (S_A and S_B) and to the effectiveness

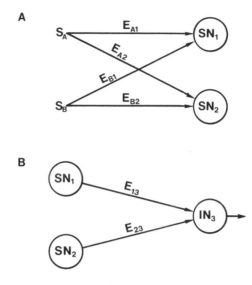

Figure 6.7
Algebra of a simple network. Inputs S_A, and S_B have effectiveness E_{A1}, E_{A2}, E_{B1}, and E_{B2} on two sensory neurons SN_1 and SN_2. These two neurons, in turn, affect interneuron IN_3 with effectiveness E_{13}, and E_{23}. Further details are described in problem 6.3.

(E_{A1}, E_{A2}, E_{B1}, and E_{B2}) of these signals on the sensory neurons (SN_1 and SN_2). Now choose values for the effectiveness (E_{13} and E_{23}) of the two sensory neurons onto the interneuron (IN_3) so that (1) the interneuron responds only to the first signal (S_A), (2) the interneuron responds only to the second signal (S_B), (3) the interneuron responds to the difference between the two signals, and (4) the interneuron responds in a way that is proportional to the average of the two signals. These same two sensory neurons could produce a multiplicity of different outputs by driving four interneurons each in one of the different ways that you have just considered. Can you describe an interacting scheme in which the interneuron responds only when both inputs are active? Your models illustrate that world conditions can be represented in different forms at different stages of neural processing. It is also important to realize that we do not yet have the ability to program computers to match the cognitive functions of daily life of a human.

Reflexes produce output pulses on motor nerve fibers in response to a distribution of impulses over sensory nerves. The motor response to sensory signals is generally not just a triggered response but depends rather on the detail of the sensory input. One might consider the output to be a *transformation* of the input. This transformation differs from one time to another dependent on the central state. In effect, much of the research effort in reflex neurophysiology has been directed at determining transformation rules for parts of the nervous system under severely constrained conditions.

Although many reflexes involve multiple combinations and recombinations of neural signals, the simple description of the end-to-end transformation can be useful. Alterations in these general transformations are often evaluated in central nervous system pathologies. Increased, decreased, prolonged, or oscillatory responses characterize many abnormalities and, by empirical observation, these alterations have been associated with specific defects.

The output of neural systems depends on the previous conditions (state) of the system as much as it does on the current input.

The combined effect of all the sensory inputs acting with the internal conditions (*state*) can be described in a formal way. This description emphasizes the fact that this state changes over time and determines all outputs. An easily overlooked fact is that the state of the system, as much as its inputs, determines the system's own future states.

Except in experimental isolation, reflexes usually operate in the context of other inputs and other responses, some of which are compatible and others of which are conflicting. The effect of multiple inputs is generally not the simple sum of the responses to separate inputs but involves interactions both within the nervous system and in its external loads. To express the combination of multiple interacting reflexes it is necessary to describe something more than a set of independent transformations. The interactions among reflexes cause the state of the system to vary over time. The path of this change (*trajectory*) is determined by a set of rules that includes the effects of interactions between the reflexes. Detailed methods for formal study of systems involving multiple interacting parts are typically found under the topic of *state variable control*. Figure 6.8 represents, in schematic form, the operations that can be used to reduce nervous system complexity to a more intuitive state description.

The strength of using a state description to describe reflexes is that it acknowledges the simultaneous presence of multiple interacting reflexes. Different re-

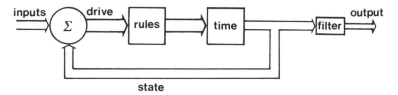

Figure 6.8
State description. The combination of inputs with the state of the system determines the total of the factors that drive the change of conditions existing in the system. This drive, acting through the system's rules, defines the rate of change of all the state terms through time. The effect of the rate of change accumulates over time, resulting in change of the state of the system. Some of the factors making up the state appear externally as observable outputs of the state.

sponses can be driven by combinations of different, but overlapping, parts of the total input. Although details of individual reflexes are hidden in such a summary, descriptions of the general properties of complex relationships are perhaps easier to follow.

In the presence of internal feedback pathways with delay and lag, it is possible to have self-generating variations of signals. With internal nonlinearities, including thresholds and saturating limits, the state trajectory of a system may traverse varying successive orbits, staying within fixed bounds but not returning exactly to any state that it has visited before. At any moment the direction taken by the trajectory in such a *chaotic behavior* is dependent on the state, input, and rules, but is so sensitive to infinitesimal differences in the state that long-term predictions of its trajectory are impossible. State variable models are useful in the study of chaotic behavior as well as in simpler responses. A potentially chaotic system can respond to inputs with a characteristic, but somewhat variable, output and even in the absence of external input can continue to produce a varying output. The internal workings of simple neuronal networks that might generate chaotic behavior will be discussed further in chapter 16.

In chapter 7 we will consider examples from motor control in which the mechanical results of one action seriously affect the rules for other actions. The state that determines motor activity includes internal conditions in the nervous system and also involves state factors that are located externally in the mechanical system.

Chapter 7

Effector Actions

The transduction, processing, and transmission of signals in the nervous system impart a survival value to the organism only after these signals have been further modified and transduced by effector organs.

The selection and encoding of information by receptors and the transmission of this information over nerve fibers are essential to the operation of the nervous system. Until this information results in a response, it is of no value to the survival of either the individual or the species. Effective neural function is not accomplished by the nervous system alone, but requires, in addition, the action of various effector organs. These effectors may act either externally or internally and their action can result in the initiation or modification of mechanical or chemical effects. As the output of the nervous system passes through these effectors, the signals are subjected to further modification through the properties of the effectors themselves. Thus effectors, and even the external influences on them, contribute to the constraints that define general neural function. The nature of external influences is often inseparable from other factors in describing neural control functions. Since mechanical loads have been the most extensively studied, this chapter will emphasize this particular external influence on an effector system.

The coordination of chemical processes probably has been a major drive toward the general development of neural communication and organization.

Some form of coordination must exist for those essential biochemical processes that use energy and materials acquired from the environment. With the development of metazoans and complex cell specializations, those species with a means of coordinating local chemical actions would have had a considerable survival advantage. In humans, the control of chemical processes is a major, although not dramatic, function of the nervous system. Most of that control is accomplished by the output of signals through either the autonomic nervous system or the intermediation of endocrine signals.

The *autonomic nervous system* is the division of the nervous system that innervates smooth and cardiac muscle and glands. Autonomic effector neurons are located peripherally in autonomic ganglia but are driven by central neurons that are, in turn, strongly influenced by sensory inputs. There is a dual innervation of many organs by the *sympathetic* and *parasympathetic* divisions of the autonomic nervous system. Frequently these two have opposing effects on a particular organ.

The two divisions of the autonomic nervous system tend to differ in the amount of their divergence and hence inversely in their ability to produce a discrete response. The parasympathetic division generally has little divergence in contrast to the widely diverging sympathetic division. This tendency for nonspecific action of the sympathetic division is especially obvious in its output through the adrenal medulla. Instead of affecting a specific organ, the adrenal medulla releases its chemical messengers into the general circulation where they have a diverse effect at many tissues.

Neural signals are responsible for modifying the rate of production, the composition, the secretion, and the transport of the products of a variety of glands.

In the early part of this century, I.P. Pavlov performed a series of dramatic experiments showing the ability of the nervous system to regulate chemical effectors. In these often-quoted classic experiments, he conditioned dogs to salivate in response to a bell. Thus an autonomic chemical effector action became associated in the nervous system with a novel sensory input. Neural signals to a variety of glands influence the composition or the rates of production or release of secreted agents. Since glandular secretions participate directly in many important biological functions, these represent an important effector action of the nervous system.

7.1.* Problem: List as may examples as you can of chemical agents that are produced and secreted in and by the body. Speculate on the different ways in which the nervous system might regulate these processes.

Chemical systems bring some unique characteristics to their role as nervous system effectors. Biological actions that use chemical effectors are generally slow. This can be due to lags in production, release, or activation of an inactive "pro" form, to accumulation or dilution within body fluid compartments, to circulatory and diffusion transport time, or to the time necessary for inactivation or removal of the chemical. The nervous system can interact at many levels in these processes, including regulation of the activity of the secretory cells, control of the chemical make-up of the substance released, or alteration of the flow rate through various body fluid compartments.

When neural signals modify the output of endocrine glands, the endocrine product forms another signal with the final result occurring in the target tissue of that endocrine agent.

Although the nervous system normally exerts control over the endocrine glands, the endocrine output does not act on a final effector but, like the action of one neuron on another neuron, is rather a link in a complex information handling pathway. Neurochemical agents, released by the nerve terminals, act on endocrine cells thereby influencing the synthesis or release of further chemical signals that will then be transmitted through the circulation to target tissues. Some of these targets are, in turn, endocrine glands rather than final effector cells. We will not discuss these pathways in detail, partly because they are traditionally assigned to endocrinology, but more important because the signal-handling dynamics of endocrine systems are not as well known as neurally driven mechanical actions.

Certainly an important function of the nervous system is what Walter Cannon (1929) called *homeostasis*. Homeostasis is a condition in which the internal environment of the body is maintained within a limited range of variability. Neuroendocrine actions are essential to the maintenance of homeostasis. To cite examples from two of the many homeostatically regulated systems, calcitonin and parathormone are hormones that respectively increase and decrease the blood calcium levels whereas thyroxin, insulin, glucagon, and the glucocorticoids are hormones that operate to regulate many aspects of metabolism. Along with an important contribution from the autonomic nervous system, the endocrine system acts as an important nervous system intermediary in maintaining the crucial balance of homeostasis.

Neurons directly control such important autonomic functions as cardiac output, vascular resistance to blood flow, resistance to air flow in bronchi, mixing and transport of materials in the gastrointestinal system, bladder emptying, size of the pupil, shape of the lens, sperm and ovum transport, and fetal delivery. These mechanical effector actions provide a second limb, with the chemical effector actions, of the nervous system's action on visceral structures.

Neural control of motor activity of skeletal muscle is accomplished entirely by the modification of muscle excitation. The response of skeletal muscle to neural excitation involves changes in muscle velocity, length, stiffness, and heat production.

Leonardo da Vinci thought that to understand motion is to understand nature. Although this may be a bit of an oversimplification, we are tempted to make the parallel simplification: to understand muscle control is to understand nervous system design. Sherrington (1941), in his book *Man on His Nature,* expresses the similar sentiment that nervous system action is meaningless until it affects a motor action.

Ultimately, mechanical efferent control through striated muscle reduces to provision of a suitable pattern of impulses, distributed in time and space over an array of muscle nerves, to cause the appropriate muscle actions. As we have already stressed, motor control is not simply the transmission of impulses from sensory receptors to muscles. A complex integration of sensory information is necessary to generate the appropriate spatiotemporal patterns that are necessary to control an effector as complex as a striated muscle. We will consider this problem from the output end, that is, what muscle must accomplish to sustain normal human activity.

7.2.* Problem: You have spent your lifetime learning how the world is represented by sensory signals. You have spent an equal time period learning how to control your muscles. Consider the processing needed to convert these sensory inputs into motor adjustments. For instance, try to describe the relationship between a particular sensory input and the activation of specific muscles that would be necessary to prepare you to catch a ball.

Muscle velocity, length, stiffness, and heat production are under the control of patterns made up of but one type of nerve impulse. In addition, there are long-term effects that modify the chemical properties of the contractile elements within the muscle and change the excitability properties of the muscle membrane. These modulatory and trophic actions may or may not be controlled by nerve impulse activity.

Not only do muscles make up about 50% of the body mass, but they require a large portion of the output of the nervous system for their control—an indication of their importance in the evolution of the nervous system. Motor nerve output acts on between 400 and 500 named muscles. These muscles are comprised, in turn, of smaller groups of units, different combinations of which are selectively activated for different tasks. The smallest element of control, the *motor unit,* is made up of a single motor nerve and all the muscle fibers that it supplies. There are about 10^5 motor units under the control of the human nervous system. These motor units are not all the same, because of appreciable quantitative differences in their size, cell metabolism, dynamic properties, and mechanical loading. The fact that there is effective control over this complex array of effectors implicates a diverse organization of excitatory elements. Some simplification of effector control results when some motor units do not act entirely independently. In such cases, groups of motor units are activated in a consistent order (Henneman et al., 1965) that produces response gradation rather than independent actions.

The type of muscle that we are discussing here is given three different, but almost synonymous, names: *skeletal, voluntary,* and *striated* are each used to distinguish this type of muscle from smooth and cardiac muscle. (This distinction is discussed further in chapter 14.) In fact, cardiac muscle has a striped appearance so it is also a striated muscle. With biofeedback techniques, it is possible to gain voluntary control of cardiac muscle and some smooth muscle so these in a sense are also voluntary. Many striated muscles are not under casual voluntary control and it takes considerable effort to gain such control. Finally, the term skeletal is not altogether appropriate, for many muscles of this type are not connected directly to skeletal structures at either end. We shall make no effort to rectify this imperfection of nomenclature and trust that our usage will be apparent from context.

Muscle contributes a major portion of the total basal production of heat in the body and is the principal source of neurally controlled heat.

An important effector action of the nervous system is the control of chemical actions that convert chemical energy into heat. A sprinting race horse can generate enough heat to raise the temperature of 500 kg of body mass by 2°C in 20 sec. The nervous system controls both the generation and the eventual dissipation of this prodigious amount of heat.

A major source of body heat is the metabolic activity of skeletal muscle (see chapter 14). Mechanical action of muscle is always associated with heat production. In fact, *thermography* is under development as a noninvasive, clinical tool for evaluation of neuromuscular disorders. In individual muscles, heat production is controlled by the activation of the same nerve fibers, using the same nerve impulses, that control the mechanical response. It follows, though, that any specific generation of heat must be accomplished by different spatiotemporal patterns of impulses being delivered to combinations of motor units.

Shivering is one instance in which skeletal muscles are used solely for heat production. Below the threshold for shivering, contraction of antagonistic muscles is employed to generate small amounts of heat without the production of external movement. At times shivering is superimposed on either postural control or controlled movement that involves the same muscles. This poses an interesting problem in control, in view of the restrictions imposed by the limited signaling capabilities of nerve fibers.

7.3. Problem: Does shivering for heat production place limitations on fine motor control? Think of examples from your experience where you spoke or performed fine finger movements while shivering. How might you determine the independence of the graded control of a specific muscle for mechanical effect and for heat production?

The force produced by muscle is the usual, but not the only, variable controlled by efferent nerve signals.

Force is an easily recognizable muscle output that is controlled by the nervous system. Nervous control partly determines the time course and magnitude of the force generated by the muscle. The force may be generated in a muscle during a period of constant, increasing, or decreasing length and it can be delivered at a small point of attachment, spread over a distributed attachment, or delivered as a lateral pressure. In any case, efferent neural control is subject to a complex interpretation before appearing as a force.

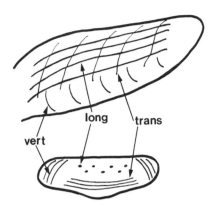

Figure 7.1
Muscles of the tongue. This schematic shows the three general groups of internal muscles that shape the tongue: vertical, longitudinal, and transverse. The tongue provides an interesting and unusual structure for muscle control because none of the muscles is attached to a bone and yet these muscles can move accurately in many directions.

As we will see in chapter 14, *isometric* (changing tensile force at a constant length) or *isotonic* (constant force during shortening) conditions are most common in experiments on muscle. Normal muscle function involves *auxotonic* (simultaneously changing force and length) conditions. The principles of Newtonian mechanics dictate that the application of forces to stop movements is as important as the application of forces to initiate movements. This then must be an important role for muscle. Muscles are also frequently employed to apply a lateral force as, for example, in the tongue or diaphragm. This is accomplished by either the hydraulic coupling between shortening and bulging of a constant volume fiber or by the vector component that is normal to tension in curved muscle fibers. In some important cases such as that of the tongue, the controlled use of a muscle may result in a change in shape (figure 7.1). External forces and work are of trivial importance in these instances. Functional results, such as speech sounds, may be even further removed from direct neural control, being related, in a complex way, to the shape of the controlled muscle.

Speech is an interesting example of the importance of configurations under muscle control. Speech sounds result from a complex interaction of air flow, tension of the vocal folds in the larynx, shape of the resonant cavity of the mouth, and the position of the tongue. A multitude of muscles regulate these parameters. The muscles of the vocal fold, tongue, and lips are not the source of the sound energy. Respiratory muscles generate almost all of the sound energy and the "speech muscles" simply modify that energy. The learned effector response is not muscle tension or length, but rather an understandable phoneme, and muscle activity is adjusted in relationship to errors in the phoneme that is heard.

7.4.* Problem: The mechanics of lateral force differ enough from those of tensile force to justify some consideration. In a muscle in which parallel, constant volume fibers constitute about 70% of the total cross-sectional area, an active tension of 10–20 N/cm^2 can be generated. Muscle fibers generally operate between 80% and 110% of their relaxed length. For a muscle with cylindrical fibers that are 35 μm in diameter and 10 cm long, how much tension would one fiber contribute? How much internal pressure would be necessary to just prevent fiber shortening? How does this value compare with systolic blood pressure? How much total compressive force would be necessary to prevent fiber bulging due to this internal pressure? How much lateral force would this pressure provide in one direction? In pennate muscles (see figure 7.7), force is delivered at an angle to the tendon. What role would lateral pressure have in the activity of these muscles? In which direction (lateral or tensile) could a pennate muscle fiber deliver the most work?

Muscles, especially when contracting strongly against a stretching force, can deliver sufficient force to tear tendons or even cause fractures. Soft tissue contusion and dental damage are not uncommon effects of extreme muscle contraction. Most muscle activities are accomplished at levels of only a few percent of maximum. Competitive sports call for some extreme motor performances but, even here, the forces delivered are usually only a small fraction of the maximum that can be delivered by any particular muscle.

Since both muscle length and its rate of change drastically affect the force delivered by an excited muscle, the result of a muscle contraction is mechanically fed back into the contractile machinery. Generally this "length-tension" feedback operates so that movement of the load by a contraction reduces the continuing force of that contraction. Thus, a particular excitation pattern will cause the muscle to deliver more force when acting on a heavy load than when acting on a light load.

Although the nerve impulses that drive a muscle are discrete events, the much longer duration of muscle twitches allows their responses to overlap and produce a relatively smoothly changing output.

The contraction of a muscle has a much slower time course than the nerve impulses that control it. This is shown graphically in figure 14.3. A reasonable approximation of a limb muscle's response to efferent neural drive is obtained with a second-order lag equation with two time constants in the range of 0.1 to 0.2 sec. When a pulse sequence similar to the pattern of impulses on a motor nerve fiber is used as the input to this equation, responses similar to neurally driven muscle forces are generated.

Whereas the impulse of a motor nerve lasts only about 0.001 sec, the resultant twitch of a muscle fiber lasts about 0.1 sec. This accounts, in part, for the response of a muscle to repetitive nerve impulses being a smooth contraction. (See figure 14.8.) This smoothing action does have a cost. Namely, when there is an abrupt change (either increase or decrease) in nerve excitation, the mechanical response follows with an appreciable lag.

The relationship between the pulse rate of excitation and the intensity of muscle contraction is a nonlinear, sigmoid function. The results of muscle excitation are determined by the mechanical properties of the load along with the forces coupled to that load.

The force developed by a typical limb muscle does not reach 5% of its maximum until the stimulus rate is above about 5 impulses/sec. The force reaches 95% of its maximum with a sustained stimulus rate of less than 50 impulses/sec. Individual fibers within a muscle vary both in their lowest limit of effective excitation and in their ability to maintain force in response to sustained excitation. Although these nonlinearities in muscle response may pose a problem for investigators studying motor control, they were faced by even the earliest nervous systems. It is reasonable to surmise that the inherent properties of muscle have played a significant role in the evolution of advanced nervous systems.

Motor control is frequently considered to be a purely kinematic problem. Even with this simplification, the relationship between changes in the muscle and the subsequent movement of the load is still complicated by the variety of changing linkages that exist between muscles and the objects that they move. Neural

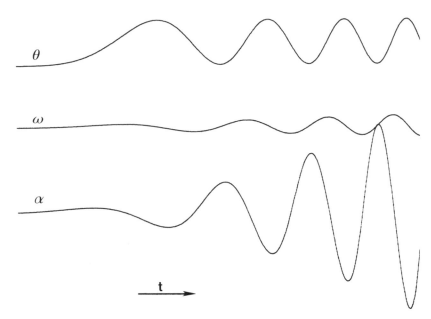

Figure 7.2
Kinematic relationships over a range of movement dynamic patterns. The top line, θ, is the angle of a joint as a function of time during a complex movement, the second line, ω, is the angular velocity, and the third line, α is the angular acceleration of this movement. Although each cycle of θ is of the same amplitude, ω, and especially α, increase with frequency.

control, however, is usually defined directly in terms of its action in the external world rather than in intermediate terms of muscle dimensions. This external action can even be extended to the action of a tool, e.g., the face of a hammer. When motor control is expanded to include kinetic control, the relationship has added to it the effects of widely differing load impedances and speeds of response. Figure 7.2 illustrates some kinematic relationships seen over a range of movement dynamic patterns. Before considering how the nervous system handles these problems, we will review the complications of a purely mechanical nature that they introduce.

Movement may be represented in terms of (1) position or angle, (2) linear or angular velocity, or (3) linear or angular acceleration. The specific terms used in a measurement will affect appreciably the appearance of a result because of the particular emphasis on low- or high-frequency components. It is thus very important to distinguish the terms that have been used when comparing different records of movement. There are published examples where specific aspects of a response have been inappropriately emphasized by taking advantage of the bias of a particular mechanical term.

Kinematics refer to the study of the changing geometric configurations that occur during a movement. Figure 7.3A shows a kinematic description of a simple bending movement such as might occur at the elbow. *Kinetic* descriptions are those that give the forces and energy exchanges involved in generating a movement. The ratio of a dynamically changing force and the resulting movement of an object is the *mechanical impedance* of that object. Impedance can combine inertial, elastic, and viscous factors. A useful principle in calculating the forces on an object is one stated by d'Alembert (described in Goldstein 1950). *The sum of the external forces and kinetic reactive forces acting on a body is zero.* This principle allows the treatment of objects, which are subject to changing movement, in the simple ways that are applicable to static balance.

The neural control of a specific movement must consider the Newtonian relationship of the force delivered and the load impedance. If two movements are kinematically the same but occur with different load impedances, it follows that not only the force, but also the muscle excitation, must have differed. Figure 7.3B shows an example of the different torque patterns required to produce a simple elbow movement under different load conditions. The nervous system must deal not only with different loads but also with the changing impedance of a particular load during a movement. Even with simple loads, if the locations of parts of the mass change with respect to the center of rotation, the inertia will change. More complex loads involve frictional, elastic, and viscous changes during the movement. Often muscle contraction does not cause load movement at all but rather modifies the movement resulting from other forces. Two examples of such actions are holding a load against gravity and stopping a moving object.

7.5.* Problem: Use practical examples to define three pairs of kinematically similar movements in which the kinetics differ because of (1) differing actions of gravity, (2) differing external loads, and (3) differing configurations of body parts resulting in alterations in inertia.

Sherrington said that the spinal cord is the cradle of the mind. His implication was that higher brain functions evolved as an extension of the functions of the spinal cord. Those motor functions that are common to both humans and phy-

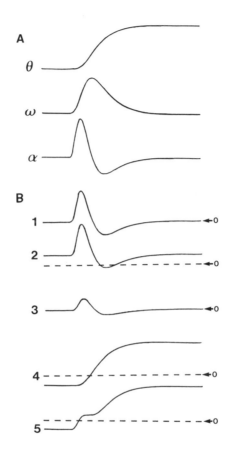

Figure 7.3
Simple kinematic representation of movement of the elbow. (A) As in figure 7.2, θ, ω, and α represent position, angular velocity, and angular acceleration. In this instance, the movement is a simple bending (for example flexing) of the elbow. (B) Forces on the hand resulting from different kinetic variations of the same kinematic movement that can occur with different loads on the elbow. B_1, horizontal movement with load in the hand; B_2, vertical movement with the same inertial load; B_3, horizontal movement with a smaller load; B_4, horizontal movement against a spring that requires an initial extension force; B_5, vertical movement against an inertial combined with a spring load. In cases 2, 4, and 5, flexor or extensor forces are required at the resting position.

logenetically lower animals probably evolved to accomplish important motor functions of those lower animals. Distinctly human motor or mental functions, such as those involved in creative art or scientific investigation, may represent a superposition of additional uses on these primitive motor pathways and neuronal functions.

When the force generated by a muscle acts on a load there is a requisite exchange of energy between the muscle and the load.

The initiation of a movement by a muscle involves the transfer of energy to the load as a force acting through a distance. Ordinarily, this energy originates in the conversion of chemical energy into mechanical energy in the muscle. On other occasions, muscle actually absorbs energy from the load. Here the kinetic energy of motion or the potential energy of position is absorbed by the muscle and, if not quickly returned from elastic storage, is dissipated as heat. The rate of energy exchange at any moment is proportional to the force exerted. In considering energy absorption, it is important to remember that rate of energy exchange (power) = force $\times$ velocity, and that total energy exchanged = $\int$ power dt.

Especially during energy absorption, the forces can reach damaging levels and a variety of strategies is invoked to limit the peak forces by extending the time over which the total energy is dissipated. "Rolling with a punch" extends the distance over which a specific amount of energy is absorbed, thereby reducing the peak force. When landing after a jump, translational energy can be partially and temporarily transferred to rotational energy. This extends the period over which the energy is dissipated. Padding in sports equipment increases the area over which forces are applied to the body and thus decreases the force that is delivered to any small area (pressure).

Muscle does not respond instantaneously to changes in the neural signal but introduces lags so that the discrete pulses of the nerve signal are smoothed into an undulating contraction. In this process, chemical energy is converted into mechanical energy that can be delivered externally or stored in elastic deformation of the contractile system. If not converted into external work, this elastic energy may be later dissipated as heat. When contracting muscle is stretched, the energy input is initially absorbed as elastic strain in both the active and passive parts of the muscle and its attachments.

The relationships among force, movement, and stimulation rate in a muscle depend only on those conditions that act directly on the muscle.

We have just described several actions of muscle, occurring after its excitation, that depend on the load and other local conditions. These descriptions have assumed the muscle's action to be independent of the specific system within which it might be working. This, like the free body diagram used in the analysis of a mechanical system, is a convenience used for the purpose of analysis. Extrapolation of information obtained from the study of an isolated muscle is based on the assumption that a muscle is dependent only on direct interactions and is not otherwise dependent on remote events. This can be called the *free muscle assumption.* In such an analysis, influences of the larger system are seen in the muscle only because of their action at the interface between the muscle and the remainder of the system. Since a muscle's response to neural signals is appreciably influenced by the load, we need also to consider the direct effects of loads presented to the muscles by parts of the body and by external objects. The magnitudes and characteristics of common loads can easily be the dominant factors in determining the muscle properties that ultimately generate the effect of neural signaling. Consequently, a particular kinematic action, accomplished under different loading conditions, must be driven by neural signals that compensate for the different load effects. We shall now turn briefly to aspects of neural control that deal with compensation for different loads.

For muscle to generate the same movement with different loads, it is necessary that the force generated by the muscle change with the load. This requires a change in neural excitation.

When a task is specified in kinematic terms, the necessary forces and the neural control of muscles are not defined until the load has been determined. The rules by which kinematic tasks are converted to motor nerve activity must be adjusted to the load. This adjustment of the rules of the controller can be described as *meta control.*

Motor function consists of the generation of patterns of nerve impulses within the central nervous system and the subsequent delivery of these impulses to sets of muscles. The muscles, in turn, respond to changes in load with feedback-like (Feldman, 1966; Partridge, 1967) or spring-like (Bizzi et al., 1982) properties that result in length-dependent adjustment of the force delivered by the muscle. This feedback property of muscle partially compensates for different load impedances. Residual errors from this compensation can be further compensated by neural reflex feedback (Berkinblit et al., 1986). Motor control includes a combination of driving signals, muscle compensation, and reflex compensation, but normal motor control is more accurate than is accountable by these factors alone.

7.6. Demonstration: Set up a motor-control task with different loads. A convenient example is packets of copier paper that must be moved from the floor to various shelves. Use an uninformed subject and have him or her move the objects, one at a time, to specified locations. The individual tasks are similar but require adjustments to compensate for the differences in starting and ending positions. Prearrange the task so that one or more of the objects are of significantly different weight. For example, fill one or more packets with styrofoam instead of paper. Observe any changes that occur immediately after the subject encounters the deviant load. Observe the following: (1) how performance is altered by the load change, (2) how quickly an adjustment is made, and (3) what changes are made after encountering the load. Redesign the experiment to avoid complications and to more carefully assess the period of adjustment.

Many motor tasks are defined with the use of visual information and are therefore in a visual coordinate system. The actual task is accomplished by muscles only after that information has been transformed from visual coordinates into muscle dimensions. As the task progresses, information about errors is returned by both visual and mechanical pathways. Information gathered about errors in one load-performance task modifies how visual information is converted into muscle control in the continuing task. As a result, future control can be precompensated. Rather than direct control of the output, this improvement requires adjustment of the rules of the controller or meta control. Meta control can cross task boundaries and refine a controller that, over a broad range of conditions, is relatively crude into an accurate controller within the narrow range of conditions currently present.

The quality of control seen in normal motor activity represents a combination of general motor programs, feedback correction of error, and the results of a continuous and rapid readjustment of the rules of the controller. The pathways and processing involved in this meta control are not well understood, although they are different from those involved in error-correcting feedback control. Meta control includes components that are fast enough to be important in walking over uneven ground. Fast meta control is not necessarily distinct from slower adjustment such as motor learning and may represent one end of a temporal continuum of adjustment of functions.

Activity of a prime mover muscle, to be effective, usually requires coordinated activity of several other muscles.

Details of the involvement of various specific muscles in normal function have been studied extensively under the topic of *kinesiology*. This is an important area of investigation in physical medicine, sports physiology, work physiology, and human factor analysis. Although kinesiology is operated through free muscle properties, it also encompasses effects of the mechanics of the involved structures and requires coordinated activity distributed over widely separated muscles (Winters, 1990).

If motor control was simply accomplished by controlling the independent muscles that affect a variety of independent loads, our understanding would already be sufficient to predict and account for most muscle activity. Few motor functions are actually so simple. Loads are not independent since the action of one muscle on its load usually affects the properties of those loads as seen by other muscles. Further, few muscle units can be activated without causing mechanical interaction with other units. Most actions also require the cooperative adjustments of multiple muscles. Joint stabilization and balancing the opposing actions of other muscles are also part of the basic motor control problem and not just secondary details. These and similar interactions show the necessary complexity of the controlling actions accomplished by the nervous system.

Following certain neurological defects, muscles that are normally only minor accessories to an important movement may become the only effector available. Even without training, a patient will often modify his or her motor control strategy and thereby take advantage of the presence of remaining control of synergistic muscles. Therapeutic training is often designed to develop this result.

Human movements start and end with muscle-controlled posture.

A large fraction of the activity of muscle is devoted to maintenance of those postures that occur between major movements. Neither sitting nor standing is a

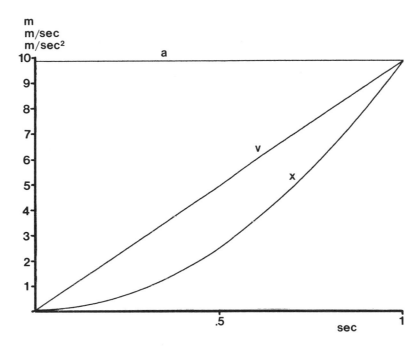

Figure 7.4
Terrestrial gravitational effects. Position, *x*, velocity, *v*, and acceleration, *a*, of an object falling without resistance in the earth's gravitational field. Note the three dimensions on the vertical axis.

purely passive act based on simple mechanical stability. Terrestrial activity occurs in the uniform acceleration field of gravity (figure 7.4). Thus the vertical bipedal posture of humans, with the center of mass above the center of support, is unstable. We might look on the standing human as an inverted pendulum. Critical balance of active muscle forces is essential even for apparently static upright postures. On the other hand, because of inertia, even a completely unsupported object will fall less than 10 cm in the first 0.1 sec.

When the body is tilted so that its center of gravity is outside the area directly above the feet, a torque exists. This torque will cause the body to begin to rotate and thus to fall. The center of gravity in this condition falls much more slowly than it would in free fall. During walking, there is sufficient time for one leg to be swung forward before there is an appreciable fall of the center of gravity. This may not be true if the speed of walking is appreciably reduced.

7.7.* Demonstration: The balance that is necessary for static posture requires that the center of gravity of the body is maintained over the center of support. To show this, stand with your heels against a wall and try to pick up an object from the floor. Describe the constraints imposed by the wall.

The upright position is not maintained as a static posture, rather there are a series of small deviations followed by small corrections. This approximation to static posture is accomplished by continuously changing the neural drive to muscles. This dynamic posture requires that the *average* balance of forces is equal to that required for a static balance. Since the deviations from vertical are small, the changes in accelerating forces are also small and, for many considerations, the forces expected in static relationships form a reasonable approximation to those in the actual case.

The control of a movement with only one degree of freedom often still requires action of a pair of antagonistically acting muscles.

Many mammalian muscles act in a tensile manner, exerting force through connective tissue attachments to rigid objects. Although this action can bring the attachment points closer together, it can neither stop that movement nor move the attachment points apart. Limbs introduce inertial loads and thus the necessity for forces to stop a movement once it is initiated. The stopping forces must come from another source such as gravity, a deformed elastic load, friction, or another muscle connected in an opposing way. Although *antagonistic* or opposing muscles are common, they are seldom arranged symmetrically on opposite sides of a simple hinged lever.

The structure of most joints sharply limits the range of possible excursion. These bony stops do not, however, normally terminate movements. The termination of movement short of its mechanical limit is generally the result of reflexly driven motor activity. In those rare individuals in whom pain pathways fail to develop, there is also a failure in development of muscle-determined movement limitation. Such patients suffer repeated joint damage and develop gross joint deformations.

Both Galen and Leonardo da Vinci recognized the need for antagonistically arranged muscles. Leonardo made a considerable point of this in experiments in which he pulled on wires that were attached to bones in locations corresponding to muscle attachments. In the mid-nineteenth century, Guillaume Duchenne

(1867) made a careful study using only muscle palpation and defined the role of most of the limb muscles. He made further observations on patients with various nerve injuries and was able to define the motor roles of many peripheral nerves and individual muscles.

Muscles do not always fall into a neat classification of antagonistic pairs. A pair of muscles that is *antagonistic* in one action may be *synergistic* in another action, and may be *supportive* in still another action. For example, muscles that are antagonistic in a single elbow flexion operate in alternating cooperation when producing a cyclic movement of the elbow.

7.8.* Demonstration: Palpate your forearm and upper arm during forcible elbow flexion and extension and identify the location, extent, and attachment of the muscles that flex and extend the elbow. Identify physical units that adequately account for the properties that you observed in palpating the arm. Make static observations at different elbow angles and diagram the geometry involved in these actions. What other actions can you identify that use some of the same muscles? Calculate the ratio of torque produced to muscle tension for each muscle at different angles. Calculate the ratio of joint angle change to change of length for each muscle.

7.9.* Problem: Compare the relative stiffness of your elbow when the antagonistic muscles are relaxed and cocontracted. The difference is clearly a function of muscle activity. If the elbow was a simple hinge joint, acted on by antagonistic muscles with equal lever arms, the angular stiffness would be related to the linear stiffness of the muscles. Write the equation that relates linear muscle stiffness to joint stiffness. Can this stiffness be adjusted between its extremes? Similarly joint torque is the result of muscle force. Write the equation that relates muscle tension to joint torque. Using Cartesian coordinates of flexor excitation and extensor excitation, plot a line from zero to maximum stiffness with no net torque on the joint. (In your first approximation make the most simple assumptions about muscle stiffness, torque, and muscle excitation.) Pick a stiffness point on this line and draw another line that joins points of equal stiffness with torques ranging from maximal flexor torque to maximal extensor torque. This is now the basis for a new coordinate system (stiffness vs. torque) that is functionally more relevant than the original (flexor excitation vs. extensor excitation). If the neural signals entering flexor and extensor motoneuron pools represented desired values of stiffness and torque, the convergence pattern might generate the appropriate pattern of muscle excitation. Describe the use of the control of stiffness and torque.

Only under very special circumstances does a muscle act against a constant force and on a constant load impedance.

As illustrated in figure 7.3, there is not a constant relationship between force and kinematic movements. Further, as illustrated in figure 7.5, the torque generated at a joint by a constant load differs with the orientation of that joint with respect to gravity. There is not a constant relationship between the kinematics of a particular movement and the neural signal that is needed to drive those kinetics but rather a large variety of possibilities depending on the load factors and the antagonistic muscle activity (figure 7.6).

The changes in load, to which the nervous system must respond, can be predictable or they can come as a surprise. The effect of elbow angle on the inertia for shoulder movement is fairly constant and can be anticipated. Likewise, we may have developed some anticipatory knowledge of the changes in force on the leg that will occur when walking in water or on sand. On first contact with an unfamiliar object, the mechanical impedance may be almost completely unknown and even the familiar loads of the body can be subject to sudden and unexpected changes of impedance. Unexpected forces are encountered, for instance when we pick up an unexpectedly empty box, or walk in a moving airplane, boat, or train. Stiff joints, produced by contraction of antagonists, are an important means by which we oppose unpredictable disturbances.

The biceps brachii muscle acts through three independent degrees of freedom rather than on a simple hinge joint, as its action at the elbow is often depicted. This muscle acts over the shoulder joint, over the elbow, and in the direction of rotation of the forearm. (Confirm this by palpating your muscle or examining an anatomy reference.) In a gravity-free situation, without external constraints, activation of the biceps would cause rotation that is partitioned among the shoulder, elbow, and forearm including counterrotation of the body. The relative size of each movement is related to the very different moments of inertia of the loads around the respective axes of rotation. During movement, elastic forces will influence the movement as will the change in moment of inertia due to the changing elbow angle. In the gravity field, the orientation-dependent forces will produce different movements in different orientations. Because of the complex

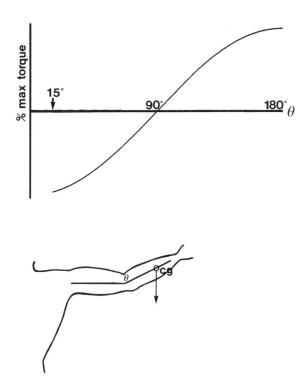

Figure 7.5
Contribution of gravity to elbow torque. The percentage of elbow torque that is exerted by gravity is plotted as a function of elbow angle when the upper arm is held horizontally. The vertical arrow at 15° represents the maximum flexion possible at the elbow. (Can you determine the scale units for this graph for your arm? What possible errors should be considered in such a measurement?)

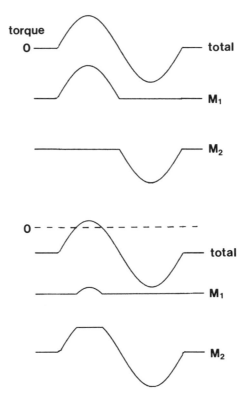

Figure 7.6
Contribution of two antagonistic muscles (M_1 and M_2) to total torque. In the upper example, two muscles contribute symmetrically, but oppositely, to the total torque at the joint. In the lower example, the same total torque is produced by asymmetric contributions of the two muscles interacting with a steady force such as gravity.

actions of this muscle, the same excitation pattern will produce different results if delivered when any of these joints are in a different condition. Successful production of a given movement requires different excitation patterns on different occasions. This includes control of the opposing muscle groups at a joint.

Load changes may be expected or unexpected, familiar or unfamiliar, and yet appropriate activation of the muscle is often necessary at just the instant when the load changes. Whereas the lag resulting from inertia usually delays any catastrophic consequences of unexpected load changes, neural compensation also suffers from lag and delays. The information that is available to the nervous system about needed adjustments can come in many forms. When the load change is expected and familiar, as in walking, it is possible to make centrally determined anticipatory adjustments in the response. With unexpected changes, however, specific new information must be acquired and used to make the adjustment. For some corrections, especially with slow movements, information about errors can be fed back while the error is occurring, to produce adjustments of the continuing neural drive. In other cases, information about the current error can provide a useful test of the new conditions and thereby help to anticipate the loading conditions of some subsequent control of that same load. For example, errors encountered in picking up an unexpectedly empty box can be used to adjust the muscle excitation in the different muscles needed subsequently to lift the box onto a high shelf.

Reactive forces, resulting from activity in one muscle, generally require stabilizing contractions in other muscles.

Because of forces used in initiating and terminating a primary movement, reactive forces are transferred to other parts of the body. These forces then must be balanced by the action of other muscles. To make any change in movement, it is necessary that there be a *reactive load* against which forces can act. Usually muscles must act to stabilize this reference part of the body. Additional muscle action is necessary to oppose unwanted movement as in the case of separating elbow flexion from forearm rotation during biceps contraction. To maintain integrity of the shoulder joint under working stresses, muscle action is required. Apparently simple movements then usually require a complex coordination of action by muscles that are widely distributed throughout the body.

Although stabilization is essential during all movement, certain more extreme cases accentuate its importance. The results of the lack of stabilizing muscle actions are one dramatic deficit seen in paraplegic patients. Often external immobilization of the body is necessary to allow these patients to execute even simple arm movements. The lack of external contact during a gymnastic vault makes it impossible for the gymnast to control kinetic energy during the flight phase. It is possible to modify rotational speed during this phase, by changing the moment of inertia of the body. When the gymnast assumes a pike or tucked position it reduces the moment of inertia of the body from that of an extended position.

A jumper or vaulter determines the path of his or her center of gravity before breaking contact with support. After that, the center of gravity moves along a well-defined trajectory. It is, however, possible to bend the body so that the center of gravity is outside the body. High jumpers take advantage of this fact and rotate their body over a crossbar although they have provided only enough energy to move their center of gravity slightly under that crossbar.

Muscles are three-dimensional, complexly organized structures whose structural details are important to their varied functions.

It is common practice to treat muscles as a set of parallel and linear tension generators acting in unconstrained space. This, however, is seldom the case during physiological function. Individual muscle fibers are packed compactly and tend to follow nonparallel, and often even curved, pathways between their ends, whereas individual fibers often terminate at intermediate points within the gross muscle. Multiple attachment points and distributed attachments are common and the separate elements of a muscle are usually connected in ways such that mechanical interactions occur between individual fibers. As muscles change length, changes in the thickness of one fiber often displace and alter the direction of pull of other fibers. *Lumbrical* muscles pull on the tendons of other muscles so that the contraction of one element alters the length and stiffness of another element. *Parallel* fibers unload each other when they contract. *Pennate* fibers change both their length and another fiber's operating angle during contraction. *Curved* fibers, such as in the diaphragm, apply a centrally directed force when they contract because of the vector sum of the forces at their attached ends.

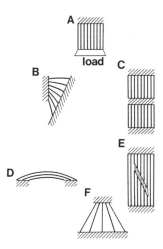

Figure 7.7
Muscle fiber arrangements. The simple arrangement of muscle fibers, attached at one end (A), that lift a load vertically is found only occasionally in nature. Some examples of arrangements actually found in animals are (B) pennate, where fibers change both their length and another fiber's operating angle; (C) series; (D) curved, where the fibers apply a centrally directed force; (E) partially series, where contraction of some fibers affects the length of other fibers; and (F) fan shaped, where the fibers deliver differently directed forces.

Different fibers in a *fan-shaped* muscle, such as the deltoid or trapezius, deliver forces in different directions with a resulting vectorial sum of forces (figure 7.7).

The rectus abdominous and cervical muscles consist of contractile segments that are connected in series but separated by connective tissue separators. The intercostal muscles have a similar arrangement with the ribs as separators. Contraction of one segment of these series-connected muscles alters the length at which other segments operate. Muscles that span two joints relate the positions of the two joints. These are often called *adjustable tendons*. When they contract they do not determine independently the angle of either joint. When the diaphragm is arched strongly it has the action of producing a difference of pressure between the thoracic and abdominal cavities. In this action it is antagonistic to the anterior abdominal muscles. In the simplest analysis, when the diaphragm contracts it flattens and produces the pressure differential necessary for inspiration. As the diaphragm becomes flatter, however, its ability to create a pressure differential becomes less. In this nearly flat position it becomes more effective in constricting the lower part of the thoracic cavity and can even develop an expiratory action.

7.10.* Problem: The fact that muscles pull and do not push should come as no surprise. The tongue, however, is a muscular structure that is attached at only one end and is capable of pushing. One need only watch children on an elementary school playground to see a popular demonstration of this statement. During mastication, the pushing action of the tongue is important in moving food to a position between the teeth. Hydraulic action converts shortening force into thickening force. Make up a truth table of the distribution of forces over longitudinal, transverse, and vertical tongue muscles that will produce (1) lengthening, (2) lateral spread, and (3) vertical thickening of the tongue.

If an excited muscle fiber that was generating 20 N of force/cm^2 of cross-sectional area (2×10^5 Pa) during isolated contraction were then to develop an internal pressure of 2×10^5 Pa, the tensile forces would be canceled by longitudinal hydraulic forces. By Pascal's law (see notes for problem 5.1), lateral *pressure* should be equal to longitudinal *pressure* with the total hydraulic *forces* generated in the two directions being proportional to the ratio of the respective *areas*. The lateral force in a muscle is divided between stretching of the cell membrane of that fiber and delivery of tensile or lateral force. In a muscle with complex geometry, individual fibers might do work in the two directions with forces that are proportional to the longitudinal and the cross-sectional areas. As in a hydraulic jack, the distances over which these forces operate are inversely related to the areas displaced. In a pennate muscle, tension on the tendon is developed in two ways. First, tensile forces in individual fibers contribute an angle-dependent effect because of shortening. Second, the reorientation of adjacent fibers because of the thickening of those fibers that are shortening can cause those adjacent fibers to pull on the tendon. This hydraulic system of constant volume fibers provides an accommodation of a muscle's action to the complex, changing loading and geometry of that muscle as different units become active during its normal contraction. Thus a muscle fiber is equally adapted to either pulling lengthwise or pushing sideways. In a muscle with complex geometry, the partition of *work* between the two types of output depends on the mechanical loading at any moment.

Muscle tension is not converted simply to torque on a hinge because of complications of articulation patterns and muscle connection geometry.

Most joints have more than one degree of freedom of action. As joints move, the direction and lever ratio of application of muscle action change. The complicated geometry of skeletal joints, where more than one degree of freedom exists, often causes movement in one dimension to change the geometric relations seen by muscles driving another movement. Thus elevation of the arm at the shoulder involves different muscle tasks depending on the degree of rotation of the arm. All three degrees of freedom at the shoulder interact in determining both muscle involvement and shoulder girdle configuration. In 1907, Lombard and Abbott made an important observation about the effect of joint angle. They observed the knee joint angle in a frog and found that, at certain angles, the rotational action of some muscles was actually reversed.

Different lever ratios and muscle lengths affect the angular and linear relationships at a joint. With a short lever to the attachment of a muscle it is possible to produce a fast joint rotation with a relatively slow shortening of the muscle. The advantage of *speed* is exchanged for the reduced *torque* that results from the short lever arm.

7.11. Problem: Ignoring air resistance, calculate various combinations of tangential velocity of the arm and release angles that will get a pitched baseball to a predetermined point. Determine a vertical "strike window" in terms of these combinations and then in terms of the time window of release.

Normal motor control depends on periods of dynamic equilibrium in positions that would not be statically stable.

A bicyclist could not stand stationary at the angles that he or she must assume to turn a corner. Similarly, most of our activity involves periods in which we deviate from positions of static equilibrium. Often, as with the bicycle, we are in dynamic equilibrium; in other cases we are actually out of equilibrium—but for such short periods of time that the resultant displacement is minimal. Between tolerable falling and dynamic balance, it is possible to accomplish many more movements than would be possible if it were necessary always to maintain static balance. Walking is a series of catastrophes narrowly averted.

7.12.* Experiment: Without using your arms to lift yourself, rise from the chair in which you are sitting. Compare your actions in rising from the chair very slowly with those associated with rising from the same chair at normal speed. Compare changes in your center of gravity, muscle stresses, and the effects of chair height and softness. Describe the dynamic factors involved in transient balances during this movement. Consider the interaction of factors that together introduce problems in arising from a chair for many elderly subjects.

To appreciate partially the problems encountered by the infirm patient, walk over a rough surface twice, first slowly and the second time rapidly. The first time walk so slowly that you always maintain static balance. If you are in static balance, you can stop on command at any instant. When walking rapidly, note the effect of speed on the energy requirement, and any differences in confidence of your balance.

7.13.* Problem: Compare walking with a wide base and with a narrow base in terms of the rotation that occurs during the period of standing on one foot while the center of balance is not over the supporting foot (figure 7.8). What body motions contribute to the dynamic balance in walking during the swing phase of one leg? Extend these considerations to a sailor's rolling gait; bipedal vs. quadrupedal vs. hexipedal (insect) walking; and climbing, dancing, or gymnastic movements.

While we are often impressed by the complexity of control exercised by an athlete, a musician, or a machine operator, we take for granted the everyday activities of walking, feeding ourselves, or throwing a stone. We seldom stop to consider the problem posed by these more mundane activities. The addition of changing loads and geometric factors between the free muscle properties and the resultant movement appreciably complicates the requirements for neural control. An even more complex control problem is the control of coordinated activity of multiple, interacting structures. Recent research into robotics has increased the general appreciation of the complexity of even the most simple controlled actions. No robot has yet been designed that can accomplish the variety of motor control that is expected of the most clumsy schoolchild. A full description of movement kinetics and kinematics in a simple robotic arm involves several pages of equations. Inspection of these equations gives one the feeling that the nervous system could not possibly solve the equations of motion for normal motor activity fast

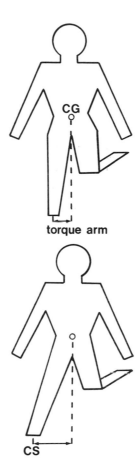

Figure 7.8
Dynamic balance. Stability is determined by the torque arm between the center of gravity (CG) and the center of support (CS). Transient instability is a necessity during walking but the degree of this instability can be different in different stances and gaits. (What are the mechanics of the "wide base" assumed by some neurological patients, the use of a single crutch, or very slow walking?)

enough to provide ongoing control. On the other hand, recent robotic developments show that simplified computations are often adequate.

7.14. Experiment: Grasp an object with two hands and, while still holding it,
examine the variety of combinations of possible joint angles of the two arms that
would allow the object to be maintained in the same position. Describe the
position of the two arms in terms of trigonometric relationships at the different
joints involved. Consider briefly a trigonometric calculation that would generate
a tracking movement in one hand from information about the movement of the
other hand. Try a few comparable arm movements without the benefit of a
connecting object.

7.15. Experiment: Stand and face a chalk board and draw a straight vertical line
a meter long. Observe the sequences of changes in shoulder, elbow, and wrist
angles employed. Compare these observations for drawing a vertical with those
for drawing a horizontal line. How many different muscle programs would be
necessary to draw straight lines at all possible different angles and positions with
respect to the body's location?

The possibility of genetic preprogramming of movement control raises interesting
questions with respect to the use of a tool. A carpenter must relate the angle,
location, and rate of approach of a hammer face to the location of a nail. This is
an example of the control of a rapid change of position of an object at an
appreciable distance from the body. It is unlikely that we have inherited the
specific trigonometric calculations to deal with the hammer dimensions and yet
we readily extend our control to the face of the hammer. In our technological
world, many of our hand and arm movements must follow specific geometric
patterns. These are, however, multilink rotating effectors driven by more or less
linearly moving muscles. Whether the nervous system uses Cartesian coordinates, torque—stiffness coordinates, or joint—muscle coordinates, some neural
transformation between representations must be made to compensate for the
mechanical transformations. These transformations need not be explicit but only
"good enough" approximations.

The positions of a multijoint system can be determined completely by muscles
that pull if there is a total of one more muscle than there are degrees of freedom
in the system. Thus, the seven degrees of freedom that exist between the shoulder
and the wrist might be controlled with only eight independent muscles. (You

might want to check this statement on a simpler system with three muscles and two degrees of freedom.) The human arm and leg are equipped with many more than this minimum number of muscles. Different muscles may be related to such refinements as movements at different speeds but, in general, it is not well established whether this structural complexity serves a specific purpose or simply represents redundancy. In the presence of multiple moving structures, the dynamic description becomes much more complex. For example, centrifugal force acts at the elbow because of arm rotation around the shoulder, and inertia for rotation around the shoulder is four times as great with the elbow extended as when flexed. As another example, the energy absorbed at the knee can be transferred to the hip by muscles that cross the two joints.

7.16.* Problem: Make a videotape of a diver, a vaulting gymnast, or a spinning skater. Use frame-by-frame measurements to determine the change of rotational velocity that occurs as the moment of inertia is reduced by changes of body shape. What reference should you use to estimate rotational velocity? (Similar measurements have been carried out on a multitude of different sports movements. Some difficulties in making these measurements are apparent when one considers that skaters have been measured spinning at up to 420 revolutions per minute.)

Braun and Fischer, in 1895, made some of the earliest measurements of body mass distributions using cadavers. Dempster, in 1961, developed tables of inertial and mass data for body parts. These tables are still in use today as parts of computer programs. More recently, similar, but more detailed, tables have been generated for use in "human factor engineering."

A single, rigid body is fully controllable in terms of six degrees of freedom. When there is a change in the configuration of control of the relationships among internal structural parts, the problem increases considerably. This is due both to the larger number of degrees of freedom and to the addition of interactions among individual parts. It is probable that these multibody dynamic problems are, in fact, never entirely solved by the nervous system. All that is necessary is an approximation that is good enough, most of the time. We sometimes fall down and the rest of the time our control need not be perfect. On close observation of walking, it appears that the control of individual steps is only close enough so that compensation within a step can approximately correct faults that have developed during the previous step along with any cumulative error.

Perhaps the acceptance of risk of error in these "good enough solutions" is what makes life possible. If we could use only correct solutions, we might never solve many critical new problems of survival. Evolution would appear to favor the gambler. Recognition of these imperfections in nervous system function is probably necessary to achieve any degree of understanding of how the nervous system operates.

Although it complicates motor control theory, a body geometry that allows alternate ways of accomplishing the same manipulation provides adaptability to variable motor problems.

The old expression that there is more than one way to skin a cat is appropriate to a multitude of motor tasks for which alternate paths to the same goal are available. If there were only one way to feed ourselves, some otherwise trivial interference could lead to starvation. An important aspect of rehabilitation after neurological damage is the substitution of alternate solutions to motor problems. Because alternate successful executions of the same motor response can take sometimes very different courses, we often solve a motor control problem by mixing parts of more than one type of solution. This mixture must be organized so that the effects of one partial solution do not introduce a major error in the effect of another partial solution.

The presence of alternate solutions to a problem adds to the difficulty in determining the solution to be used in a specific case. Since arm movement has more than six degrees of freedom, there are, to take one example, alternate ways to position a cup. Put another way, there is not enough information in stating the desired location of the cup to define how the arm should be positioned. (Convince yourself that there are more than six degrees of freedom in your arm movement.) The successful locating of a cup shows that additional information, beyond merely cup position, is present in the control of arm position.

Even the isolated spinal cords of frogs (Berkinblit et al., 1986) can control different sequences of leg movement in successive attempts to remove an irritating object from a specific skin location. The task appears to involve an underdetermined solution, a situation often called "Bernstein's problem" (Bernstein, 1967). Since the neural signals are produced that are necessary to generate alternate patterns, this calculation must not require the complex and extensive circuitry of supraspinal motor centers.

Perhaps the degrees of freedom available for motor tasks are not excessive. One practical example illustrates how we can find the extra constraints to solve another simple motor problem. To turn on a light switch it is necessary to reach a particular point in space and then to move a switch to a specific position. You can do this with any one of a multitude of strategies—stretching to reach the switch, using a ruler to reach the switch, walking first to the vicinity of the switch, or even activating a robot's movement. However, the existence of alternate solutions shows that there are extra degrees of freedom in possible solutions. The selection of a particular strategy introduces extra information. When you choose one strategy you have made several other possible adjustments irrelevant. If you choose to walk to the vicinity of the switch, you have partitioned the horizontal position problem into two separate problems—the point to which you walk, and the position of your hand relative to your body. You have added two dimensions of initial information, namely the coordinates that are needed to specify your walking goal. In other cases, there are irrelevant dimensions that can be left to chance or gravity and need not be controlled.

7.17. Experiment: Visual inspection of an object involves excess degrees of freedom in determining the orientation of the eye. Both neck rotation and eye rotation produce about the same effect on eye orientation. Although the two movements cannot be determined separately, the object's relative location provides information to determine both. Design an experiment to record head angle with respect to the body and object positions, and eye position. (Electrical recording from electrodes at the outer corner of each eye can be used to measure eye rotation and there is considerable literature describing methods to be found under the topic of "eye tracking.") Locate several sound-producing devices at various angles around the head. Have the subject look at a sound source as quickly as possible after a sound is heard. Calibrate and measure eye and head angles and calculate the combined effect on eye orientation during responses. Before doing the experiment predict the expected results and plan as many control tests as are necessary. After making a preliminary plan, find references to similar studies of eye movement. How is your plan better or worse than experiments that have been reported before? Now refine, and do, the experiment. Try to decide what information is available to the nervous system to make a coordinated movement using a combination of the two separate activities. How might your data mislead you in developing an explanation? What questions are unanswerable from your experimental plan? How could you deal with these questions?

There are not only alternate quantitative methods of accomplishing some simple motor tasks but alternate quantitative methods of partitioning the same task. In the simple action of using a hammer to drive a nail, there are different ways of partitioning the hammering action and the aiming action. For instance, when using a 1.5-pound carpenter's hammer, the hammering action is usually done with wrist motion and the aiming is accomplished by shoulder and elbow movement. With a 4-pound blacksmith's hammer, the elbow is used for hammering and wrist and shoulder adjustments provide the aiming. With a 16-pound "double jack," the driving of a railroad spike is largely done at the elbows and shoulders, and feet, trunk, and hands are used in aiming.

If the motor system actually deals with motor control by solving the problems as we have described them, then the neural controller must be very complex indeed. On the other hand, it may be that motor control is organized in some mathematically less tractable form but one that nonetheless results in a simpler practical control. Although it has been traditional to describe motor control in a largely linear way, it is known that the nervous system and muscles behave nonlinearly. There are reasons to think that some of these nonlinearities impart to the neural controller useful properties that cannot easily be accomplished in a linear manner.

Chapter 8

From Reception to Perception

> Perception is based upon anticipatory attention and the integration of many sensory mechanisms and it represents their final synthesis. The integration is experienced subjectively as a percept.
>
> William James (1890)

Both the motor response to and the perception of the environment involve central processing of information about the world that has been transduced into signals on sensory nerve fibers.

The reception, encoding, and transmission of information about the internal and external world lack value until that information leads to an outcome different from the one that would have otherwise occurred. Practically, the utilization of neural information always involves some modifications even if no more than delay and relocation. Other chapters consider the transformation of input signals into an output driving form (reflexes), processing patterns (learning), the internal generation of signals (emergent responses), or signal encoding and transmission. This chapter will emphasize the relatively complex combinations and processing of input patterns that result in new but specific patterns of neuronal activity.

The stream of neural impulses that enters the nervous system by way of the 10^7 sensory fibers relates to the conditions outside the nervous system. That stream of impulses, after interactions within the nervous system, leads to both effector drives and to the subjective phenomena of perception. Although there is no compelling evidence that the nature of the processing in these two cases is in essence any different, effector responses often follow fewer steps of processing to an output that is much easier to measure and to study. Since processing of sensory information is the basis of all of our knowledge of the external world, the study of responses in another individual is subject to any vagaries of our own perceptive processes. Reliance on our perceptions is further complicated by various indications that significant perceptual deviations from external reality do occur. Having thus discredited our whole basis, we will now proceed in this chapter to examine the phenomenology of neural processing of information. This includes the discriminatory processes that lead to perception and others that appear to use similar processing to generate effector responses.

For the nervous system to provide useful adjustments in response to either conditions within the body or in the external world, it must differentiate among those conditions. Sometimes information about the time-varying magnitude or intensity of a single variable is sufficient. In other cases, the critical information involves differentiation of separate objects and relationships in an environment that is composed of many objects. Neural functions identify not only objects but relationships among objects, changes in the relationships among sets of objects, and changes in the relationships between the objects and the individual. Many events are part of continuing processes that predictably produce future events. Utilization, in higher nervous systems, of this continuity and pattern provides a survival advantage.

Sherrington (1906) was instrumental in establishing quantitative methods in the study of central processing. These studies, using spinal reflexes, related the magnitudes of inputs to the temporal patterns of output intensity. Later he and his associates (Creed et al., 1932) did much to define how simple combinations of inputs could produce a pattern in a single output dimension.

In functionally primitive nervous systems, fragments of information about the magnitude and rate of change of certain relevant variables are processed so that the response is quantitatively determined by the input. A similar quantitative processing of essentially unidimensional information is also found in some human neural function, as, for example, in motor and visceral reflexes. From such primitive function, evolution seems to have emphasized the development of facilities for more and more complex processing of neural signals. Thus, although humans do not necessarily excel in either sensory resolution or in strength or speed of motor responses, we use our nervous systems for especially effective interactions with the environment. In humans, information processing by the nervous system underlies the subjective phenomena of perception, awareness, and self-consciousness. At which level of neural evolution these first appear is difficult to determine since the answer depends more on how the terms are defined than on any discontinuity in the evolution of function. In this chapter we will not differentiate between processing that leads to those outputs that are selected or scaled by an input pattern and processing that leads to perception with no recognized effector activity.

8.1. Debate: Either alone, or with an enthusiastic forensic antagonist, debate the following statement. "Consciousness, awareness, and perception are unessential epiphenomena that emerge from functionally important information processing in the nervous system." Choose either the pro or the con position but also prepare your rebuttal of expected arguments of the other side.

The identification of an object in sensory space results not from discretely localized information but rather from a spatiotemporally distributed pattern of incoming nerve impulses.

Different receptors respond to different types of impinging energy and these energy exchanges often relate to multiple objects in the environment. Consequently, the activity pattern on a sensory nerve fiber is likely to be ambiguous with respect to the particular exchange of energy that initiated the sensory input. This ambiguity can be reduced by comparison of the activity within a set of receptors, each with different response characteristics. We can infer that to get enough sensory information to identify a particular object, the nervous system must use the activity of multiple receptors. Object representation by sensory receptors is ordinarily distributed both spatially over different receptors and temporally over each individual receptor.

Pulse-encoded signals are in common use in technology, using a variety of different encoding rules. Examples of various methods of encoding using seven separate conductors are shown in figure 8.1. An *integer analog* encoding rule is used to generate the bar graph analog representation of an integer value in some speedometers (figure 8.1,A_1). A *local discrete* code is used to select specific locations for a visual imitation of a hand on a watch (figure 8.1,A_2). Digital computers usually communicate integer values in a *binary* code (figure 8.1,A_3). Some digital displays show numeric symbols by a pattern of activation of seven segments (figure 8.1,A_4). Telemetry of continuously varying measurements can be accomplished with a *pulse rate* code in which magnitude is represented by the repetition rate of pulses (figure 8.1,B_1 and 8.1,B_2). Except for the binary code, the nervous system makes use of some variant of each of these types of encoding. (See also figure 9.7.)

8.2. Problem: Compare the efficiency of pathway usage, fault tolerance, and speed of communication that results from different pulse-encoding rules. Consider the types of encoding shown in the examples used in figure 8.1 including the different patterns seen in the pulse rate encoding in examples B_1 and B_2. Identify combinations of fibers in B_1 and B_2 that carry information about intensity, enum-

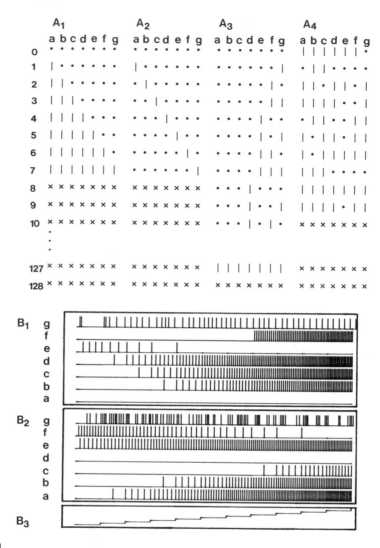

Figure 8.1

Examples of ways in which impulse codes are used to represent information both in technical applications and by the nervous system. a–g represent parallel signal pathways. (A) •, a point without an impulse; |, a point with an impulse; and ×, an out-of-range value for which the selected code lacks representation. Each horizontal line can represent either magnitude values or other enumerated information. The codes represented in A_1–A_2 are illustrated as being carried simultaneously on seven parallel pathways (a–g) but could be carried on a single pathway at seven designated points in time. The encoding in A_1 (integer analog) and A_2 (local discrete) can designate 8 discrete conditions, that in A_4 (seven-segment symbolic) can designate 10, and that in A_3 (binary) can designate 128. (B) Two illustrations (B_1 and B_2) of ways in which the same seven fibers (a–g) might encode two different stimuli that increase stepwise in time as in B_3. Objects and events in the world are ordinarily reported to the nervous system in sequences of impulses on parallel but differently encoded pathways.

erated input, or are symbolic of the particular input in a way that resembles parallel signaling in examples A_1, A_2, and A_4. Consider how pulse rate encoding of magnitude could be combined with multiple pathway signaling of other information about the stimulus world. Discuss the encoding benefits from simultaneous activity on the seven fibers responding to graded intensities of two different stimuli shown in B_1 compared to those shown in B_2.

The information content of a pulse rate code is theoretically infinite but practically it depends on how well the receiver is able to distinguish differences in the continuously variable interval between individual pulses.

Actual neural signals carry more information on a single fiber than is possible with the synchronous binary codes that are often used as models. The content of these signals is also harder to analyze. Theoretically there is no limit to the detail that could be represented by a continuously variable impulse rate. However, the ability of the recipient neuron or muscle to resolve differences in impulse rates of arriving impulses sets a limit on the effective information content of those signals. The continuous nature of neural signals causes the information to be approximate rather than either clearly right or wrong. Error ratios depend on how both total information and the error are defined rather than being intrinsic to the signal-encoding process. Objects are then represented by relationships among multiple inexact signals.

8.3.* Problem: Consider the simple task of differentiating visually between triangles and other geometric objects. A preschool child easily learns to make this distinction. Begin with information from an array of visual point receptors such as are found in the central part of the human retina. Define the specific operations that would lead to a "true" response for all the parts of figure 8.2 that are triangles and a "false" response for all the parts that are not. List the problems that you encounter. Would your processing accept or reject a three-dimensional object that is triangular when viewed from one direction but not from others? Are there any cases in which your perception is different from your formal analysis? How would you have to extend your processing to join these identifications to the recognition of the meaning of the spoken word "triangle?"

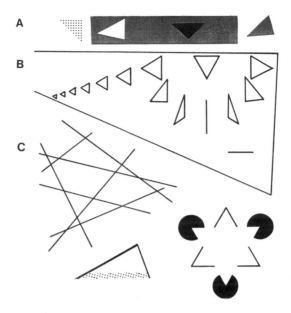

Figure 8.2
Triangles. (A) Six triangles distinguished by different relationships of contrast with their backgrounds. Are they all triangles? Define a single rule by which a computer might recognize any triangle. (B) Enclosed in a triangle too large to be shown completely are 15 representations of the same triangle each from a different view point. (C) Various triangles that are defined by differing types of boundaries. Does your rule select the same examples as your perception? If not, which is correct?

Events that involve changing relationships among objects depend on spatial and temporal information about object identification and interobject relationships.

8.4.* Experiment: With a cooperative subject in a moderately lighted location, abruptly shine the light from a pen light into the subject's eye and hold the light there while you observe the resultant pupil diameter changes. (This is a common neurological test for CNS function.) Write a description of exactly what you saw. With the light at a different distance (to alter intensity) repeat the test and observations. While the light was held steadily on the eye, did you observe any oscillations of the pupil diameter? Was either the pupil response speed or amplitude affected by the intensity of the light? Graph sufficient information from this experiment to account for the observations. Construct a family of time graphs of light intensity falling on specific areas of the retina in *your* eye as you made the observations.

During the occurrence of any event, many of the observer's sensory fibers will be actively transmitting time-changing patterns of nerve impulses. Many of these patterns are totally unrelated to the event of interest. Most of the remainder will be responding to that event but their inputs also will include other sources of stimuli. Although some fibers may carry more important signals than others, there is no reason to expect that the relevant signals appear only on specific fibers or carry another identifying tag that would allow isolation based on some central nervous system property. Part of the task of identification of a particular event involves isolation of the relevant information from the irrelevant information that arrives with it. Since extraction of the relevant information amounts to discarding the irrelevant part of the total input, this process could introduce serious conflict in sensing multiple simultaneous events.

The utilization of current information to predict future conditions is critical to the function of the nervous system.

Identification of some transient events provides no information about what will happen in the future. Other classes of events are a part of an ongoing process so that current conditions can be used to predict what is to be expected in the future. For these processes, the nervous system might manipulate information in a way that is parallel to, but leading, the external process and thereby develop a response that is adjusted to meet future conditions. Movement of an inertial object is a common example of a process in which fixed rules permit prediction. Continuity rules in other processes can be complex and are not even necessarily stable. Stored information about past occurrences of presumably comparable processes is important to many predictions made by human nervous systems.

   Three practical limitations to making a prediction of the future state of a system from the current state and the known rules are (1) the rules are generally not known exactly, (2) the system may be subject to unexpected external influences, and (3) the system is often so sensitive to current conditions that minimal imperfections in the knowledge of current conditions will have an appreciable effect on future conditions. On the other hand, most real systems do not change instantaneously but require time for effects to develop permitting accurate predictions for a short period into the future. As the time of prediction is extended, the accuracy deteriorates until all that can be predicted is the range of possible conditions. If the information about state is continually updated, then continuing short-term predictions are possible. Engineering prediction may be improved for future use, by adjusting the predictive rules because of errors that are observed in current results. The nervous system deals with similar problems, is subject to similar limitations, and profits by adjustment of rules (*meta control*).

8.5.* Problem: Choose some familiar sporting activity that involves returning a ball, such as tennis, ping pong, handball, or baseball. Obtain information about the appropriate ball velocities (i.e., published data, videotape measured flight times, or oscilloscope measurements of the interval between sounds). Calculate the distance that the ball will travel during the period that it takes an individual to respond to visual information about the approaching flight. What part of the flight path is available to predict the contact point for the ball. How much error in striking location can be tolerated if an acceptable return is to be accomplished? What is the required accuracy of information and what are possible sources of useful information other than that concerning the last moment velocity and position?

The "interception problem" in engineering seeks to control the trajectory of one object so that it either intersects, or avoids intersection with, the trajectory of an observed object. The inertia of the controlled object and the accelerating force available limit the magnitude of the trajectory changes that are possible. If the observed object is in ballistic flight, its course is predictable from the observed data and even if it can maneuver, the extent of the deviations of its trajectory will be limited by inertia. A biological application of this problem can be illustrated in American football. Catching a pass and avoiding contact with a free ball are examples in which the independent object obeys ballistic rules. Making or avoiding a tackle are cases in which the independent object is maneuverable. These examples, although biologically trivial, are parallel to problems that probably played an important part in the survival of our ancestors.

Ordinary cognitive processes are developed through experience and are based on stored information as well as on recent sensory input.

To this point, we have generally been able to describe the rules for the utilization of sensory information. Many cognitive processes, common to human activity, are not readily related to specific sensory inputs. Common activities such as language comprehension and generation probably involve different information processing from one individual to another while still producing results that agree tolerably. We have no basis to presume that different personal logical constructs represent different principles of neuronal function, but we know little about the operations that are actually involved. Some of the problem in trying to relate these processes to sensory information results from the fact that they commonly use information obtained over a long period, stored in an unknown way, and accessed by unknown means.

In the preceding chapters, we have seen that individual receptors are sensitive to different fractions of the quantitative detail of their physical environment. This selective sensitivity determines the information that is represented by the impulse pattern on specific sensory nerve fibers. The specificity that this imparts to the signals on a sensory nerve fiber is sometimes shown by describing these fibers as *labeled lines*. Many outputs of the nervous system are similarly carried by labeled lines. Output labeling is imparted by the discrete nature of the anatomical sites of action of individual fibers and by the specificity of the chemical or mechanical conditions that result from the activation of individual effectors.

In the most thoroughly understood cases of reflex responses, information on labeled input lines is combined in a rather fixed way onto output neurons. A similar tracing of "perception" signals has generally been impossible and, as a result, indirect information about the process of combination of input information has been used to develop theories for perception. One example is speech perception where the relationship between the perception and the receptor activation can be estimated from the characteristics of a *spectrogram* (*sonogram*) (figure 8.3). A speech spectrogram is a three-dimensional graph with time plotted on the abscissa, sound frequency plotted on the ordinate, and intensity represented by density. It is not theoretically possible to resolve precise frequency information while simultaneously deriving details of fast changes in intensity. So, when a narrow band filter is used to resolve frequency detail over a relatively long time, it conceals details of brief changes of intensity. A broad band filter, on the other

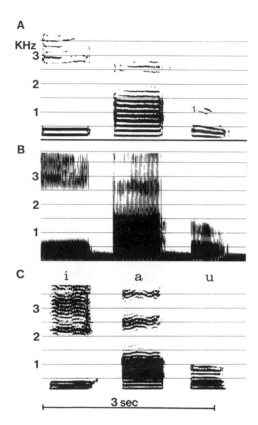

Figure 8.3
Spectrograms of three different vowel phonemes, *i*, *a*, and *u*, showing the involvement of multiple formants as components of each sound. (A, C) Narrow band (50 Hz) spectrograms of the same three phonemes as uttered by two speakers, showing good resolution of frequency detail. (B) Wide band (300 Hz) analysis of the same sounds as shown in (A) showing fine temporal detail. See figure 3.4 for corresponding waveform records. (Recorded by Donald S. Cooper.)

hand, resolves transient intensity changes but loses details of frequency. Auditory perception includes both frequency detail and brief intensity changes and presumably the perceptual process must carry out these two types of filtering simultaneously.

Object recognition may result first from recognition of individual features and then from recognition of a combination of these features.

In studies of subjective aspects of perception, objects are often described by their characteristic combination of features. A specific speech sound or *phoneme* (e.g., *e*) is characterized by the pattern of constituent frequencies or *formants* of which it is composed. Perception depends on some result of the pattern of activity on multiple frequency-labeled lines in the cochlear nerve. Other patterns lead to the perception of other phonemes. Perception of other types of features as, for example, in visual recognition also involves excitation patterns of multiple receptor units. Recognition of each feature involves pattern recognition in time and across multiple sensory nerve fibers. Specific attributes elicit characteristic subsets of the neuronal activity patterns that underlie the perception of that particular feature. The perception of an object is represented as the combination of multiple identified features.

An individual auditory receptor cell responds to a limited range of sound frequencies; a speech spectrogram is roughly equivalent to the information carried on the labeled lines in the cochlear nerve. The variations of density on a horizontal line across the spectrogram approximate the varying intensity of excitation of a single auditory hair cell and other horizontal lines represent other hair cells. Each detected formant (frequency band) in the sound is, in effect, a feature of the particular phoneme sensed. Changes in pattern are also features and are especially important to consonant phonemes. A vertical line on the spectrogram shows the vector of intensity terms that describes the stimuli to all the individual receptors at a single moment in the speech sound. The whole spectrogram shows the time-varying vector of stimuli to the cochlea. The neural interpretation of this spatiotemporal vector is the basis for perception of spoken information.

Certain vowel phonemes can be differentiated from information of only the first two formants (Peterson and Barney, 1952). Figure 8.4 shows three easily distinguishable vowel sounds in a plot of the frequency of the first formant against that of the second formant; in these dimensions, these vowels have nonoverlap-

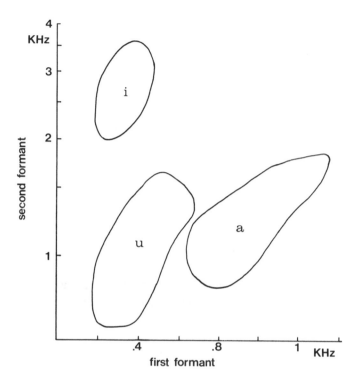

Figure 8.4
Location of the bounds of variability in frequency of vowel sounds of *i*, *a*, and *u* on a graph of their first formant against their second formant. These bounds enclose points determined on repeated utterances by 76 different speakers. (Redrawn from Peterson and Barney, 1952.) The vertical height at any frequency of the first formant and the horizontal width at any frequency of the second formant show the tolerance of variation for the frequency component of the related formant. The diagonal spread of a bounded region indicates constancy of the ratio of the two frequencies while producing the same perceived phoneme at different absolute values of frequency.

ping ranges. Some other vowel sounds are not as well separated within these two dimensions, and when spoken are more subject to misinterpretation. In these cases, dependable separation is attained when at least one more formant is considered. In contrast to vowels, the physical identification of consonant phonemes usually requires additional information about the sound.

8.6.* Problem: A pulse rate code, carried on a single pathway, can transmit magnitude information about only one dimension. If a particular feature, with its attributes, is handled as a multidimensional signal, that signal must be carried on multiple fibers. Choose an example of a feature with associated attributes and describe different ways in which the information might be encoded by central neurons. How might several unidimensional, local representations of the input information deal with this encoding? Define a distributed scheme of signaling in which each unit carries multidimensional information. Describe an encoding scheme that would retain the multidimensional information and yet involve only single unit signals for any one condition. Describe the availability of information in these different forms and consider the number of units that are required to encode it.

Two types of clinical study suggest that visual information is processed through successive stages of refinement. First, subjective reports of visual experiences when electrical stimuli are used to excite artificially some parts of the visual system demonstrate an orderly progression of the development of perception. Second, lesions at points in the visual pathway suggest a similar order. With electrical stimuli at successive points, starting from the receptor, flashes of light are succeeded by patterns, and finally even recognizable forms. Lesions at sites from receptors to central neurons cause successively total blindness, only pupillary constriction to light, avoidance responses, unconscious object recognition, object recognition without the ability to assign a name, and finally seemingly normal perception. Some of these defects have been called "blindsight" (Cowey and Stoerig, 1991).

Many important studies (including three that led to Nobel prizes) have included investigations of the response of individual neurons to visual stimuli. Hartline and Ratliff (1957) showed that in an array of visual receptors, adjacent units interact to increase the effect of spatial contrast of light level. Granit (1955) showed that information from visual receptors is combined to produce not only three different spectral distributions of intensity but also local brightness information that is somewhat independent of color. Hubel and Wiesel (1962) found individual cells in the visual cortex that respond to bars of light with particular sensitivity to a limited range of orientations and other cells that respond to oriented bars and edges but are insensitive to their location in the visual field. In addition, cells have been identified that respond best to directional movement of oriented bars or edges (Barlow and Levick, 1965). These cells exhibit characteristics of feature detectors followed by successive recombination into more complex representations.

8.7.* Problem: In a series of studies conducted at Bell Laboratories, Harmon (1971) used photographs to evaluate the relationship between identification of different faces and the characteristics of those faces. Features and attributes were tabulated and related to reliability of differentiation. Make a table of various features using the photographs in figure 8.5. Provide space to indicate both the observability of the feature in each of the four photographs and the attributes of each feature. Which photographs have the most features in common and which the least? Can the individuals be distinguished by differences in the features present? Do the two photographs of the same individual have the most features in common? Can you state in advance a formal basis for comparing a new set of photographs to distinguish those of the same individual?

8.8.* Problem: Reconsider problem 8.3 and figure 8.2. Define a means of processing pictil information that will generate a response to the various lines. Use summation (both positive and negative) and a threshold characteristic so that a response is produced only when the pattern tested is a line. In figure 8.2, which lines are not easily detected? Are there differences between your perception of lines and your detector's identifications? What is the most difficult logic problem that you encountered in accomplishing this identification?

Percepts in the nervous system can exist only as patterns of activity distributed over many neurons.

A convincing case can be made that perception ordinarily depends not on local information but on information that is distributed over neurons with diverse inputs. That is, there is no "Grandmother cell" in the nervous system that is either necessary or sufficient to recognize your grandmother. Although individual

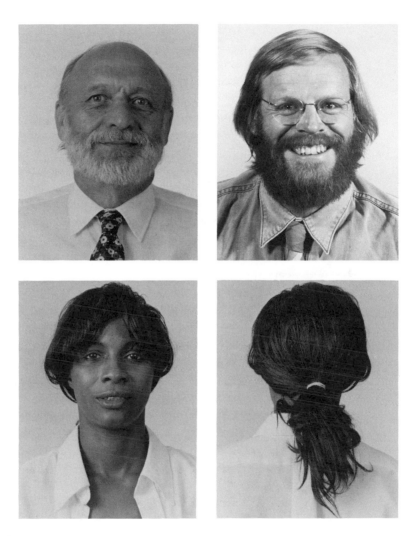

Figure 8.5
Four photographs of heads for feature and attribute identification. See problem 8.7.

receptors respond to a combination of inputs, seldom do responses relate closely and uniquely to any of the things that we would classify as features. Motor responses to the recognition of objects also appear as activity that is distributed in time over many motor neurons without evidence for the isolation of individual input features in the response. Although perception may be accomplished by parallel feature identifications followed by simple logical combinations, sometimes this interpretation may inappropriately constrain our thinking about all neural processing.

Individual neurons in the central nervous system have been shown to have receptive fields that include mechanical stimuli to well-separated skin locations in combination with responses to stimuli to visceral organs (Fields et al., 1970). Although these may be superfluous signals in the nervous system, these neurons do supply as much information about existing conditions as that supplied by any other neuron. If these receptive fields represent a feature, it is not very like the features proposed in studies of cognition.

While studying activity in individual neurons that carry information from the frog retina to the frog brain, Lettvin and his colleagues (Maturana et al., 1960) found individual neurons that had a selective response to small dark spots that moved against a stationary background. They speculated that this response is the signal that provides a "good enough identification" of food (a bug) present in the frog's visual field. This "bug detector" function most certainly requires that the neuronal circuits of the retina perform more complex functions than the simple extraction of features or the simple combination of identified features.

In a study of the amount of information involved in distinguishing different faces, Harmon (1973) divided continuous tone pictures into a set of rectangles of uniform size. Then each rectangle of the original picture was replaced with a rectangle with uniform density that approximated the average density in the corresponding part of the original picture. Following this manipulation, a face could still be identified when the picture contained only a small fraction of the information present in the original picture (figure 8.6). Even when the rectangles were so large that the edges demarking features of the original picture were eliminated, and even when edges that were not in the original picture were introduced, it was still possible to recognize specific faces. Face recognition, in these cases, must use some sort of global analysis rather than feature extraction in the usual sense.

8.9.* Math Problem: Data that originally supported conflicting theories sometimes no longer pose a problem after a new unifying theory appears. Provide a simple

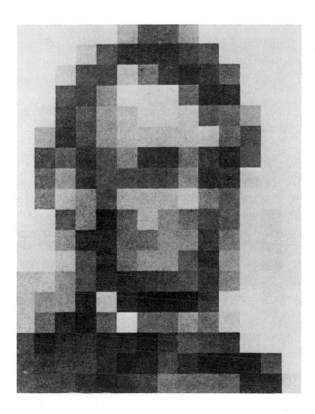

Figure 8.6
A picture reduced by computer analysis to an array of gray squares 13 wide by 18 high. Each of the 234 squares was assigned one of 16 gray levels to correspond to the average gray in the corresponding part of the original picture. View the figure first with good resolution (good light, normal reading distance, and good focus) and then with poor resolution so that the square edges are not resolved. What are the differences in available information and perceived detail in the two cases?

interpretation that will unify the explanation of (1) the data showing simple feature identification, and (2) unified processing of more global data at individual stages of neural function. What cannot be explained by your model? Is your model realistic from what you know of neural function?

The limitations imposed by computer models have biased current interpretation of the nervous system.

Computer development over the last half century has had a profound influence on our understanding of how signals are combined in the nervous system. Not only have computers become an essential tool for the measurement and analysis of data from biological systems, but computer models of those systems have biased the way in which the biological systems are interpreted. Ideas about computation and its terminology have been widely transferred into the neurosciences. Sometimes these transfers have led to new understanding, but, in other cases, they have added only new terminology to old ideas or they have even obscured known neural properties where computers do a similar process by a different means. As computer methods have been developed to do tasks that once were done only by humans, we have learned much about the problems but little about how the nervous system actually deals with them.

One of the first serious attempts to relate digital computing to neural function appeared as a series of papers by McCulloch and Pitts (1943). These papers brought to the attention of neuroscientists the important fact that an array of very simple logical operators could produce complex and useful results. However, the applicability of this work to neural function was limited by major differences between actual neurons and their binary "neuromimes" that were based partly on the then current theories of how neurons were synaptically excited.

The representation of multiple factors in the response of a single neuron, in simultaneous processing by different neurons, and in the orthogonal structure of some parts of the nervous system has led many investigators to describe neural processing in terms of vectors and matrices. More recently, the more specific "tensor transformation" (Pellionisz, 1988) has been used for these representations. There is some debate over the justification and merit of this type of terminology for application to neural function. At least when linear assumptions are avoided, the shorthand of matrix notation can be useful for a compact description of ideas about real neural systems. Those descriptions of neural function that use matrix notation provide a direct path to computer simulation, which can then be evaluated for unrealistic implications.

8.10.* Math Problem: Using matrix notation and making the assumption that linear representation is valid, write equations for two stages of neural processing including receptors and second-order neurons. Start with an m-dimensional source of stimulating energy acting in various combinations and with various degrees of effectiveness on n sensory receptors. (Do not, at this time, include the complication imposed by the discontinuity of pulse codes.) The n sensory signals are then distributed with various weightings onto p central neurons where the combinations determine individual output signals. Consider the effect of the relative size of m, n, and p on the maximum dimensions of information that might be available at various levels. Next make the assumption that there exists a 1% unidentifiable variability in the scaling of each receptor's response. How does this "noise" affect the maximum amount of information about the world that could be reliably retrieved from an individual central signal? What additional assumptions did you need to make to quantify this answer? Would noise, at other points in the processing sequence, be equally detrimental?

Models, by definition, are simplifying representations of the systems that they model. Computer models of nervous system function have revealed inconsistencies in previous theories and have generated unexpected effects that have clear relevance to the real system. On the other hand, current attempts to simulate "higher brain function" are so inadequate that one suspects that critical qualitative defects must still exist in the models that are being used. In the well-defined, but very limited, task of playing chess, only recently have computers been able to produce respectable competition to human players (see Hsu et al., 1990). Other restricted tasks, such as reading handwriting, interpreting speech, manipulating diverse objects under optical control, and moving over visible terrain are all near the limits of current computer technology.

Many new computing methods are currently being explored that bear more resemblance to human neural function than did the earlier "von Neuman" machines. In these computers, it is common to have more than one processor running simultaneously. Some massively parallel processing systems use numbers of processors that are comparable to the numbers of neurons found in very simple nervous systems. Sometimes these parallel architectures are used in a way that is presumptuously called a "neural net." They can be programmed for single tasks over thousands of training cycles by a self-adjustment of the weight of their connections. Other experiments incorporate analog computing elements for speed and, in so doing, mirror some continuous aspects of real neuron function. Special programs are now available to estimate "good enough" problem solutions when the input information is neither reliable nor complete, a task faced more often than not by real nervous systems. Other programs are provided with large amounts of general information about specific classes of problems and are organized to combine parts of this stored information with input data to make decisions. As many aspects of the difference between human and machine function are diminished, we will eventually face the question of whether these developments can ever impart consciousness to machines.

8.11. Math Problem: If the neural information on which perception is based represents a transformation of sensory transductions of world energy information, then the identification of external world properties from central signals results from some sort of inverse transform in the central signal. Consider those mathematical conditions that determine the existence of a unique inverse transform for a particular forward transform. What kinds of transforms have no inverse? Do neural transformations include some for which inverses would not be expected to exist? How are illusions related to inverse transforms?

The relationship between sensory input and internal signals is shaped by connections that are determined by genetics and then modified by experience.

For a central neuron's response to reflect the pattern of an object's activation of a set of sensory receptors, pathways must exist that carry the information from the receptors to central neurons. Since only a few of the total array of receptors connect to any one central neuron, the *lack* of pathways is a major determinant of the sensory drive to any neuron. For those connections that do exist, effect (excitation, inhibition, modulation), dynamics, and effectiveness (weighting factor) for the individual signal's action further shape the relationship between the total sensory excitation and the response in a recipient neuron. Ultimately both motor responses and perceptions operate from information that was first molded by this structural and functional input filter.

Since the number of neurons in mammals does not increase after birth, any changes in connectivity must represent either changes in weighting of signal pathways or their elimination. Such local modification of signal combinations must underlie the shaping of functional responses. Genetic information determines what molecules can be synthesized, whereas local conditions modify both the amount synthesized and the postsynthesis fate of the molecules. Local environment can influence how genetic information produces gross structure and, thereby, like learning, leaves a trace of the past environment in each function. In addition, both the basic structure that constrains later learning and the processes by which learning modifies local function are dependent on genetic information. Genetics and environment are inseparably linked throughout life in determining neuronal function.

The receptive fields that drive activity in many central nervous system areas have been mapped and have frequently been found to have a spatial distribution that resembles the spatial distribution of the receptors. Thus, different pitches of sound are represented on the corresponding part of the cortex in a *tonotopic map* with a unidimensional, pitch-dependent sequence, similar to the locations of specific frequency sensitivities along the cochlea. As is common in several other sensory maps, the auditory cortex has more than one map of the same family of receptive fields.

8.12.* Problem: What functional significance might be attached to the presence of a tonotopically organized mapping of receptive fields within the auditory system? Contrast this with other sensory modalities in which a similar processing of signals might be useful but would not benefit by the processing area being organized as a map of spatial distribution of the sensory receptors.

Two-dimensional locations on the retina are mapped onto the visual area of the cortex in a distorted way. Central parts of the visual field occupy a considerable proportion of the cortical area and so provide resolution of the finest detail. Further distortion arises because the retinal and cortical surfaces are of a different shape. Still another distortion arises because optically corresponding halves of the two retinas are mapped in near superposition on individual cells in the cortex to provide an additional replication of the map of the central visual field.

Since the skin is a closed envelope that is represented with a body position map (*somatotopically*) on the cortex, a distortion is introduced into the cortical map This distorted map with giant fingers and face and a minuscule torso is called a *homunculus*. As in a planar map of the world, a discontinuity is unavoidable at the edges of the somatotopic map. (Consider some experimental studies that you might use to evaluate the possible perceptual importance of this structural discontinuity.)

Perhaps the simplest functional mapping is that combining the sensory with the motor map with only minimal processing to produce a reflex. In the spinal cord, individual muscles are represented by clusters of motoneurons ordered like the muscle locations along the limb. Since monosynaptic reflexes generally originate in the muscle on which they operate, this is also a muscle-based map of terminations of sensory input from muscle spindles.

In a variety of reflexes, different individuals respond in approximately the same way to a given stimulus. These responses may represent the result of a genetically determined connection pattern, but recent evidence does not entirely support this assumption. The alternative is that similar reflexes have been learned in different individuals because of the similarity in their independent experiences.

The *vestibulo-ocular reflex* is the reflex by which a stimulus to receptors of the (vestibular) *semicircular canals* in the inner ear produces predictable eye (ocular) movements. During brief head rotation around any axis, this reflex leads to eye movements that tend to maintain the image of stationary external objects at a constant position on the retina. Each semicircular canal responds to components of movement in a specific (Cartesian) plane. Similarly, individual extraocular muscles produce eye rotations in a fixed direction with respect to the head. One can correlate eye movement with semicircular canal stimuli to predict presumed connections of the vestibular nerves to the motor nerves that innervate specific extraocular muscles. It can be demonstrated, however, that the same connectivity diagrams do not apply to all animals. Rabbits, with their eyes oriented differently with respect to the semicircular canals, have a different functional relationship between a semicircular canal and the extraocular muscles. It is now clear that this functional relationship is not based on fixed anatomical pathways but is subject to modification with experience. By wearing special eyeglasses with inverting prisms, individuals can be subjected to visual worlds that have been reversed from the normal. This reversal of the visual field makes the normal vestibulo-ocular reflex adjustment of the eye position counterproductive. During several days of continuous use, subjects learn to perform visual tasks well in spite of the reversed fields and actually affect a reversal of the vestibulo-ocular reflex. The supposedly rigid connectivity-based response is rather plastic and can adjust within hours to altered functional relationships. Many well-known reflexes have developed under uniform circumstances so that learning of the same response is rewarding to all individuals. Common patterns of experience can produce a similar learning of input relationships, thereby forming the basis for similar perceptions.

8.13.* Problem: Consider the relationship that exists between a vestibular stimulus and the corrective eye movement that occurs when rotating the head while wearing corrective glasses. How is this relationship affected when the glasses have positive (farsighted) or negative (nearsighted) corrective lenses? How is this relationship altered by bifocal glasses? Use a pair of bifocal glasses and check your prediction by rotating your head from side to side while observing a stationary object first through the near focus lens and then through the far focus lens. Would a person who wears that set of lenses regularly find that the image appears stationary in both cases if the vestibulo-ocular reflex were completely corrective? When riding in a car, view a twisting road in front through a pair of binoculars. What effect does this have on the angular disparity (retinal slip)?

Many effects of signal combination that are essential for perception are comparable to combinations known in reflex function.

Neuronal processing of sensory information ranges in complexity from the simple unidimensional transfer of sensory input into motor response that is found in insect tropisms and human stretch reflexes to the most involved cognitive interpretation of the world. Intermediate between these extremes is a variety of perceptive and reflex processes that are only partially understood but that may be made up of the same operations that contribute to the more complex operations. Further consideration of and investigation into the mechanisms at this level may be both feasible and productive in advancing our understanding of still more complex functions.

Any neuron that is driven by signals from multiple receptors deals with a combination of spatially distributed signals. Beyond the summation of signals of contiguous receptors that simply increase reflex responses, these responses depend on more complex functions of multiple receptors, often including signals from different types and combinations of receptors that make use of the information in the specific location or type of stimulus to the individual receptors. For example, Magnus (1924) showed that the stretch reflex, which causes extensors in the leg to contract, is more effective if the plantar skin of the foot is in contact with a continuous surface. Semicircular canal stimulation accentuates the response of stretch reflexes in the legs, but if the neck is moved simultaneously the vestibular effect is reduced (Kim and Partridge, 1969). Similarly, simple combinations of signals from different receptors are thought to be the source of perception of localized burn sensation when pain, hot, and tactile receptors are simultaneously activated.

8.14. Questions: Under what circumstances would a vestibular stimulus occur simultaneously with stretch of leg muscles? How would the circumstances differ depending on whether neck bending also occurred? Both color perception and the perception of specific odors are called *synthetic senses* because they arise only as an interpretation of the relative activation of more than one type of receptor. For example, the smell of "cake" is produced by some combination of such odors as "butter" and "vanilla." In the visual system, it is possible to produce the same color sensation with different spectral distributions acting on the three receptor subtypes. The combination of two spectrally pure colors in different ratios will produce a continuous range of different perceived colors. How might this continuous range be represented in the central nervous system in a way that is unique for the different sensations?

When perception or motor response varies with the input in a discontinuous way, the processing of signals must include a partitioning that selects which response will be initiated. For a response to be effective, it must act for some minimal length of time. This is true even if the stimulus falls on the borderline between those that would drive different types of response. A toggle or hysteretic action has been observed in a variety of discontinuous response patterns so that once a particular response begins (e.g., respiratory inspiration) it often continues for an effective period before any shift to the other response (respiratory expiration) occurs.

One well-studied example (Creed et al., 1932) is the scratch reflex in the dog whose spinal cord has been isolated from the influence of higher neural centers. Using two "electric fleas," in different locations, it was shown that spinal processing was sufficient to direct the scratching action to the location of the active stimulus. When both stimuli were applied simultaneously, the reflex "decision" was not to scratch a point intermediate between the two stimuli, but rather to scratch at the location of one or the other stimulus. Sometimes the scratching changed to the second point after a period of scratching at the first point. This choice is accomplished in the relatively simple pathways supporting the local reflexes of the spinal cord. Complex inputs can initiate a change in location of a quadruped. The result can be effected by a multitude of forms of locomotion (creeping, walking, trotting, galloping, or running), but a continuous variation in gaits is never seen. Many dichotomous decisions in perception have been studied; a simple example in speech recognition is illustrated in figure 8.4.

As with spatial convergence, the temporal sequence of successive impulses onto a neuron influences the response of a simple reflex or perception.

Although certain sequences can generate a perception of continuing excitation, differences in the patterns of impulses over time generally underlie more complex processing. Time must be represented in the processing in either the intensity sequence or the time intervals. Perceptive event recognition suggests storage of some representation of the event from which different responses can be generated subsequently by different matches or mismatches.

A time-varying signal is unidimensional if only instantaneous values are extracted from it. On the other hand, if the pattern of the time variation is considered, more than one dimension is being extracted from the signal. The practical dimension of the signal is dependent on how much information is extracted. In engineering systems continuous signals are often subjected to an infinite series analysis (such as Fourier, LaGuerre, Walsh, or Lee and Schetzin analyses) and these theoretically infinite series are truncated to a few terms that provide an adequate description of the signal. In the nervous system, information about those parts of a signal that originate at successive times is distributed spatially over different neurons in a network, which is similar to mathematically partitioning frequency components. Once converted from a temporal pattern to a spatial pattern, temporally separate parts of the signal can be independently processed. Temporal relationships, once distributed over space, can be treated in a manner similar to spatial patterns.

Temporal variations of the intensity of a sound with a constant pitch can lead to recognition of different patterns in time. Variation of sound that is continuous in both time and intensity produces a distinctive perception. In these cases, there must be some way for the comparison of the present input with previous signals and the generation of some recognition of time intervals that are related to the intensity variation. The 40 different sound patterns that are the building blocks of human speech are short segments of sound of varying intensity, distributed

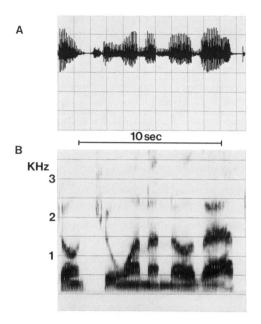

Figure 8.7
Two recordings of the sentence "Don't you want to know that." (A) A direct record of sound
(as in figure 3.5). (B) A spectrogram of the same utterance. The important details of such
speech include changing formants, relationship among formants, high-frequency noise, interruptions, and initiation of sound and sequence of these changes. Individual words are not
always separated by interruptions of sound. (Record made by Donald S. Cooper.)

over multiple frequencies and including noise elements without any characteristic
frequency. Transitions are essential features of some phonemes. To interpret
speech, it is necessary to deal with patterns in both frequency and time (figure
8.7). Often the interpretation of one segment of speech sound is not clear until
subsequent details are included.

Neural function makes exchanges between the temporal and spatial patterns of neural activity.

Spatially distributed inputs can generate temporally distributed sequences of
motor actions. Temporally distributed inputs can drive multiple motor units
whose spatial distribution depends, in a complex way, on the temporal distribu-

tion of the input signals. In still other cases, temporal information is used inter-changeably with spatial information to produce a single result.

During the visual or manual exploration of an object, information about sta-tionary relationships among points on the object is converted into a spatiotem-poral pattern of sensory inputs. To restore information about the spatial organization of the object being explored, the spatiotemporal pattern must then be organized into a perception of space. It is, thus, necessary to call on infor-mation concerning all the body movements that contributed to the exploration and this information must be combined with spatial information about the location of the stimulus on the receptor surface over the same period. Similarly in visual information, the retinal image must be reconciled with eye movements and neck and body movements.

8.15.* Problem: How might information from motoneurons be useful in the pro-cessing of information resulting from the exploration of an object? Describe the relationships between each type of input and the pattern that is derived from exploring a cubic object. How can a particular piece of information be represented alternatively by a spatial signal, a magnitude signal, or a temporal pattern?

8.16.* Experiment: Assemble a group of equal-sized cards with images of objects of several levels of complexity. In a dark room, choose a card from a shuffled pack and place it in a convenient location for viewing. Using a photoflash gun, light the object briefly and note how much detail you can recognize during a single flash. Flash illumination eliminates exploration of the object by eye move-ment. Redesign your image set to determine whether object details are derived from an essentially stationary input or by activating available memory patterns with partial information.

Recognition of a change of visual or tactile location or the change of pitch of a sound requires a spatiotemporal signal that carries information about the order of activation of a series of receptors. The visual information associated with movement toward or away from an array of identifiable points is complex and produces a sensory experience called a *flow field*. As an observer moves forward, a point directly in line with the movement will maintain a constant visual location. The visual angle between the movement path and objects off that path will increase as the movement continues. This results in movement of the retinal image of those objects away from the stationary target image and suggests a flow of space away from the target position. The rate of change of these directions is dependent on movement velocity, distance to the observed objects, and the distance of these objects from the movement path. The location of the target can be extrapolated from information in parts of the flow field that do not include that target. The information in a flow field is characterized by the order of activation of groups of visual receptors. The sensation of objects flowing away from a given point requires the processing of information that might come from any part of the visual field and that might move in any direction and with any velocity. The processing system requires access to very distributed information. A typical flow field provides redundant information about both static and moving geometry. One important use of flow fields is to provide depth information beyond the 5-m range of binocular depth perception.

A stationary point in a flow field is important to a pilot in estimating the point of touch down on landing or to a driver in recognizing the direction of motion of a car. When the observed object is moving instead of the observer, points on the object produce a sense of movement that is related to a flow field. A calculation of the appearance of movement of points in a flow field, similar to those in figure 8.8, is the basis for the computer graphics used in movies where it is desired to give the impression of rapid movement through a star-filled space.

8.17.* Problem: Use a graphic construction to decide what information is available about the geometry of a system from the apparent movement of one, two, and several off-center points. Would observation of the apparent movement of a single off-path point in the visual field provide as much information as is available from the apparent movement of more than one point? From flow field information, can you theoretically determine the direction of travel, with and without a visual target? Can you find the velocity of movement and the relative distances to different objects?

Because perceptions are usually relative rather than absolute, current details are associated with a transient frame of reference.

The personal significance of the location of objects in the world depends on where those objects are with respect to the individual. When an individual changes location his or her frame of reference, within which locations are evaluated, moves. In addition to spatial dimensions of a stimulus source, many other

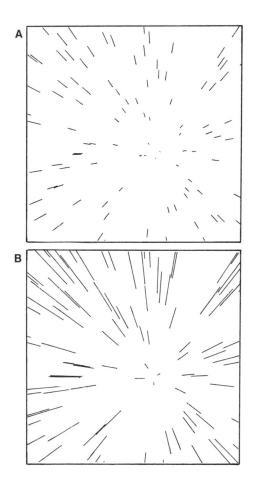

Figure 8.8
Flow field representation of the distributed information about visual objects during movement. Line lengths are proportional to the velocity of apparent movement of points at various locations. (A) Line lengths show flow of points on a plane during a period when the distance to the plane is decreased by 10%. (B) Line lengths, from the same starting positions, showing flow during a reduction of distance to the plane by 30%. For objects at different distances, the percent change of distance caused by a particular movement will vary.

sets of information about the world are relative rather than absolute. This necessitates shifting and rescaling of the reference frame to interpret the stimulus dimensions. Our perceptions, and even our reflexes, operate in variable frames of reference over a variety of dimensions. A changing frame of reference is a familiar experience in visual perception. It is important that the perception of objects does not change with the character of the lighting under which the objects are viewed. Although a piece of coal reflects more white light in the bright sun than does a sheet of white paper in candlelight, our frame of reference changes with the lighting conditions but the two objects are consistently distinguished as black or white under both viewing conditions. Somewhat less familiar is the shift of color perception. The face of a person sitting in the shade on the grass will reflect a high level of green light but we ordinarily perceive the person's face color in a frame of color reference that is shifted in a compensatory way. Only when we view color slides taken under those conditions is the increased green apparent.

The frame of reference is central to the perception of motion. A normal individual when moving has a frame of reference for motion that matches his or her recent average velocity and local variations can be easily recognized. A patient suffering from Ménière's syndrome has, in effect, an altered frame of reference in which a stationary position is perceived as a pronounced movement. Carnival rides take advantage of tricks that alter the rider's frame of reference for movement, often with bizarre results. A familiar central nervous system–based shift of our frame of reference is the "waterfall phenomenon." Observing a flow in which different parts of the visual field involve different movement velocities will, within a minute or two of constant observation, lead to a changed perception of movement. On turning away, solid objects will appear to flow in the opposite direction. This effect can have important consequences in the industrial setting with constantly moving machinery parts.

The reflex or perceptive outcomes of particular stimuli depend on the state of the nervous system at the time of arrival of the stimulus.

Responses to stimuli generally differ between comatose and alert attentive states of an individual. Between these two extremes, individual details of the state of the nervous system at the time of arrival of a particular stimulus can significantly alter the response that is expected. Part of the information converging on the information-processing system is not from external stimuli but rather is internal to the nervous system itself.

One example of the dependence of a response on the state at the time of arrival of the stimulus was given the name *precedence of stimulus* by Gesell and Dontas (1952), who showed that a stimulus to a respiratory nerve produced a prolonged inspiration if delivered during inspiration but produced prolonged expiration if delivered during expiration. In a second example, Shik et al. (1968) showed a similar effect of the state at the time of a stimulus in a cat walking on a treadmill. If the cat's foot encountered an obstruction, either the stance phase would be prolonged or the flexion phase would be increased, depending on the cat's phase of walking at the time of contact. In these cats, the distinction could be made by the remaining nervous system even after much of the brain had been removed. Finally, a simple perceptive analogy has been studied under the name of *set* in which a general subject, when introduced before a specific input, strongly influences the interpretation of that input. One example is the inability to recognize a phrase in one language if another known language has been suggested in advance.

8.18. Problem: In this section, we have associated pairs of perceptive and reflex observations with the implication that they may be accomplished by similar neuronal processes. Our pairings are only suspected and are not proven cases of parallel function. From your background experiences, try to identify additional perceptive patterns and perhaps also reflex examples. Put together a new and instructive combination of a possibly parallel reflex and perception. Do you suspect that any of our pairings are probably not parallel?

Perceptual processes can be conveniently described using the concept of perceptual basins.

The simplest (and most studied) reflexes and perceptions have been described as a fixed response to a combination of stimuli that meet a certain criterion. In somewhat more complex cases, the response varies quantitatively with a range of stimuli. In either case there is a transformation of the input pattern into a response according to a constant rule relating output to input. As we consider more typical cognitive activity, we find that the relationship between the sensory input pattern and the resulting perception becomes more variable. The whole range of inputs that separately evoke a particular perception can be considered to fall within the *basin* of that perception, just as rain that falls in the area that feeds a particular river falls within that river's basin. We have encountered an example of a basin in the range of formant combinations that are perceived as a particular vowel phoneme (figure 8.4).

Sherrington recognized the convergence of diverse inputs that activate a particular motor unit. He spoke of the motor unit as the *final common pathway* of diverse reflexes. The perceptual basin is also a final common pathway, in this case, responding to different distributed patterns of input but producing an output that is much more complex than results from the activation of a single motor unit.

The basin terminology merely describes a group of observed relationships without explaining how they are accomplished at the neuronal level. Since different input patterns fall within the basin of a particular perception, that perception, by itself, does not uniquely identify which input pattern was activated. Very different inputs can activate the same perception. Knowledge of the occurrence of an event is not an assurance that you experienced it directly. Dreams and hallucinations evoke complex perceptions for which there is no immediate external basis. In this instance, signals from the internal state may override the effect of current sensory input in activating the basin involved.

On different occasions the same percept may be extracted from the total sensory inputs that contain not only different critical information but different background information.

Except under laboratory conditions, a given set of stimulus conditions is unlikely to be encountered twice. The same or equivalent objects are, however, frequently encountered under conditions in which it is essential to recognize their correspondence from the varying stimulus patterns that they provide. The basin terminology describes the appropriate identifications of objects with the necessary exclusions of the background. Figure 8.9 represents schematically a few variations of basin relationships.

We take for granted the activation of a given perceptual basin when, on different occasions, the presenting features are different. This occurs to some

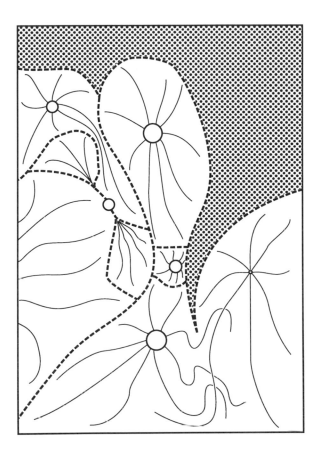

Figure 8.9
Various types of perceptual basins in two input dimensions. An individual basin includes all
the combinations of inputs that feed into a particular perception (represented by a small circle).
These include basins that vary in size, are compact (entirely contiguous), or partitioned (are
separated by sharp sepatrixes—dashed lines), or overlap in the displayed dimensions. Some
combinations of inputs are not further identified with only these two dimensions. Large circles
show perceptions with more recognizable attributes.

degree when viewing an object from different directions so that the features are subject to different degrees of visual foreshortening or occlusion (e.g., see the triangles in figure 8.2B). In the extreme, a different viewpoint may present a totally different set of features but will still activate the same basin (e.g., figure 8.5).

8.19.* Problem: How many ways can you identify the object *cat*? Identify pairs of examples in which

1. The same group of receptors is used but the information is only partially identical.

2. The object pattern is entirely different but uses the same set of receptors.

3. The same information, processed through the same logic, activates the basin but the signals originate in an entirely different set of receptors.

4. Entirely different information and receptors are used for the basin activations.

5. The cat is involved in an event so that the same set of receptors is subjected to a radically changing input pattern without alteration of the resulting identification.

6. Two quite different objects are mistakenly identified as the same cat.

7. The source of the stimuli is the same cat but the cat is misidentified.

The receptors activated and the response intensities that define a particular phoneme are different when it is spoken at a different loudness or pitch. If spoken by different individuals, differing "irrelevant" frequencies are also present. Thus basin activation for a particular phoneme is based neither on an absolute intensity nor on a specific input pattern but on particular relationships falling into a special range of variations of input patterns over time.

   The activation of a particular basin by various input patterns occurs when an excess of receptor signals is delivered into the basin, and then, when the total combined input reaches a complex threshold for identification, the appropriate response is generated. When no irrelevant sensory inputs are delivered to the basin, then interference will not be a problem. The minimum set of inputs needed to activate that basin is likely to be a very small fraction of the total receptors providing input to a basin. Other objects may activate sensors that overlap with the total set that is required for a minimal basin excitation and if the correct object identification still occurs some more complex mechanism must explain basin performance.

When a sound pattern is delivered to opposite ears, activating hair cells in opposite cochlea, or when an object is viewed under different light levels, activating only rods or only cones, the receptor sets that are activated are entirely different. However, the two sets correspond very closely and can produce the same perception by a simple convergence of the two signal arrays onto the same network of interpretative neurons. For visual inputs, rod and cone receptors have pathways that converge within the retina. On the other hand, when a specific object is recognized by its tactile and by its visual input, no simple correspondence exists in the patterns of receptors that are excited. In such cases, there is no obvious basis for the convergence of these separate signals onto the same perceptual basin.

Sometimes, similar sensory inputs are sharply partitioned and excite different perceptual basins depending on small but critical temporal or spatial details.

In some cases quite different input patterns may represent the same object; in other cases only slight differences in input patterns signal different source objects. Perception of the differences in objects requires the patterns to be partitioned so that different basins are activated. The partitioning may depend only on differences of pattern in space, intensity, or time of input to the same receptor set. Frequently, the differences of inputs that activate a single basin are greater than the differences between an input that activates that basin and those inputs that activate another basin. This is apparent when comparing the photographs in figure 8.5. Research in *human factor engineering* examines the means of widening the difference between inputs that activate different basins. For example, it is important to separate the basins to differentiate the controls for wheel retraction from those for the throttles in an aircraft cockpit. Examination of these studies can be instructive in understanding the nature of, and differentiation between, perceptive basins.

Since the response of individual neurons to their input is altered by blood gas levels, drugs, central activity, temperature, and so on, changes in these agents might be expected to shift some *separatrixes* that divide particular basins. A shift of the division between response basins is one explanation for the changes in judgment that occur at high altitude, during fever, or under the influence of drugs or emotions.

During normal activity, multiple objects and events are usually present simultaneously. They may be sensed by independent or overlapping groups of receptors. Sometimes activation occurs in multiple basins simultaneously (e.g., when a conductor evaluates simultaneously the performance of members of an orchestra). Individual receptors contribute to more than one basin and the basins must, in some way, share those input pathways. In other cases, basins with overlapping inputs are mutually incompatible (e.g., the basin that identifies an animal as a cow but distinguishes this from the basin identifying an animal as a horse). Contention between basins may occur at the unit level if different distributions of activities within a single array of neurons distinguish the two basins. If the two basins are made up of independent arrays of neurons, then some reciprocal action between the basins is necessary. The activity of basins is seldom a final static result; both the input pattern and the perception are frequently subject to changes.

Interpersonal variations of the reported perception of a specific stimulus range from variations that are considered normal to deviations that may have serious adverse consequences for the individual. Some variations stem from faults at the receptor and others occur during processing of the signals from the receptors. Although some atypical responses may be considered as secondary to psychotic disorders, others are not considered pathological and represent minor variations in basin activation. Such deviations are much better known than understood.

Commonly used clinical tests of both visual and auditory function will identify certain defects, but patients often experience difficulties that are not shown by these tests. In auditory testing, one standard test has long been a measure of the frequency-dependent threshold for sound perception in a quiet environment. Audiometry tests deficits in receptor level processing but is a poor predictor of performance in speech comprehension in a noisy environment. In assessment of the visual system, one performance test uses symbol identification under good lighting to decide the minimum visual angle that can be perceived and many optical defects are identified by such acuity tests. However, individuals with equal visual acuity often do not have equal ability to discriminate details in complex environments or under varying lighting conditions. The processing of sensory information is not thoroughly evaluated by current methods and better testing may require a better definition of what is accomplished by normal neural processing.

Diverse inputs activate individual basins the uniformity of which is shown by the constancy of the perceived objects.

The output of a basin is either that ethereal thing called a perception, or a more concrete motor response, or both, that occurs in answer to the input pattern. When a basin is activated, the total response that is generated can include details that originated in past inputs and may not result from any part of the current input. Clearly motor response is driven by neural activity that is distributed in space and time and presumably perception is also associated with certain characteristic neural activity. Although it is not clear how perception is derived from the pattern of neural activity, we will consider both the neuronal patterns and the perceptual or motor effect to be the outputs of an active basin.

Since whenever a basin is activated the same perception is produced, there is a constancy in the interpretation of the whole variety of possible activating stimuli. If the inputs that activate the basin are appropriately organized, then this constancy of interpretation parallels a constancy of the object in which the differing stimulus patterns originate. The source events or objects are then recognized to have constancy of some properties.

Although the input that activated a basin may have included signals that originated from only a small fraction of the properties of the source, to the extent that the source is constant, the unobserved properties can be assumed to be present. Once an identification has been made, then many unobserved attributes may be properly attached to the perceived object. Thus, when you recognize the presence of a person that perception is automatically extrapolated to include eyes, ears, nose, mouth, arms, and legs without the necessity for a current sensory basis. When a discrepancy between the expected and the observed is noted, there is a tendency to develop an increased attention to sensory detail. A person, seen from different distances, subtends different visual angles and excites different sized arrays of receptors. Such differences could be the basis for recognizing differences in the size of objects, yet the viewed person is generally interpreted as an object of constant size at different distances. Similar constancy is also found in the color of objects under different spectra of ambient light and in objects viewed from different directions. Phonemes, spoken at different pitches and at different loudness, are also perceived with constant meaning. Witnesses of a brief event will often later add to the event unobserved elaborations that dependably fit the expected pattern. Such extrapolation is a significant source of error, not only in reports of legal witnesses but also in clinical and scientific observation.

The important neural function of recall of information that was acquired in the past can be described as an extrapolation following activation of a basin. Any of the input patterns that have been attached to a basin can activate that basin with the consequent retrieval of unobserved details that had been previously associated with that basin. This is the reason that a student desiring to remember course information is advised to develop as many associations with that information as possible by activities such as listening in class, making notes, reading a different presentation, manipulating the information, and discussing the subject. These associations should increase the number of inputs that can activate the basin within which the desired information is accessible. Clues that can activate a basin may be details that just happened to overlap in time with the observation of interest. For example, when a class is divided to take an exam in different locations, there is an advantage for those who take the exam in the location in which they heard the lectures. It appears that sensory inputs from the room become part of the access to those basins within which critical information is embedded. In the extreme, a set of information around a notable event can be *imprinted* in memory so that any entry into the basin of the event leads to retrieval of extensive detail of associated objects and events.

An active basin presumably amounts to a characteristic activity pattern within a set of neurons. Multidimensional information requires multiple neurons. Generally, studies of units that might be involved in a perceptual basin have centered on the search for particular neurons or a particular temporal activity pattern that can be associated with specific objects or events. In a few cases, patterns have been found in the average of many repetitions of the same stimulus, although these patterns are not apparent on a single test of the same input. We know of no instance in which different input patterns that drive a single perceptual basin have been shown to produce a consistent pattern of activity in a specific neuron.

Studies of the brain regions involved in olfaction have not uncovered temporal or spatial patterns that differ with specific odorants. What has been observed is the distribution of activity over a whole region that is related to the specific odorant (Freeman, 1989). If basin activity is ordinarily organized in this way, it would seldom have been observed because there have been few studies that were analyzed in a way capable of demonstrating such activity.

The rules by which a sensory input is converted to a response are plastic. On different occasions the same input can activate different basins or one basin can be activated by different inputs.

The characteristics of a basin are relatively constant over short periods of time but tend to change over longer experience. The underlying plasticity of neural function is evident as changes in both the set of stimulus patterns that can activate a basin and in the details of the response that results from that activation. Sometimes the boundaries are expanded and new stimulus patterns are added; in other cases, the basin is reduced by the elimination of some previously effective inputs. In either case, the definition of the basin is altered, becoming either more general or more specific. These changes can provide improved function, adjustment of function to new conditions, or even degradation of function.

When I.P. Pavlov conditioned dogs to salivate in response to a bell, he was adding a new territory to the basin that recognized the arrival of food. On meeting a strange person you may first generate a recognition basin responsive to their face and then rapidly add new, and rather different, areas to that basin including name, voice, pattern of walking, or personality traits. Reduction, instead of extension, is seen when a child, having been taught "ball" with a particular ball, may have to remove the stimulus "red" from the acceptable routes into the basin "ball." One way in which perception of the world changes is by change of the range of patterns of sensory activity that elicits the same final interpretation.

Often, following a central nervous system lesion, some function that is lost is restored over time. Initially this may reflect the return to the normal function of surviving neurons as acute effects subside. However, neurons responsible for a specific transformation may be permanently lost. The replacement explanation would require that their function be completely replaced by other pathways requiring those new pathways to take on both the connections and the transformations of those that were lost. Using the basin interpretation, the loss of part of an entry pattern into a basin does not necessarily alter the response of that basin, although its usual activation may be prevented. Recovery of lost basin function may require only the normal refining changes of the basin input. Because of these refinements, residues of the original input may be adapted to become acceptable patterns for activating the old basin. Such modification of basin activation relies on only the recognized plasticity of the nervous system.

Refined appreciation of the world around us often comes through the subdivision of our perceptual categories. Sometimes a new basin is needed to identify a class of inputs that was originally lumped with others. This partitioning requires extra information that is necessary to make the distinction. In other cases, refined identification defines new subbasins within a still-useful original basin. Perception subbasins are a case in which the river analogy is inappropriate since basin activation often feeds into the more detailed identification of the subbasin, unlike the flow direction from tributaries into a river.

A child that calls all animals "doggie" soon learns to move horses into a new classification that is not just a subclass of dog. Sometimes the background for an inappropriate inclusion in a basin may be obscure. So a child having been told that something was purple while coincidentally hearing Beethoven's fifth symphony may require considerable further instruction to remove purple as an attribute of that music. A different partitioning occurs in the new bird-watcher who first learns to separate the family of sparrows from other birds and then, with considerable effort, partitions that family into species such as Lincoln and Song sparrows.

In the operant conditioning paradigm introduced by B.F. Skinner, the subject is presented with an unchanging stimulus while responses that approach the desired target action are rewarded in order to gradually change the response in that direction. This reshapes the response side of the basin. Repeated motor responses to a repeated input pattern often encounter different loads. These load changes commonly elicit short-term alterations of the motor response that compensate for the load changes. In perception, it is common to alter the content of the response to the identification of a particular person. Activation of a basin for a new acquaintance elicits recall of very few traits but, with more familiarity, that same input recalls many more attributes. Through the whole sequence of changes of output, the input boundaries of these basins may or may not have been subject to change.

Alterations of basins may require changes at a few specific locations in the nervous system. The basin is altered by changes in the effect of specific signals and these changes must occur along pathways dealing with those signals. If the basin modification follows an experience that involves a specific stimulus pattern, the locations for change become labeled by the route taken by the activity produced in that experience. It is not so obvious how the location for changes is identified when the basis for modification is taught without a direct experience.

The naive brain, exposed to neural inputs from sensory stimulation, must organize its own activity in a way that discovers the existence of consistency in the source of and relationship among these stimuli.

Although the simple tropisms of an insect can occur because of genetically determined connections in the nervous system, the understanding of a specific human language certainly does not. Genetics provides the basis on which languages can be built, but not the specific language itself. The array of patterns of nerve impulses arrives within a naive nervous system with no labels attached. With this flood of impulses, and a nonspecific network of interacting neurons, the nervous system must discover the existence of regularity, the importance of pattern, the effect of reinforcing and nonreinforcing responses, and the bases for combination and response modifications.

At birth, a certain set of reflex functions is already operational, but even the foundation for more complex function is not apparent. Sucking, respiratory responses, and other responses of importance to survival are normally present. Beyond a few primitive properties, the human nervous system must be self-organizing (see Yates, 1987). The external manifestations of the progressive organization of this information processing have been studied extensively in developmental psychology. Those functions that are dependent on the accumulation of factual detail require, of course, time to develop. Equally important is the necessity for an extended development of the methods of dealing with information. The complexity of the neural processing performed by individuals increases from birth at least through the mid-teen years.

The newborn human does not initially recognize the existence of objects. Pattern recognition, developed during the first few months of life, permits specific responses to the neural signals from particular objects. It takes roughly a year to develop the ability to recognize that an object continues to exist even when it is no longer observable. Only later does the child recognize a clear distinction between "self" and "world." It takes several years more to recognize such generalizable ideas as the conservation of matter as is shown by the child's response to questions related to the transfer of water among different shaped containers. (Conservation of energy is often denied by adults!) Ideas about specific cases develop a decade before individuals can appreciate abstract ideas and their relationship to specific cases.

A succession of additions of more refined operations to the repertoire of the nervous system is one way that complex function can develop in an originally naive nervous system. Such a progression is not only conceptually attractive but it is supported by observations. It is, however, not without cost. The time course of development implies that individuals must live for an appreciable period depending on only primitive stages of development. At all stages of development, the existing organization must work well enough to permit survival. It may not be possible to build the most efficient final system by simply making additions to functionally acceptable subsystems. We should not attempt to explain observed function based on the most efficient processing without consideration of how that result could have developed in the biological system.

8.20. Problem: Development of the use of a tool has been studied for the case of a spoon. This surprisingly complex task is easily observed in children of the appropriate age. Organize your observations of a child's grappling with this problem by means of a written record of observations or with a videotape. Your record should include several details regarding each trial. Record possible locations of contact with the spoon, orientations of the spoon, parts of the hand used in the contact, ways of approaching the food with the spoon, and disposal of the food from the spoon. You will need plenty of room for notes. The task of setting up the record is instructive with respect to the information that needs to be learned, but observation of the number of trial variations is more informative. After accumulating a set of data, put together your summary of how the skill is acquired. Before you conclude that the initial problem comes entirely from lack of general motor control, make some observations on yourself as you learn some new skill (e.g., learning to use chopsticks, knitting needles, or a musical instrument.)

It is natural to study neural function in instances that are simple enough to offer some hope for understanding. On the other hand, there is a tendency to forget that those cases we have discussed represent only a selected subset of all neural functions. The simplest or even the moderately complex reflex responses that have been extensively studied do not offer some of the operational challenges to the nervous system that characterize our most human cognitive processes. If these higher functions are simply elaborations of the operations that occur at the simple level, then it is not obvious how that elaboration is organized. The student of neuronal function, in developing theoretical explanations, should not concentrate on simple processes to the extent of forgetting that these more complex operations also exist and must have some functional basis. It may be expedient to design our experiments to isolate simple details, but our theories should aim for compatibility with the most complex extensions.

Chapter 9

Information Storage

The ability of humans to learn and remember facts is indeed impressive. William Shakespeare drew from a vocabulary of about 30,000 words to write his plays and sonnets. A good maitre d'hotel will know the names and favorite dishes of hundreds of regular customers. A.R. Luria discusses the remarkable memory of a mnemonist in the very readable little book, *The Mind of a Mnemonist* (1987, p. 12): "Experiments indicated that he had no difficulty reproducing any lengthy series of words whatever, even though these had originally been presented to him a week, a month, a year, or even many years earlier." Most of us can add examples to such a list of feats of memory. Although neuroscience is still a long way from explaining these abilities, considerable strides have been made in recent years toward understanding how neurons are modified by experience and how those modifications are maintained for extended periods of time.

9.1.* Questions: Try sampling your memory. How well can you describe your kindergarten class? Can you remember names, relationships of objects, or smells? How valid do you suppose those memories are? Try remembering the same things from your senior year in high school. Do you suppose that these memories are more valid? Try remembering the details of the most momentous event in your life. Is this memory more detailed than other memories from approximately the same time in your life? What did you have for breakfast this morning? How detailed is that memory?

9.2.* Questions: What is a memory and what constitutes learning? Is a brief visual afterimage a memory? Does persistent modification of reflex activity constitute memory? Does learning include avoidance of food that once made you nauseated? Did you learn what you had for breakfast? Compare your experiences of *cognitive learning* (e.g., understanding the concept of a derivative) with those of *motor learning* (e.g., becoming proficient at riding a bicycle or typing). Are the necessary number of learning trials similar; is the forgetting time course similar?

The experimental study of learning and memory in humans dates to the work of Hermann Ebbinghaus in the late nineteenth century. His technique, used first on himself, was to make up long lists of three-letter nonsense syllables. (His syllables consisted of two consonants separated by a vowel.) From this list he would randomly pick shorter lists to memorize. His studies included investigations of the effect of the number of repetitions and list length on retention and the effect of time on the ability to remember a memorized list.

9.3. Experiment: Use Ebbinghaus's method of nonsense syllables to demonstrate some characteristics of learning and memory in yourself. Although these straight-forward experiments require a minimum of equipment, they do require careful data collection and a period of days to complete. (1) Use a short list (e.g., 10 items) to find the relationship between the number of learning trials and amount retained for a given time. (2) Use equal length lists and the same number of learning trials to assess the time course of your forgetting. A convenient method to measure forgetting is to measure the number of repetitions necessary to relearn an old list. Does the forgetting curve show separate short- and long-term components? Would you expect there to be an effect that depends on whether the syllables are phonetic (pronounceable) or not? Be sure to design your experiment to take this effect into consideration.

We will presume that memory resides in the effectiveness of the interactions between neurons.

In his *Discourse on Method* (1637), René Descartes proposed that there exists a sharp distinction between mind, a uniquely human attribute, and matter, the *automata* of the human machine. Although it is not our intent to discuss this dualism of philosophy here, it does conveniently introduce the basic tenet of this chapter. Restating Descartes's dualism in the form of a more restrictive question, we might ask: Are learning and memory emergent properties of the cellular structure of the nervous system, or are they measurable physical properties of the neurons and their interconnections? The working hypothesis of this chapter is the reductionist approach that learning and memory reside in changes in the morphology and biochemistry of the synapses between neurons. Functionally this implies a change in at least one of the following: release of neurotransmitter, delivery of neurotransmitter to its receptor site, the effectiveness of the receptors for the neurotransmitter, or the location of neurotransmitter release. (The details of synaptic transmission will be considered in chapter 13.)

The evidence for a specific location for memories within the brain might seem to have been well established by the experiments of the Canadian neurosurgeon Wilder Penfield. In surgeries to remove centers of epileptic activity from the brains of patients, he electrically stimulated specific brain regions. His patients reported having vivid recollections of events in their lives that he called "experiential illusions." Often these illusions were similar to the auras that the patients experienced before an epileptic seizure. Are these specific brain locales the site of memory storage, or do they simply evoke retrieval? Are other parts of the nervous system capable of storing information? As early as 1906, Sherrington had noted that repeated activation of spinal reflexes causes them to become less effective, or to habituate. Habituation persists for a considerable period and thus represents the storage of information within the nervous system. Probably most regions of the nervous system can be modified because of experience. These modifications can range from transient alterations of the time course of electrical potentials to long-term memory.

Learning leads to changes that increase or decrease the effectiveness of impulses arriving at the junctions between neurons and the cumulative effect of these changes constitutes memory. Since memory includes either avoidance or enhancement of particular parts of a response, the consequences of previous experience must be evaluated to select the needed direction of specific changes. Such an evaluation implies some standard of judgment that may, in turn, have been learned from some previous experience that had been evaluated by still more primitive values. Ultimately, the chain of developing standards for judgment must rest in some inherited primitives.

Often a particular pattern of neural activity leads to a result that occurs some time after that activity has ended. Learning in such cases must be related to the activity of neurons involved in the already completed neural activity. This requires some means of relating the activity that is to be changed to the evaluation that can be made only after the delayed consequence.

Memory is the maintenance over a period of time of an alteration of function as a consequence of previous experience.

In this chapter on information storage we will use the term memory as a specific subdivision of the more general process of *hysteresis*. We borrow the word hysteresis from physics and give it the general definition of any modification of future actions because of past actions. We will use a generally accepted definition for *learning,* that is a change in neuronal response resulting from previous experiences with a given stimulus. *Memory* is then the maintenance of this change over time.

Specific parts of the nervous system are capable of specific types of learning, different animals have different learning abilities, and animals are capable of learning some particular things at only specific times in their lives. Simple spinal reflexes can be conditioned even when the spinal cord has been totally isolated, whereas higher brain centers are necessary for the learning of language. Chickadees can learn the location of hundreds of hidden seeds, whereas humans can learn only about 12 such locations. Food aversion, which most of us have experienced, is an example of a specific predilection for learning. The ability to learn a pairing of taste and nausea is much stronger than the ability to learn a pairing of taste and pain or of a visual stimulus and nausea. Young children are predisposed to learn to walk at a specific time and to talk beginning at another specific time. There is a critical period, to about age 2 in children, in which learning deficits result from metabolic disease or from nutritional deficiency. An absolute identification of the physical basis for learning disability caused by undernourishment is difficult to establish but the evidence supports the notion that certain aspects of brain development during this critical period are essential for future learning potential (Tizard, 1974). Although learning can continue throughout life, there is a critical aspect of this early period in children.

Not only is there a unique learning potential in children, but children's memory capability is different from that of adults. This is exemplified by the condition of *infantile amnesia,* the lack of recall by adults of early childhood events. Young children can register and recall memories at the time, but have much more limited ability to recall these memories later in their lives than would be expected for the time elapsed. Perhaps the changes in neural processing that result from early learning modify the function so much that early memories are corrupted beyond recognition.

Human learning represents a specialization into certain specific areas of a general ability of all animals.

Although there is a tendency to limit our consideration of learning to humans, important experimental evidence about the mechanisms of learning and memory comes from studies of such animals as the arthropod *Drosophila* and the mollusc *Aplysia*. Most of the important aspects of neuronal excitability and plasticity probably arose very early in evolution and have since been highly conserved. There is no reason to expect that the cellular mechanisms of learning and memory elucidated in these animals are not also used in humans.

One can make a case for a correlation between the ability to learn in lower animals with their ability to evolve to higher animals. An important impetus to evolutionary change in a species is a change in the environmental conditions experienced by that species. If individuals are not able to learn behavioral strategies to deal with the altered environment, the species will not survive the long time periods required for genetic modifications to produce permanent adaptation. The fruit fly, *Drosophila,* has long been an important subject of genetic studies. Recently, identified gene mutations have been found that lead to an impairment of learning, memory, or memory retrieval. Because the gene products of these mutations are known, we are at the point of understanding some of the cellular processes potentially involved in learning and memory.

Learning that involves the association of two stimulus patterns is distinguished from learning of the specific properties of a single stimulus pattern.

Psychologists generally subdivide learning into two categories. (1) *Nonassociative learning* occurs when the organism learns specific properties of a stimulus. This category includes *habituation,* in which the animal decreases its level of response to a repeated, non-noxious stimulus, and *sensitization,* in which a novel stimulus increases the response to a second or continuously repeated, nonnoxious stimulus. (2) *Associative learning* relates two stimuli and includes, in turn, two subcategories: *classical conditioning,* in which the animal learns the relationship of one stimulus to another, and *operant conditioning,* in which the animal learns the relationship of a stimulus to the animal's own behavior. Many animals are good at learning the association between events that reliably occur together in time. This ability is generally better for shorter time intervals. The ability to learn other types of associations, such as spatial associations, is much more variable among different animals or individuals.

A useful, albeit not usual, approach to categorize these types of learning makes use of the basin concept presented in chapter 8. Classical conditioning uses modification of basin inputs whereas operant conditioning results from modification of the output from a basin.

Short-term memory lasts for only a period of conscious awareness whereas long-term memory can last a lifetime.

There are two general overlapping categories of memory in humans, *short-term memory* and *long-term memory*. As the names imply, short-term memory has a maximum effectiveness measured in minutes to hours, whereas long-term memory can last years. Clinical data from trauma, seizure, and coma further delineate the distinction, since long-term memory can survive several hours of silent electroencephalogram (EEG), whereas such an insult eliminates short-term memory. (See chapter 10 for a discussion of the EEG.) There appears to be an active consolidation process necessary to convert short-term memories into long-term memories (figure 9.1). There are well-known cases of patients without consolidation capability. These unfortunate people can maintain short-term memory for many hours of conscious use, but once their attention is transferred the memory is lost. Neurologists classify many types of memory loss as *amnesia*. Two important types of amnesia are (1) anterograde amnesia, loss of memory for some period following a traumatic event, and (2) retrograde amnesia, loss of memory for some period preceding a traumatic event.

Short-term memory relies on functional modifications of the synapses between neurons.

As mentioned above, trauma can eliminate short-term memories without affecting either long-term memories or the consolidation process. The immediate aspect of short-term memory is obvious, and cellular mechanisms have been elucidated that operate on a time scale appropriate to this process. There is a second, longer aspect of unconsolidated memory that probably results from the self-reinforcement of these same processes. In the neurophysiological literature, two mecha-

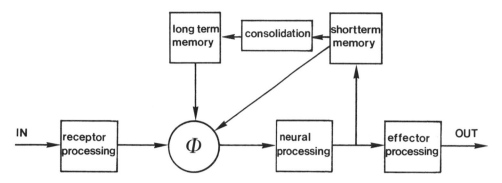

Figure 9.1
Schematic representation of memory processes. All sensory information is subject first to receptor and other neural processing before becoming available for memory storage. Storage is initiated as short-term memory that can be later consolidated into long-term memory. All memories can interact with incoming sensory information and it is the result of this interaction that determines the output of the nervous system.

nisms for short-term memory have been discussed extensively, reverberating excitatory activity in unmodified existing neural circuits and rapid modifications at the synapses between neurons. There is no good evidence that short-term memory occurs without concurrent modification of the biochemistry of the synapses between neurons.

Lorente de Nó, in 1933, demonstrated an anatomical basis for the possibility of functional reverberating circuits (figure 9.2). These anatomical circuits have been evoked by many physiologists to explain various forms of information storage in the nervous system. For instance, Sir John Eccles stated in 1953: "In continuously circulating around any particular chain of neurones, the impulses would give a specific pattern of activity in space and time, which of course could form the basis of specific sequelae, e.g., conditioned reflexes or memories." More recently the idea that short-term memory exists as activity in reverberating circuits has fallen out of favor for two reasons. First, there has been no definitive observation of brief pulses of electrical activity repeatedly cycling in anatomically identified closed loops; and second, all the observations of short-term memory can be explained by known modifications of synapses. The approach taken here will be to develop the idea that short-term memory results from modifications of the ion channels and neurotransmitter receptors of neurons. The idea of maintenance of electrical activity in existing circuits, however, needs another com-

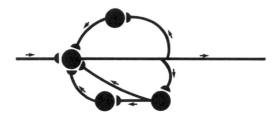

Figure 9.2
Reverberating circuits. Anatomically demonstrated closed loop pathways called reverberating circuits were considered, probably incorrectly, to be the basis of short-term memory. One problem with this theory is that only fatigue could account for the termination of an extended response.

ment. In circuits that produce positive feedback, transient electrical events can be considerably prolonged.

The time over which a single pulse has an effect in any circuit depends on the time constants of the rise and fall of that pulse. The effectiveness of a single action potential cannot exceed a few tens of milliseconds (see chapter 12), and the effectiveness of a group of action potentials does not outlast the final action potential by much more. In a neuronal circuit that displays positive feedback with a gain of less than one, these time constants can be considerably increased (figure 9.3). By this means, then, a single action potential or, more dramatically, a group of action potentials can have an effect in a neuronal circuit for an extended period. Such an effect may be important in initiating the changes that lead to short-term memory.

Synaptic efficacy can be modified transiently by many different biochemical processes.

It is worth delineating the various rapid hysteresis processes that exist within the nervous system. Although the delays inherent in action potential propagation and synaptic transmission affect temporal relationships, they do not, per se, affect future actions and therefore do not cause hysteresis. We will assume that simple delays do not produce information storage. The most rapid hysteresis processes, lasting less than a second, are often called *iconic memory*. In this category are certain direct processes of sensory receptors, such as visual afterimages. Somewhat longer hysteresis-producing processes require circuits using the synapses

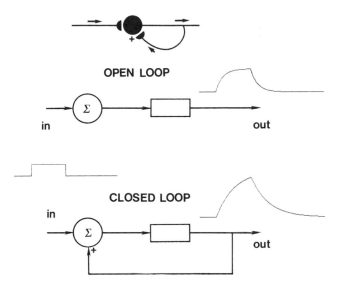

Figure 9.3
Positive feedback. Closed-loop dynamic circuits result in positive feedback and are capable of greatly increasing the time constant and time course of pulse responses.

between neurons. Synapses, as we will see in chapter 13, are the junctions between neurons that serve as the most important sites of integration of information in the nervous system. The input to the synapse is the impulse pattern in a *presynaptic* neuron that releases *neurotransmitter.* This neurotransmitter acts, through *receptors* in the membrane of the *postsynaptic* neuron, to produce the output of the synapse. The most rapid modifications of synaptic activity are phenomena such as *positive feedback, posttetanic potentiation, disinhibition, presynaptic inhibition,* and *presynaptic facilitation.* Processes in this category result from changes in postsynaptic sensitivity or in presynaptic neurotransmitter release mechanisms. At the longest extent of the rapid hysteresis-producing processes are *long-term potentiation, long-term depression,* and *activity-dependent presynaptic facilitation,* where there are maintained modifications of presynaptic proteins or changes in postsynaptic receptor activity. Short-term memory most probably uses various combinations of these processes.

The marine mollusc *Aplysia californica* has been an exceedingly useful experimental preparation for the study of short-term memory. An advantage of experimental study of simpler nervous systems, such as that of *Aplysia,* is that the specific identifiable cells responsible for individual behavioral actions can be submitted to electrophysiological and biochemical studies. The gill withdrawal reflex in these animals is a protective reflex in which the delicate gill is withdrawn when a mechanical stimulus is applied to it. If repeated, nonnoxious mechanical stimuli are applied, the withdrawal will become less vigorous; that is, the reflex *habituates*. If a strong mechanical stimulus is applied to another part of the animal, *sensitization* occurs and the previously habituated gill withdrawal reflex will return to, or exceed, its original vigor.

Habituation in *Aplysia* occurs when sensory neurons release progressively less neurotransmitter from their presynaptic terminals onto the postsynaptic motoneurons. Sensitization results when an additional facilitating neuron releases a neurotransmitter to receptors on the sensory neuron's presynaptic terminal, causing an increase in the amount of neurotransmitter released by that sensory neuron. The facilitating neurotransmitter acts through a sequence of events that ultimately causes the addition of a phosphate molecule to ion channel proteins in the presynaptic membrane of the sensory neuron. This modification of the ion channels lengthens the electrical response of the sensory neuron's presynaptic terminal, causing the sensory neuron to release more neurotransmitter onto the motoneuron. Since the phosphate molecule remains attached to the protein for some time, the enhanced synaptic transmission and, therefore, sensitization persist (figure 9.4). Sometimes these pathways can be self-reinforcing, thereby extending the period of protein phosphorylation considerably beyond the time when the neurotransmitter occupies its receptor. The phosphorylating reactions will eventually end and the proteins will subsequently return to their original state.

One important mechanism by which short-term memory can occur is through the alteration of existing protein molecules.

Neuron function depends ultimately on the actions of protein molecules in the cell membrane. All proteins in animals are produced by the *transcription* of the genetic code of DNA into RNA and then the subsequent *translation* of the RNA code into the amino acid sequence of protein molecules. The action of protein molecules is often modified by chemical changes that occur after the synthesis of the amino acid sequence. One very important way in which such a *posttranslational modification* occurs is, as we have been discussing, through the addition of a phosphate molecule to the protein. One pathway by which protein phospho-

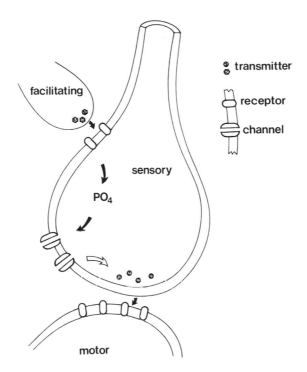

Figure 9.4
Sensitization. Sensitization at the sensory neuron-motoneuron junction in *Aplysia* results from
the action of a third, facilitating neuron. Transmitter from the facilitating neuron, at its receptors
on the sensory neuron terminal, initiates a sequence of second messenger steps that causes
phosphorylation of ion channels in the sensory nerve terminal. Phosphorylation of these ion
channels results in a lengthening of the presynaptic electrical event, thereby causing more
transmitter to be released from the sensory nerve terminal in response to a sensory impulse.
(Thus the parameter that scales the response to a sensory signal is increased.)

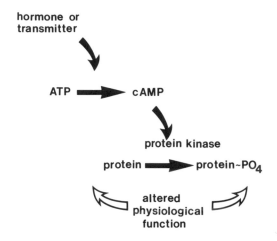

Figure 9.5
Protein phosphorylation. One very important second messenger system by which hormones or transmitters exert an effect on a cell's function is protein phosphorylation. In this process, the membrane receptor, when occupied by a hormone or transmitter, initiates a process that causes ATP to be converted to cyclic AMP; this molecule then activates an enzyme, protein kinase, that adds a PO_4 molecule to specific proteins. The presence or absence of PO_4 on protein molecules is important in determining the physiological function of the protein in the cell. Excellent discussions of protein phosphorylation can be found in most biochemistry textbooks. A discussion that relates specifically to proteins in neurons is in *Neuromodulation, the Biochemical Control of Neuronal Excitability,* edited by L.K. Kaczmarek and I.B. Levitan.

rylation occurs begins with a hormone or neurotransmitter causing the conversion of the metabolically important molecule ATP into the intracellular messenger molecule cyclic AMP. Cyclic AMP is then capable of activating the enzyme, protein kinase, that is responsible, in turn, for protein phosphorylation. Finally, because of phosphorylation, the physiological function of the protein is significantly altered. Of particular significance is that phosphorylation of the proteins that form ion channels can affect whether the channel will open or close (figure 9.5).

Short-term memory has been studied in mammalian brains by investigating the phenomenon of *long-term potentiation.* Following an appropriate brief repetitive stimulus, there can be a persistent 50% increase in the size of the postsynaptic response in certain synapses. An important aspect of this phenomenon is the entry of calcium ions into the postsynaptic cell during the repetitive stimulus. The calcium can have several functions; two possibilities are that it may increase the number or the responsiveness of the postsynaptic receptors or that it may signal the presynaptic cell to release more neurotransmitter.

This mechanism of short-term memory depends on a change in the action of existing protein molecules. New protein is not synthesized. Although these effects are typically transient, they can last potentially for the lifetime of the modified protein molecules.

We can, at this point, make several generalizations about what we expect for a mechanism of short-term memory. (1) It is not necessary to hypothesize the creation of new neuronal pathways. Plasticity within existing pathways can account for most of the observations and short-term memory occurs too quickly for it to require any major modification of neuronal pathways. We should not, however, eliminate the possibility of changes in the morphology of the existing synapses between neurons. These effects also might occur through changes in the number of *active* postsynaptic receptors for neurotransmitter and by rapid modification of areas of synaptic contact between neurons. (2) Short-term memory probably does not result from nerve impulses reverberating in closed loop neuronal circuits. Increased time constants resulting from positive feedback of summating neural signals may be important in the initiation of short-term memory. (3) There is convincing biochemical evidence that no protein synthesis is necessary for short-term memory. The modification of existing proteins is most certainly important, but new proteins are not synthesized. Protein modification can occur rapidly by direct cyclic nucleotide-mediated posttranslational effects on ion channel proteins. Somewhat longer effects are realized through self-reinforcing activation of the cyclic nucleotide synthetic machinery so that the enzyme reactions are maintained for longer periods of time.

Memory consolidation depends on arousal and stimulus repetition and probably requires protein synthesis.

A dramatic example of the role of consolidation of memory is the case of the patient H.M. (described by Milner et al., 1968). In an attempt to control his epileptic seizures, this patient underwent removal of a specific brain region (the hippocampal formation). Following surgery his intelligence remained above average, he had normal short-term memory, and he had normal long-term memory for events that occurred before the operation. He was unable, however, to make any further consolidation of short-term memories into long-term memories. He could learn new tasks and use those new memories as long as he continued to concentrate on the task. Once his attention was diverted, though, it was necessary for him to relearn the task. In his words, "Every day is alone in itself, whatever enjoyment I've had, and whatever sorrow I've had."

The process by which long-term memories are produced from short-term memories is a specific and obviously important process. We will consider two important characteristics of *memory consolidation.*

First, the ability to consolidate memories depends on the state of arousal of the brain and/or on the number of repetitions of whatever is being learned. Two often-quoted examples are that most people who remember the shooting of President Kennedy or the Challenger explosion have a vivid long-term memory (flashbulb memory) of the entire surroundings within which they heard the news. By contrast, our long-term memory of the multiplication tables depends on endless repetition when we were in the third grade, with very little emotional arousal and little memory of associated detail.

The thousands of trials required for "learning" in the computer systems that have been called "nerve networks" leads us to suspect that biological learning must have a more efficient means of making the necessary adjustments than has been developed for these artificial networks. When our theories of biological learning have been duplicated in these artificial systems, the result has fallen far short of what is observed in the original biological system. Repetition in synaptic networks is probably necessary to adjust connections and scaling, but the specific details of this process are not currently understood.

Second, the ability to consolidate memories requires protein synthesis. Consolidation and learning are interrupted when inhibitors of protein synthesis are applied during and immediately after the experience occurs; they have no demonstrable effect when applied 1 hour later.

Long-term memory persists through alterations of consciousness and depends on protein synthesis.

It is well established that long-term memories are resistant to sleep, anesthesia, coma, electroconvulsive shock, and other alterations of the state of consciousness. Although amnesia may immediately follow trauma, the long-term memories are usually recovered. This suggests that the amnesia may represent a retrieval problem rather than a problem of memory.

In 1911, the neuroanatomist Ramón y Cajal proposed that long-term memories represent morphological changes in the genetically determined connections of the brain. He thought that use of neuronal circuits caused changes in the morphology of the neurons being used. A similar activity-based morphological change was espoused by E.D. Adrian in 1947. He proposed that memory traces were initially encoded in reverberating electrical signals but that long-term memory represented a modification of the circuits over which these signals passed.

There are several very active areas of current research investigating the mechanisms of long-term memory. One area is that of classical conditioning in various invertebrates, most notably the gill withdrawal reflex of *Aplysia*. The second area is a phenomenon called *long-term potentiation,* which occurs in the mammalian brain, most notably in the region called the hippocampal formation.

The same gill withdrawal reflex of *Aplysia* that has shed so much light on the short-term memory process of sensitization also can undergo long-term conditioning or long-term behavioral sensitization. The mechanism responsible for these long-term effects appears to be the maintained activation of protein synthesis because of gene induction. In *gene induction,* an existing gene is activated so that it continues to produce a protein, specifically a type of ion channel. In addition, morphological changes occur that result in an increase in the size of the synaptic contacts between the sensory and motor neurons.

Long-term potentiation can be observed to persist for weeks in neurons of isolated slices of mammalian brains that are maintained under conditions similar to those used for cell culture. In these sites it has been found that inhibitors of protein synthesis disrupt long-term potentiation. The proteins synthesized may be any of a number of components involved in the action of either the pre- or the postsynaptic neurons.

The mechanisms underlying long-term memory depend on the regulation of protein synthesis. This may be the synthesis of ion channels, of neurotransmitter receptors, or of other proteins involved in synaptic morphology. Synaptic terminals, however, tend to be on remote processes of neurons, far from the nucleus that contains the DNA. The mechanism by which events at remote synapses initiate changes in protein synthesis in the nucleus is not currently understood. One interesting idea, suggested by the work of P.M. Laduron (1987), explains the synaptic regulation of gene activation by the transport of vesicles up and down the nerve axon. The presynaptic terminals of synapses that are capable of being modified have receptors for modulatory neurotransmitters (neuropeptides). It appears that bits of the presynaptic membrane containing both the receptors and their attached neurotransmitters are pinched off to form vesicles within the presynaptic terminal. These vesicles are then transported from the synaptic terminals back to the cell bodies by the normally present process of fast axo-plasmic transport. At the nucleus the occupied receptors serve to activate genes for protein synthesis. The newly synthesized proteins can then be transported back to the presynaptic terminal where they could cause changes in synaptic function (figure 9.6).

We can draw two conclusions about the mechanisms of long-term memory. (1) Synthesis of new DNA is not necessary or even possible. Since neurons (except for olfactory receptors) do not undergo mitosis, there is no potential for synthesis of new DNA. This does not, however, preclude a change in the transcription from existing DNA to RNA. In fact, it is quite certain that new RNA is necessary for long-term memory. (2) Protein synthesis is necessary for long-term memory.

Long-term memory is dependent on the regulation of genes that control continued protein synthesis. The synthesized proteins can be channels that affect the electrical properties of neurons and therefore the release of neurotransmitter, or postsynaptic neurotransmitter receptors that affect the effectiveness of released neurotransmitter. In either case, the effectiveness of transmission between neurons is modified in a way that outlasts the life span of the proteins found in neurons. In addition, long-term, but local modification of synaptic efficacy can occur because of morphological changes in synaptic terminals.

Human memory retrieval is associative and distributed.

Inputs, related to pieces of the stored information, are necessary cues to retrieve an entire memory, thus memory is associative. Present cues are used to reconstruct past events through comparisons, inferences, or suppositions. Associative memory has striking similarities to that proposed in 1949 by Hebb. According to his description, "The child's development in the first few years will consist of establishing separate systems in the brain, groups of brain cells that will act together and reinforce one another's activity." (As is all too often the case, we must use the same word in two contexts. The word "associative," used earlier in this chapter in defining types of learning, does not necessarily relate to its use for types of memory retrieval as discussed in this section.) Memory is distributed in that one neuron is not used as an address to store one memory. At the very least, memories are stored in the interconnections between neurons. Multidi-

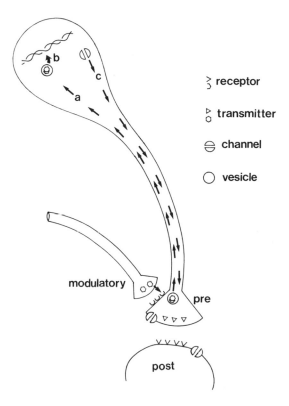

receptor

transmitter

channel

vesicle

modulatory

pre

post

Figure 9.6
Long-term memory through regulation of gene function. In a mechanism suggested by the work
of P.M. Laduron (1987), neurotransmitters attached to their receptors are transported in vesicles
to the cell body (a). The occupied receptors then activate genes for protein synthesis (b).
Specifically, ion channel proteins could be produced (c), and these channels, when inserted
into the cell membrane, would subsequently modify the electrical activity of the neuron.

mensional memories must be stored in multiple synaptic pathways that are probably shared with other memories.

Standard computer memories are sequential and are separate from the processing machinery, in these ways they provide a poor model for neural memory. In a sequential memory, each bit of information is placed in a register (like a mailbox) with a specific address. It is necessary to know the address to retrieve the memory information from the register. With an error of even one bit in the address, there is no a priori reason that the retrieved information will have anything to do with that sought. An exception is the special case in which the stored information is sequential in time, and there does exist a correlation between the contents of sequential memory addresses. Associative memory, on the other hand, takes part of the stored information and uses that as a cue to find the rest of the stored memory. Such content-based retrieval requires extensive special processing in a computer but in the nervous system appears to be intrinsic to all memory retrieval. In neural function, the more information that is initially available, the better the retrieval, but good retrieval can be obtained with even a small amount of the total information. A further important characteristic of associative memory is that even when errors in retrieval occur, the incorrectly retrieved information is often related to the correct information. To use the basin terminology of the previous chapter, associated events are the inputs to the basin of a stored memory.

Recent advances in computer technology have led to machines that can potentially operate more like human memory. Some parallel distributed processing computers use not only a distributed memory but have a redundancy of the computation and storage elements. There are currently some experimental computers called connectionist machines that act more like the nervous system in processing information. These computers store information and process it in a complex distributed network. Furthermore, the processing is relative and does not depend upon an inflexible absolute logic.

An important premise in this chapter has been that memory storage depends on distributed changes in synaptic connectivity between neurons. This premise is supported by both the physiological changes in synaptic efficacy that we have been discussing and the morphological changes that have been observed coincident with learning in neuronal synapses.

A network of elements can be constructed with functionally simple nodes that allow associative retrieval of information that has been stored in a distributed manner.

During the 1940s Warren McCulloch and Walter Pitts made a series of important observations about the properties of networks. This far-reaching work set the stage for a considerable body of subsequent work in the modeling of neural networks. In one simple model of associative memory storage, memories are stored in the interactions between nodes in a circuit where the strength and sign of the connection are dependent on the succession of pieces of information being stored. When part of one piece of information is applied (i.e., when some nodes are activated) the rest of the information is retrieved with a high degree of accuracy. This type of computer model may give insights into biological storage and retrieval processes. Appendix H gives a simple example of a computational circuit that shows some aspects of distributed and associative information storage.

9.4. Problem: Try to devise an associative memory scheme that incorporates as many characteristics as possible of neuronal memory mechanisms. You may want to use a digital computer to test the effectiveness of your scheme. Can you devise any tests of the biological applicability of your scheme?

9.5. Demonstration: Take several simple sentences and ink over individual letters or whole words. How effectively can another person reconstruct the original sentence. How is associative memory used in reading? How might associative memory be related to specific reading errors?

The genetic code provides an effective memory of ancestral experiences.

This chapter has been concerned with neural mechanisms of memory, but brief mention needs to be made of other means by which information related to behavior is stored in individuals. We have already mentioned those forms of information that we defined as hysteresis rather than memory. These are, however, generally other neural processes. Obviously the genetic code stores information over generations and this information is continuously being retrieved every time a new protein is made. Those traits that are inherited represent acceptable behavior of ancestors, whereas those traits that are missing can include those that have not been tried but also those that have been excluded from the genetic pool by death of cohorts of the ancestors. Thus, all neural function depends ultimately on information retrieved from genetically stored information. A central point of this chapter is that experience can modify the content and the way in which this information is retrieved.

More than one-half of the perhaps 10^6 human structural genes code for RNA that is translated into proteins in the nervous system. Many of these are related to the ion channels, neurotransmitters, and receptors that determine synaptic function. The bounds of the behaviors that can be controlled by a nervous system are set by "hard-wired" neural circuits that are genetically defined. Important examples of behaviors strongly influenced by this "hard-wiring" include instincts, autonomic reflexes, all learning primitives, fixed action patterns, and some central motor programs. A more general view is that general connections are established between neurons by genetics, but these are enhanced or diminished by learning.

Studies of mutations in the fruitfly, *Drosophila,* reveal that certain ion channels are necessary for learning and memory to occur. Songbirds learn songs from their parents, but only at certain times in their development. The release of gonadal hormones is, in this case, responsible for regulating the bird's ability to learn. Clinical evidence from identical twins who were raised apart from each other show that they tend to have similar IQs despite differences in their education. These data point to there being a genetic memory not only for behavior but also for the ability of an animal to learn.

Learning and memory have intrigued natural philosophers down through the ages. Neuroscience now has the legacy of that tradition and has begun recently to provide a wealth of answers about how information is stored in the connections between neurons of the brain.

Chapter 10

Neuroelectric Phenomena

In an issue of the proceedings of the Bologna Academy and Institute of Sciences and Arts dated 27 March 1791, Luigi Galvani published an article that was to be a milestone in the world of physics and physiology. He began this paper, which was entitled *De Viribus Electricitatis in Motu Musculari Commentarius,* with the following description. "I dissected and prepared a frog and placed it on a table, on which was an electrical machine, widely removed from its conductor and separated by no brief interval. When by chance one of those who were assisting me gently touched the point of a scalpel to the medial crural nerves of this frog, immediately all the muscle of the limbs seemed to be so contracted that they appeared to have fallen into violent tonic convulsions. But another of the assistants, who was on hand when I did electrical experiments, seemed to observe that the same thing occurred whenever a spark was discharged from the conductor of the machine." With these words, Galvani launched an extended controversy in both the physical science community and the field of electrophysiology. In this chapter we will be concerned with the antecedents of Galvani's work, stimulation and recording of electrical activity in excitable cells—a pursuit that has given science and technology many of its methods of electrical recording and impulse generation.

Physiological excitation of nerves and muscles in the body originates either spontaneously within that cell, from sensory receptors, or from other nerves. Direct electrical stimulation of a nerve fiber is not a normal occurrence. Electrical stimulation of nerves and muscles is used experimentally in many situations where the parameters of the stimulus must be known or controlled accurately. Several clinical diagnostic and treatment procedures use direct electrical stimulation of nerve or muscle fibers.

In tissue, electrical current is carried by the movement of charged ions in opposite directions with the arbitrary designation of current direction being that of movement of positively charged ions.

An electrical principle, important in the stimulation of excitable cells, is that *current must flow in a circuit.* Whenever we stimulate a nerve or muscle we must provide both a *cathode* and an *anode* connection so that current can both enter and leave the tissue in a pathway that moves charge through the membranes of the excitable cells.

Michael Faraday first used the terms cathode and anode in the early nineteenth century when referring to electrodes in electrolyte solutions. The negative electrode is called the "cathode" from the Greek καθοδοσ meaning a downward way. The positive electrode is conversely the "anode" from the Greek ανοδοσ meaning an upward way. When current is passed between electrodes through an ionic solution, positively charged ions or *cations* migrate toward the cathode and negative ions, or *anions,* are attracted to the anode. Since ions are actually moving in both directions, current direction is arbitrarily defined as moving through the solution from anode to cathode. Biological currents are regularly defined using this convention. In a metal conductor, current is carried by the movement of electrons the direction of whose movement is opposite to the direction designated for current. (Current in semiconductors can be carried by electrons moving in one direction or by "holes" moving in the opposite direction.) Current through any region is a measure of the total charge transfer, which is dependent on the driving forces, the charges on the carriers, the numbers of carriers, and the mobility of the carriers.

In some situations, both the cathode and the anode are placed close to the excitable cells so that the current flowing at each of these electrodes will have a direct, and opposite, effect on those cells. In other situations, either the anode or the cathode is placed close to the excitable cells and the other electrode is placed far away. When this is the case, although current flows to or from the distant electrode, its path is so broad that it has little direct effect on the excitable cells. In this latter type of stimulation, called *focal stimulation,* the electrode placed near the excitable cells is connected to be the stimulation focus.

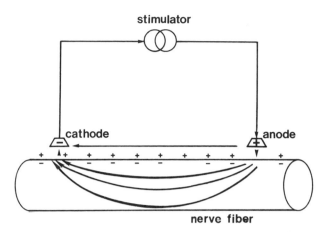

Figure 10.1
Bipolar stimulation. Current flows from a stimulator to an anode, through the nerve to the cathode, and then back to the stimulator. The current flowing across the cell membrane at the external cathode causes excitation.

Current flowing outward across the membrane of an excitable cell tends to stimulate that cell.

We will discuss the excitation of nerve fibers in greater depth in chapter 12 but will begin now with two points about this process. (1) Current must flow across the membrane of a neuron in order for it to have an effect on that cell. (2) Current flow in one direction across the membrane is excitatory and current flow in the other direction necessarily counters excitation.

Figure 10.1 shows a typical bipolar stimulation arrangement with a cathode and an anode close to a nerve fiber. The stimulator attached to these electrodes is a source of current that, by convention, flows from the anode to the cathode. As part of the current path, some current will flow across the membrane into the nerve fiber at the anode and that same current will flow out across the membrane to return via the cathode to the stimulator. This transmembrane current is a *capacitive current*. The current at the cathode flows in such a direction as to discharge the existing charge on the cell membrane, which acts as a capacitor. Discharge of this capacitor is the requisite first step in the process of excitation. Current flowing to an external cathode causes excitation. The effectiveness of a current in causing excitation depends on the current density, which, at any point in a tissue, is dependent on total current, electrode size, and the distance of the electrode from the excitable tissue.

10.1.* Problem: In many experimental stimulation situations the nerve being stimulated and stimulating electrodes are covered with oil to prevent tissue drying. Draw an equivalent circuit including two stimulating electrodes and a nerve and use this diagram to explain why it is advantageous to bathe the nerve in oil rather than in physiological saline.

A corollary to the external cathode being the site of excitation is that an external anode causes depressed excitability of the nerve. This process is often called *anodal block*. Whenever a nerve fiber is stimulated with bipolar electrodes, one electrode will excite the fiber and the other electrode will depress excitation. A commonly used technique to avoid blocking impulses before they are effective is to place the cathode nearest to the recording electrode or point of action of that fiber. To further complicate the situation, early in the history of electrical stimulation of nerves, it was observed that although the cathode is usually the site of excitation, sometimes excitation occurs at the anode (Pflüger, 1859). One case in which this is true occurs after a long pulse of stimulus current, a condition called *anode break excitation*. We will establish the mechanism responsible for this phenomenon in chapter 12 but in anticipation we can state here that anodal (or hyperpolarizing) currents can make the membrane more capable of being excited because they decrease sodium channel inactivation.

During normal functioning of the nervous system it is the presence of sensory receptors at the ends of certain fibers and the existence of chemical synapses between neurons that specify the direction of impulse propagation. Electrically stimulated nerves, however, can propagate an impulse in either (or both) directions from the site of stimulation. *Antidromic* describes propagation in the direction opposite to that of normal conduction and *orthodromic* describes propagation in the direction of normal conduction of a fiber.

Electrical stimulation of excitable tissue in the clinical setting is usually accomplished by the delivery of current between an external anode and cathode so arranged that part of the current passes across the excitable membrane.

In older textbooks of physiology, considerable time is spent in explaining the details of how nerves are excited with extracellular electrodes. Figure 10.2 shows

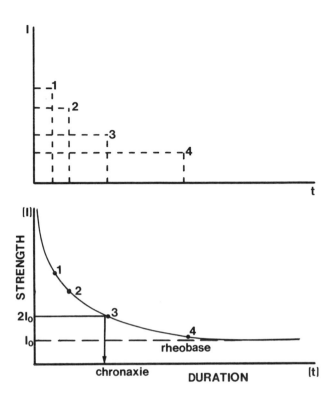

Figure 10.2
Strength-duration relationship. The upper graph shows the relationship between stimulus current and pulse duration of four stimulus pulses that are just sufficient to stimulate a particular nerve. These points are used to produce the strength–duration curve in the lower graph. The asymptotic value of this relationship is called the *rheobase* and the stimulus duration necessary to stimulate the nerve at twice rheobase is defined as the *chronaxie*.

one relationship that defines stimulus conditions. This inverse relationship between the amplitude of stimulus current and the duration of the pulse of current is known as the *strength-duration* relationship. In 1926 L. Lapique defined two terms that characterize the relationship between stimulus strength and duration. These terms are *rheobase,* the minimum current that can cause stimulation, and *chronaxie,* the stimulus duration necessary to stimulate the nerve or muscle at twice rheobase current. These two values give an approximate determination of the whole strength-duration curve. Although these techniques are not as important in modern neurophysiological research, they still are the method of clinical stimulation.

An instructive equation is obtained from the strength-duration relationship for a specific nerve fiber in the limiting conditions where the current is large and the pulse duration is short. Under these conditions, the relationship is approximately hyperbolic, implying that the product of the independent variable (duration) and the dependent variable (strength) is a constant.

$$(I - I_0) \times t = \text{constant}$$

where I is the stimulus current and I_0 is a constant (rheobase) current. From physics, we know that the product of current and time is charge. Under these conditions, stimulation of a nerve requires that a fixed amount of charge is removed from the membrane capacitor near the cathode. This amount of charge can be obtained by passing a small amount of current for a long time or a large amount of current for a short time. Another way of saying this is that excitation is initiated when the membrane capacitor is sufficiently discharged.

The strength–duration relationship approximates a hyperbolic curve only for short durations and large currents. A more accurate representation of this relationship is obtained from the equation

$$\frac{I}{I_0} = \frac{1}{1 - \exp(-t/k)}$$

where I is the current amplitude, t is its duration, I_0 is the rheobase current, and k is a constant that is characteristic of a specific nerve. The actual relationship between strength and duration is complex and was once the subject of much analysis (see, for example, H.A. Blair, 1932).

10.2.* **Problem:**   Over what range of values for stimulus duration does the exponential equation given above predict an approximately constant product of $(I - I_0) \times t$?

Muscles characteristically have longer chronaxies than nerves. If stimulating electrodes are placed near the synaptic junction of a nerve and a muscle, one will normally measure the chronaxie of the more excitable nerve. If the nerve has been chronically damaged, though, the muscle can be stimulated directly and the chronaxie for the muscle will be obtained. Regeneration of the nerve will cause the chronaxie to decline toward the low value characteristic of the nerve (see, for example, Ritchie, 1944).

When the stimulus current is increased slowly rather than being applied as a sudden pulse, a complication is observed. The slower the onset of the current, the more current is necessary to stimulate the nerve. Nineteenth-century German literature spoke of this as *einschleichender Strom,* literally "sneaking-in current." Today we refer to this process as *accommodation* and understand its basis to be a result of the process of sodium channel inactivation. Differences in accommodation and thresholds between classes of fibers can be exploited to allow selective excitation of only certain classes of fibers in a mixed nerve.

10.3. Problem: How would accommodation affect measurements of the strength-duration curve?

The effectiveness of extracellular electrodes in eliciting a response depends on the diameter of the nerve fiber being stimulated. The threshold for extracellular stimulation decreases with increasing fiber diameter. Since direct electrical stimulation of nerve fibers is not a natural occurrence, there is probably no physiological significance to this relationship. In fact, for synaptic inputs to neurons, small diameter neurons have thresholds lower than larger diameter neurons. The relationship between threshold and fiber diameter for an extracellular stimulus is important in physiological experimentation and in clinical procedures since nerves contain fibers of different diameters. One can take advantage of the differences in threshold to stimulate selectively only those fibers of larger diameter. Transcutaneous nerve stimulators (TNS) are used clinically to stimulate peripheral nerves. Selective stimulation of large fibers is used to produce analgesia from certain forms of pain. By taking advantage of the variation in threshold with fiber

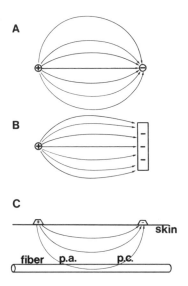

Figure 10.3
Current flow in a volume conductor. Current, defined as the movement of + charge, flows from the anode to the cathode. The effectiveness of this current in stimulating an excitable cell depends on the current density. Current density is represented by how close together adjacent lines are. (A) The pattern of current flow between two point electrodes found in an unlimited field. (B) Pattern of current flow between one point electrode and a second large (indifferent) electrode in an unlimited field. (C) Pattern of current flow from electrodes placed on the skin surface and used to stimulate deep structures. The actual points where the current enters and leaves the excitable tissue are called the *physiological anode* (p.a.) and the *physiological cathode* (p.c.).

diameter, large fibers can be selectively stimulated when the stimulus current is adjusted to the minimally effective level.

The variation of current density in different parts of a volume conductor can be used to localize the tissues that will be most effectively stimulated.

Figure 10.3B shows the pathway of current flow between two electrodes in a volume conductor. The effectiveness of a current in stimulating an excitable cell is, in part, dependent on the density of that current. This figure demonstrates, by the closeness of the lines of current, that the current density is greatest in the region near a small electrode. Focal stimulation takes advantage of this because

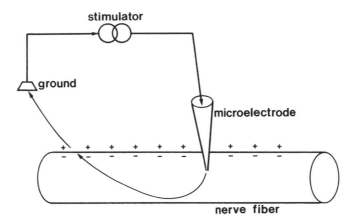

Figure 10.4
Intracellular stimulation. Current flows from a stimulator, through a microelectrode, to the
inside of a specific nerve fiber, out across the cell membrane, to an indifferent (or ground)
electrode, and then back to the stimulator. Current flow outward across the membrane, as is
shown in this figure, will excite the neuron.

in this case only one electrode is close to excitable cells. If this electrode is then
made sufficiently small, and the total current is appropriately adjusted, only cells
within a small region will be stimulated. The earliest use of focal stimulation of
the brain was by Fritsch and Hitzig (1870). Their discrete stimulation of specific
brain areas provided the first demonstration that there is a topological representation of specific movements at discrete locations in the cortex. This technique
is used frequently today in experimental neurophysiology to excite neurons in a
specific region of the brain and in surgery to localize functional areas.

Misleading measurements can be obtained when stimulating a nerve or muscle
with electrodes located on the skin and some distance away from the excitable
tissue. As shown in figure 10.3C, only a fraction of the stimulus current actually
passes through the excitable tissue. The point of greatest current density in the
excitable tissue, called the physiological cathode, will be displaced toward the
anode when compared with the locations of the skin electrodes. This affects any
measurement that is based on the location of the stimulating electrodes or on the
strength of the stimulus current.

An alternate, and more discrete method of stimulation uses an intracellular
microelectrode to stimulate a single cell (figure 10.4). Here current is passed from
the intracellular electrode across the membrane to an external (ground) electrode.

The charges that either accumulate on, or are removed from, the cell membrane cause the cell either to be made less excitable (hyperpolarized) or to be stimulated (depolarized). Since this method is localized and stimulates only one neuron, the response is usually very limited. Sometimes, however, activity of a single neuron can elicit a significant, observable behavior in an animal.

10.4.* Problem: Since cells are exceedingly small, it is usually possible to insert only one intracellular microelectrode. To be able to use this microelectrode for intracellular recording and simultaneously for passing stimulating currents, it can be incorporated into a Wheatstone bridge. Draw the circuit that would allow a single microelectrode to be used for stimulating and recording intracellular potentials and explain how such a circuit would work.

Although electrical stimuli can be used to excite either sensory or motor nerves, it has been extremely difficult to generate and deliver appropriate spatial and temporal patterns of activity to substitute for defective physiological excitation.

Since the mid-nineteenth century development of hand-cranked electrical stimulating devices, there has been much publicity and enthusiasm for the possible use of these stimuli as a replacement for defective neural function. These efforts have been especially concentrated on muscle control and in replacing defective peripheral auditory and visual receptor function. Following a century of false promises, prosthetic stimuli are only now achieving some limited clinical application and are the subject of intense current research. (A recent review of developments in this field is found in Loeb, 1989.)

Current technology makes it possible to measure important auditory or visual information using compact and reasonably economical devices. This sensory information, to be useful, requires the considerable amount of processing that is normally accomplished at or near the sensory receptors. Although we still have only a limited understanding of this processing, enough is currently known so that rudimentary instrumental processing is now being accomplished and there is cause for optimism about future possibilities. The biggest current problem with sensory prostheses lies in delivering the information to the central nervous system. One current solution is to deliver the information indirectly through an array of points on the skin of a limb or the trunk. This technique is very limited both in its speed and in its spatial resolution. Some success has been achieved with auditory prostheses that directly stimulate the cochlea in the inner ear and these results are actually more effective than would be predicted from current theory. Direct stimulation of the auditory or visual cortex is still fraught with major problems. For example, to replace fully the signals carried on a single optic nerve by artificial pulses would require a minimum of 10^6 independent connections to specific neural units.

Loss of motor function can result from injury to muscle nerves, loss of motoneurons, loss of pathways from the brain to the motoneurons, or loss of cortical motor function. Muscles are commonly stimulated electrically using *functional electrical stimulation* or *FES* to maintain strength during temporary loss of peripheral nervous innervation. There are major problems in permanent muscle stimulation both with delivering the stimuli to the muscles and in picking up appropriate motor control patterns from the central nervous system. There is currently a major effort in laboratories, especially in the United States and in Yugoslavia, to solve these problems.

Although methods of delivering stimuli to individual muscles are well developed, one problem lies in delivering the stimuli appropriately to specific muscle fiber types. A simple increase of the stimulus strength recruits the different fiber types in a peripheral nerve in an order that is the inverse of that seen in normal function. (Large fibers have the lowest threshold for electrical stimulation and small neurons have the lowest threshold for normal synaptic excitation.) Furthermore, it is difficult to drive any muscle fiber to produce a weak, but sustained, contraction. Various tricks using accommodation and timed anodal block have been used to attempt to solve these problems.

Appropriate input signals are a prerequisite to the generation of motor control stimuli.

The most accessible signals from which motor control stimulus patterns can be generated are mechanical signals. These signals have often been overlooked in prosthetic development. Mechanical signals can replace both sensory feedback and its reflex processing. One case in which use has been made of mechanical signals is in compensation for loss of control of dorsal flexion of the foot. In walking, a simple switch on the heel activates a stimulator to stimulate muscles to raise the toes during the forward swing of the foot. Slightly more complex mechanical drive to grasping muscles has been devised for patients with partial paralysis of the arm.

Since many quadraplegics have some residual control of neck, shoulder, or even arm muscles, this control is often used as a basis to control other muscles. An array of electromyographic electrodes can be used to identify multidimensional signals from these muscles. Processing this array of control vectors is theoretically easy but practically difficult. Only highly motivated and persistent patients have had much success in learning to use these control signals for practical purposes. The challenging problem here is learning how to use an existing pathway for alternate communication.

Acquisition of signals for detailed control across a spinal lesion is both important and difficult. Direct electrical output from the brain might provide voluntary control signals. Task-related electrical signals have been shown in the brain but present analysis methods are far from adequate to provide a basis for using these signals for prosthetic control. We do not know enough about brainstem and spinal processing of these signals to allow substitution for that processing. The dense packing of fibers with different roles and the fact that specific control functions may be distributed across intermingled fibers stymie efforts to obtain access to these signals. Besides biological repair of interrupted pathways, the technological bridging of gaps is probably the most desirable solution. It is, however, the solution that is furthest from current realization.

The activity of excitable tissue results in local currents and potential changes.

Luigi Galvani used electrical stimulation in his experiments and took as his indicator of nervous activity the resultant muscle contraction. His indirect evidence for electrical activity in muscle was that a nerve could be stimulated by muscle activity associated with a contraction. Local recordings of the actual electrical activity of excitable cells required sensitive measurement devices that were not available until the middle of the nineteenth century. Much of the progress of recording of electrical activity reflects the progress in developing faster and more sensitive recording devices. Emil du Bois-Reymond (1848) used a galvanometer to measure currents in muscles, Edgar Adrian and Yngve Zotterman (1926) used a tube amplifier and capillary electrometer to measure single nerve impulses, and Herbert Gasser and Joseph Erlanger (1922) used a cathode ray oscilloscope to record the actual time course of the action potential. Further progress came with the introduction of intracellular potential recording and the measurement of transmembrane currents in the middle decades of this century by Gilbert Ling, R.W. Girard, Kenneth Cole, Alan Hodgkin, and Andrew Huxley. More recently, advanced amplifier and electrode technology allowed Erwin Neher and Bert Sackmann (Hamill et al., 1981) to record the current through single ion channels in the cell membrane.

Temporally overlapping activity in multiple nerve or muscle fibers generates local voltages that result from the addition of the separately generated currents in the shared volume conductor.

The varying overlap of naturally generated impulses produces summing and subtracting effects that depend on the timing of different unit activities with a complex external record that is called an *interference record*. The activity in such records tends to increase with the square root of the density of activity in the tissue from which the response is being recorded. The recording from a nerve trunk that has been stimulated artificially shows the effect of different conduction velocities of the different fibers and is called a *compound action potential*. (The recording from a single active fiber is a *unitary action potential*.)

The details of current flow during an action potential are a subject for chapter 12 but a few points are important here. Most important is that the peak of the propagated impulse is associated with the flow of current into the interior of the nerve fiber; this moving region is called a *current sink*. The propagated impulse is preceded by, and followed by, regions of outward current flow or *current sources*. The time course of the extracellularly recorded potential depends on the location of the recording electrodes with respect to the passing current sources and sinks.

The time course of the recorded action potential from a single nerve fiber depends on changes in differences in potential between the two electrode sites as the nerve impulse moves along the fiber.

The electrical signals recorded with remote extracellular electrodes are small, usually measured in microvolts. Since it is often difficult to shield the recording electrodes, the measured signal is frequently contaminated with unwanted noise (most notably in North America 60-Hz or in Europe and Asia 50-Hz interference from power lines). One method of minimizing this is to use a differential amplifier whose output is proportional to the difference between the two inputs. An interfering signal from a remote source will be received with the same amplitude by both electrodes. The difference will then be just those voltages generated between the two electrodes.

Differential amplifiers used in extracellular recordings have a (+) input and a (−) input. Three different types of recordings can be made, depending on where these two electrodes are placed with respect to the nerve (figure 10.5A). As an action potential propagates past a point, the moving current sink is registered by the extracellular electrode as a region of relative negativity. Similarly the smaller current sources become regions of relative positive potential along the outside of the nerve.

Biphasic recording is obtained when both of the electrodes are placed close to a nerve along which is propagated a compound action potential. The major event seen here is the negativity associated with the propagated current sink. If the electrodes are arranged with the (+) electrode in the direction from which the impulse is arriving, then the amplifier will register first a negative deflection as the action potential passes the (+) electrode and then a positive deflection (negative times negative) as the action potential passes the (−) electrode. If the electrodes are far apart, the arrival of the impulse at the two sites will be more separated in time. If the two electrodes are at the same location on the nerve, the two deflections will change together so that no difference will be recorded. At any intermediate spacing of the electrodes, there will be varying degrees of overlap of the two deflections, thereby producing a biphasic compound action potential.

10.5. Problem: Calculate the (spatial) length of a propagated action potential under the following three conditions: (1) a large, rapidly conducting nerve fiber with a conduction velocity of 100 m/sec and an action potential duration of 0.5 msec, (2) a small slowly, conducting fiber with a conduction velocity of 1 m/sec and an action potential duration of 2 msec, and (3) a muscle action potential of 10 msec duration conducted at a velocity of 5 m/sec. What would a compound action potential look like in these three cases if the extracellular recording electrodes were in contact with the active fiber and separated by 1 cm? How would the records differ if they were recorded from a volume conductor with some distance between the electrodes and the nerve fiber?

Monophasic recording is a somewhat simpler situation in which both electrodes are on the nerve but the nerve is rendered inactive under the second electrode

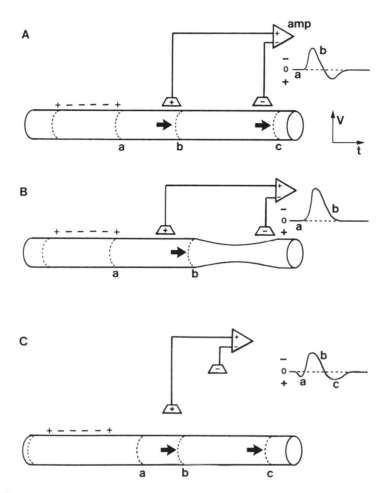

Figure 10.5
Extracellular recording. Extracellular recording electrodes attached to a differential amplifier produce a signal that is proportional to the difference in the potential recorded by each electrode. (A) With two electrodes placed close to an active region of a nerve, the differential recording is *biphasic*. (B) When the nerve fiber is crushed (but not transected) between the recording electrodes, the differential recording becomes *monophasic*. (C) If one of the electrodes (indifferent) is placed at a distance from the active region, the differential recording is *triphasic*. This figure follows the established convention of extracellular recording in which negative deflections are displayed upwards.

(figure 10.5B). Here the propagated action potential and its concurrent wave of negativity affect only the active (+) electrode and thus only a negative deflection is recorded by the amplifier. The simplest method in which a recording such as this is obtained is when the nerve is crushed between the two recording electrodes. Monophasic recordings, where it is practical to record them, reveal more of the characteristics of the propagated compound action potential since no second deflection is being subtracted from the initial one.

The triphasic recording situation is established when the second (−) electrode is placed at some distance from the active nerve (figure 10.5C). The distant electrode is called an *indifferent electrode*. In this type of recording, even the active (+) electrode is often at some distance from the current sources and sinks of the propagated action potential. The effect of the current source preceding the action potential now becomes more apparent as does the effect of the second current source following the action potential peak. The compound action potential now is registered as a positive deflection followed by a negative deflection followed by another positive deflection.

It is important to keep in mind that in each of these cases, the recorded potentials are the result of current flow in the extracellular space around the active nerve fibers. The compound action potential from many fibers is useful in understanding many important characteristics of nervous activity, but it does not reveal all the details of the potential change inside of a single nerve fiber.

The spatial and temporal distribution of the electrical event of an action potential are related by the conduction velocity of the nerve impulse.

The propagation of action potentials in nerve fibers is an involved process not at all equivalent to the propagation of an electrical pulse on a metal wire. Because of this, nerve conduction velocities are considerably slower than the speed of light. Typical conduction velocities for nerve fibers fall between 1 and 100 m/sec and can be easily measured with extracellular recording techniques over a moderate length of nerve.

10.6. Problem: Just for illustration, calculate the above range of nerve conduction velocities in miles or kilometers per hour.

Conduction velocity is a measure of distance traveled by a nerve impulse in a given time, usually calculated in meters per second. The most accurate means of measuring conduction velocity is to stimulate a nerve at one point and then to measure the times of arrival (t_1 and t_2) of the compound action potential at two points that are as widely separated as possible. One then needs to measure the conduction distances (x_1 and x_2) from the site of stimulation to the two recording points. Conduction velocity (v) is then obtained from the relation:

$$v = \frac{x_2 - x_1}{t_2 - t_1}$$

10.7.* Problem: To assess the conduction velocity of the superficial peroneal nerve in a patient with diabetic neuropathy, the nerve was stimulated and the compound action potential was measured at two locations along the nerve. The peak deflection, at a distance of 50 mm, occurred 3.2 msec after the stimulus was applied, and at 200 mm, the peak was at 6.3 msec. What is the conduction velocity in this nerve? See if you can obtain a reference to normal values for this nerve and determine whether this patient has a normal conduction velocity.

Several pathological conditions lead to alterations in peripheral nerve conduction velocity. Some important examples are Guillain-Barré polyneuropathy, a demyelinating disease, Wallerian degeneration, an aftermath of nerve injury, compression injuries, ischemia, and cold injury.

With the introduction of the cathode ray oscilloscope by Gasser and Erlanger (1922) it was possible to study the rapid details of nerve action potentials. Using this tool, these investigators showed that the action potential of the bullfrog sciatic nerve showed multiple peaks. Figure 10.6 shows the results of such an experiment in which a nerve is stimulated and the compound (monophasic) action potential is recorded at five points along the nerve. From the preceding discussion, it should come as no surprise that the compound action potential arrives at successively later times at each point. What might be surprising, though, is the change of shape of the compound action potential. At more and more distant recording points a shoulder appears on the falling phase of the action potential and then separate peaks break off to form a second and third elevation. This nerve contains three distinct groups of fibers with fast, intermediate, and slow conduction velocities. Just as the legendary rabbit leaves the tortoise further and further behind as the race becomes longer, so the separation of the three peaks becomes more pronounced when the conduction distance is longer. For those interested in the historical development of electrophysiology, it is well worth

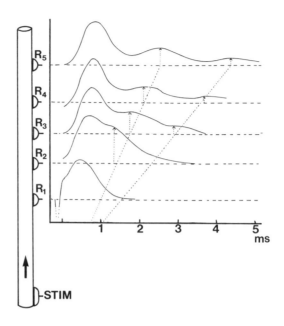

Figure 10.6
Compound action potential propagation. The compound action potential is made up of contributions of fibers with different conduction velocities (see table 10.1). If a nerve is stimulated
at one end (STIM) and the compound action potential is recorded at various points (R_1, R_2, R_3,
R_4 and R_5), one or more slower peaks will emerge as the conduction distance is increased. The
slope of the line relating the arrival of a specific peak to the conduction distance is the conduction
velocity of that peak. The records in this figure are the published tracings from some of the
first oscilloscope records of compound action potentials. (From Erlanger and Gasser, 1924.)

reading Erlanger and Gasser's book *Electrical Signs of Nervous Activity* (1937)
in which they describe the methods and results of their Nobel prize-winning
studies.

One often-used method of classifying nerve fibers is based on groupings of
conduction velocity. In this classification, nerve fibers are specified as types A
(α,β,γ, or δ), B, and C. Another classification system that has been used with
sensory nerves takes excitability as the criterion for classification. This system
specifies fibers as group I, II, III, or IV. Table 10.1 gives some characteristics of
the different nerve fibers within these classification systems and shows the approximate relationship between the systems.

Just as is true with stimulus threshold, nerve conduction velocities depend on

Table 10.1
Characteristics of Nerve Fibers[a]

Type	Group	Diameter (μm)	Conduction velocity (m/sec)
Afferent			
A	I	12–20	70–120
	II	6–12	40–70
	III	1–6	5–40
C	IV	~1	0.5–2
Efferent			
Aα		12–20	70–120
Aβ		14–16	40–80
Aγ		2–8	10–50
Aδ		1–6	5–30
C		~1	0.5–2

[a]See Somjen (1972).

the diameter of the fiber. The larger the diameter of a fiber, the faster its conduction velocity. For many types of nerve fiber, this relation is linear with very little deviation between individual measurements. The function of many nerve fibers is also related to fiber diameter, velocity, and excitability.

The most precise measurements of the electrical properties of excitable cells come from single cell recordings.

The earliest intracellular recordings made in the laboratory of Alan Hodgkin (Hodgkin and Huxley, 1939) used a 50-μm capillary electrode that was inserted into the 500-μm squid giant axon. With the subsequent development of microelectrodes, and then of whole-cell patch clamping, intracellular recordings have been made from many different types of nerve and muscle cells.

10.8.* Problem: The dimensions involved in some of these measurements lead to some surprising results:

1. Suppose you are using a microelectrode with a tip diameter of 0.5 μm to pass a stimulating current of 10 μA. Calculate the current density at the tip in amperes per square centimeter.

2. Suppose you wish to measure the voltage drop between two points that are 100 μm apart with an amplifier that can measure down to 10 μV. What voltage gradient (volts per centimeter) is necessary for detection?

The potentials recorded intracellularly in excitable cells are different from the extracellularly recorded ones that we have been discussing. In the first place, it is possible to record maintained potentials and not just the transient potentials that result from changing current sources and sinks. It is then possible to measure the constant *resting potentials* within these cells. In the second place, the potential changes within a cell can be large in comparison with the potentials measured extracellularly. The intracellular action potential in a single neuron or muscle cell is a potential change of about 1/10 V. Intracellular recordings are invaluable for understanding the properties of a single cell. Further important contributions to the understanding of the electrical properties of single neurons come from utilization of the technique of *voltage clamping*. This technique is based on the fact that intracellular potentials can be predictably changed by passing current of the proper magnitude and direction into the cell. When the current that is passed is regulated by a feedback circuit it can be used to determine the conductance (or permeability) of the cell membrane to various ions under a variety of conditions. Membrane permeability is regulated by specialized ion-passing channels in the membrane. Voltage clamping allows the experimenter to measure these processes, which are the underlying basis of all electrical activity of excitable cells (Hodgkin et al., 1952).

A primary problem in making intracellular recordings lies in measuring potentials through small electrodes with their inherently high electrical resistance (figure 10.7). (Microelectrode tips are often <1 μm in diameter with a resistance in excess of 10 MΩ.) Since the intracellular voltage is divided between the voltage drop through the electrode and that measured across the amplifier input resistance, this requires an amplifier with a high input resistance. Furthermore, the amplifier must be capable of rapid responses to register accurately the rapid events associated with the action potential. Voltage clamping imposes additional problems inherent in the negative feedback control of intracellular potential accomplished by passing current into the cell. Patch clamping, as we will see in chapter 12, carries the amplifier requirements even further to accomplish the goal of passing picoampere currents into small cells or even through individual ion channels. Widespread interest in the area of intracellular recording, though, has

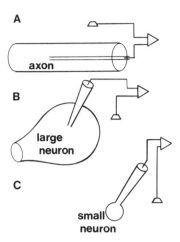

Figure 10.7
Intracellular recording. Intracellular potentials are measured with a differential amplifier that receives inputs from an electrode inside the cell and an indifferent electrode placed in the extracellular bathing solution. Intracellular potentials are measured in large axons (A) by inserting wires or capillary tubes into the axon, in large cell bodies (B) with microelectrodes that are inserted through the cell membrane, and in small neurons (C) with patch clamp electrodes that are sealed onto the cell membrane before a small hole is broken in the cell membrane.

created enough economic impetus so that these electronic devices are commercially available.

Muscles are a second category of excitable cells whose electrical activity is commonly measured.

Electromyography (*EMG*) is the clinical technique of recording electrical activity in muscle cells. The simplest electrodes used to measure the electrical activity of muscles are metal discs that are placed on the skin (distance recording). There are two important problems found in using external recording electrodes. First is the problem of polarization in the connections to tissue. The conversion from ionic conduction in tissues to electronic conduction in metallic wires is one source of polarization. This source is often minimized by using so-called nonpolarizing electrodes such as silver–silver chloride surfaces. Another common source of polarization is the fact that different ionic carriers do not all have the same mobility. For this reason KCl solutions (K^+ and Cl^- have very similar mobilities) are often used as a bridge to tissue. The second important problem is the resistance at the tissue interface. High resistance in this junction will drop the source voltage before it can act on the recording instrument. Various low-resistance "electrode pastes" are used to minimize this problem.

A second technique for EMG recording is to use needles placed within the muscle to record locally, albeit extracellularly, from muscle fibers. It is this second clinical approach to electromyography that gives the most discrete information about muscle activity. With needle electrodes, it is possible to identify the activity of individual motor units during weak and moderate contractions. The recording arrangement using needle EMG electrodes is similar to that previously described for triphasic compound action potential recordings from nerves. The needle electrode is the active (+) electrode and the indifferent (−) electrode is placed nearby on the skin. A useful alternate technique for placing electrodes is to put two fine, teflon-coated wires with small hooks at their ends in a single hypodermic needle. The hypodermic is inserted into the muscle and the hooks on the wires allow them to remain even when the hypodermic is removed. Electrodes inserted in this manner will remain in place, even during exercise, for many hours. These recordings reveal *motor unit activity,* that is, compound action potentials in a group of muscle fibers all of which are innervated by a single motor nerve and are thus synchronously excited. Clinical diagnoses are based on the timing and the nature of the recorded activity.

EMG activity, recorded from a needle electrode, is normally absent when the muscle is at rest, but there is a gradual increase in both the number of active units and the firing rate of those units when the muscle is voluntarily contracted. There are several pathologic conditions that can be revealed with the EMG. Abnormal activity can occur in spasticity when the muscle is at rest. Sharp spikes, or *fibrillations,* are recorded in the spontaneous discharges of single muscle fibers following loss of innervation. Broad spikes, or *fasciculations,* that are spontaneous discharges of whole motor units result from disease of motoneurons or irritation of peripheral motor axons. During peripheral nerve regeneration, the reduced number of nerve fibers takes over muscle fibers that have no innervation so that during voluntary contraction the motor unit activity is of greater amplitude. Patients with muscular dystrophy have high-frequency repetitive discharges in the EMGs of abnormal muscle fibers; these are called *myotonic potentials*. These distinctions are most easily recognized when the amplified voltage is used to drive a loudspeaker and distinction made on the basis of the sound of the activity.

Local activity in the brain produces a low voltage that changes relatively slowly. Recordings of these potentials can be valuable in evaluating certain aspects of brain activity.

In 1929, Hans Berger placed metal electrodes on his son's head and attached these to a double coil mirror galvanometer. He measured electrical potential waves and attributed them to activity of the brain. His interpretation was subjected to much criticism and even today many questions exist regarding the exact source of the electroencephalogram. Clearly, nerve fiber activity contributes little, while cell body and dendritic slow potentials make significant contributions to the recorded potential. There are many situations in which potentials can be measured at a distance from excitable cells. This requires, however, that large numbers of excitable cells have a regular organization in space and that their electrical activity is rather synchronous.

Electrical activity can be measured on the scalp or, with surgical exposure, on the surface of the cortex, yielding the *electroencephalogram* (*EEG*) and *electrocorticogram* (*ECoG*), respectively. In either case, the recorded potentials result from current sources and sinks in an appreciable volume of the densely packed (10^4 to 10^5 neurons/mm^3), regularly oriented, cortical neurons. Generally, an array of electrodes is affixed to the scalp and potentials are measured between various pairs of these electrodes usually, but not always, with both electrodes over areas of neural activity.

Figure 10.8 shows, in a simplified diagram, the current flow in a cortical neuron. Excitation typically occurs through a synaptic input in the region of the neuron nearest to the cortical surface. For an excitatory synaptic input, this point becomes a current sink yielding a negative potential at the extracellular electrode. If this current was flowing only in a single neuron, there would be no measurable potential at the distant electrode. In some circumstances whole groups of neurons receive externally or internally generated inputs simultaneously and the resultant current flow causes a measurable summed potential. The potential waveform, recorded as the EEG, is dependent on the locations of the current sources and sinks within the cortex and in the timing of the synaptic events that modify the current sources and sinks.

In its simplest form, the externally recorded potential is simply the product of the current flow at the active current sink and the resistance of a part of the external solution.

$$E = I_{\text{sink}} \times R_{\text{ext}}$$

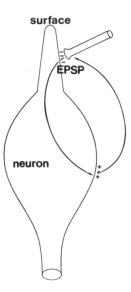

Figure 10.8
Current flow in a cortical neuron. Excitatory synaptic input (EPSPs), near the cortical surface, initiates an intracellular current flow to deeper regions of the neuron and subsequent extracellular current flow back to the region of excitation. An electrode placed on the scalp near the cortical surface will measure the transient negativity that results from this current flow.

Although the current is increased when it results from a group of synchronously active neurons, the external resistance is typically small so the sum is also small. The potentials measured with EEG electrodes are generally in microvolts.

Normal EEGs have several common patterns that are more or less correlated with various states of brain activity. The EEG waves are generally classified with respect to their frequency (1–35 Hz) and their amplitude (20–100 μV). Table 10.2 gives some typical EEG wave patterns and their associated brain states.

EEGs are useful as a diagnostic tool for several pathologic conditions. Unconsciousness is reflected in a general slowing or disappearance of the EEG activity. Localized lesions of the cortex yield a localized slowing or silence of the EEG. Irritative lesions including epileptic foci reveal themselves in several specific EEG characteristics. Focal seizures give a sharp electrical spike, known as an *EEG spike,* over the region of the focus. Generalized seizures produce synchronized activity from many regions of the cortex. EEGs are useful in psychiatric

Table 10.2
Typical EEG Wave Patterns

EEG wave	Frequency (Hz)	Amplitude (μV)	Brain activity
α	8–13	~50	Awake, relaxed (adult)
β	13–30	<20	Intense mental activity
θ	4–8		Common in children
δ	<4		Deep sleep

diagnosis to eliminate specific focal brain lesions in a diagnosis, but are generally not useful in diagnosing specific psychiatric disorders.

EEG spikes should not be confused with nerve or muscle action potentials that are also often called spikes. Nerve action potentials originate in a single neuron and are 5% or less of the duration of an EEG spike. Muscle action potentials also originate in a single cell but are of a duration similar to EEG spikes. Action potentials from muscles of the head can be a troublesome interference in EEG recording.

10.9.* Problem: How might you use Fourier analysis in the interpretation of EEG activity? Can you speculate about a way in which EEG analysis might be automated?

Recent advances in superconductor technology have made possible the measurement of the magnetic fields produced by the currents flowing between cortical neuron sources and sinks. This technique is called *magnetoencephalography*. Although this technology is still specialized and of limited general usefulness, this measure of cortical electrical activity has some appealing possibilities since magnetic fields are not distorted by the skull and thus can be accurately localized.

Synchronous peripheral stimuli produce characteristic and local electrical changes (evoked responses) in the cortex that can be extracted from the underlying EEG activity.

Another type of neuronal response that can be recorded over specific sites of the cortex is the response to a synchronous sensory input. These are most commonly recorded following an impulsive stimulus to the skin, eye, or ear and are called *somatosensory, visual,* or *auditory evoked potentials.* Evoked potentials have been used experimentally to map areas of the brain that receive sensory input from specific locations. They are also useful in interpreting the location of deficits in the transmission of sensory information through the various junctional points in the central nervous system. The light flashes or clicks used to elicit evoked potentials, although offering simplified analysis, are not very representative of normal inputs. Recently, changing checkerboard and other patterns have proven useful with evoked potentials for visual diagnosis. Probably more complex inputs also will be developed for initiating auditory and cutaneous sensory evoked potentials.

Evoked potentials are commonly so small that they cannot be individually identified within the background EEG activity. There are several techniques that have been used to extract a repeating pattern of response from the background, but the common method currently in use depends on a procedure called ensemble averaging. A period of time following an impulse stimulus is divided into an ensemble of successive short time windows. Starting at the time of the stimulus, a sequence of voltages occurring during each window is digitized and the results are stored in successive bins in a computer memory. A succession of stimuli (often thousands) is delivered and the corresponding ensembles of values are added to those already in the bins. The resulting set of summed values is proportional to the average response at a set of times after the points of stimulation. Because the long-term average voltage of the EEG is zero and its pattern is not synchronous with the stimuli, successive contributions of the EEG to individual bins will generally cancel. On the other hand, any part of the electrical potential that is initiated by the stimulus will tend to have similar values in the same bins of successive responses and the stored value will grow in proportion to the number of stimulus cycles recorded.

Summed electrical activity can be recorded from many other sites associated with excitable cells. Although the greatest use of most of these potentials has been in neurophysiological research, some of them do provide clinically useful information and could perhaps be useful in the development of sensory prosthetic devices. We will list here only a few examples of these potentials. The *dorsal root potential* is recorded on the dorsal surface of the spinal cord following certain sensory stimuli. The *electroretinogram* or *ERG* can be recorded with electrodes near the retina of the eye following a bright light flash. The *cochlear microphonic* can be recorded with an electrode near the cochlea of the inner ear and it gives a faithful representation of auditory inputs to the ear.

10.10. Problem: This chapter has been largely concerned with various techniques associated with the electrical activity of excitable cells. It is perhaps appropriate to end the chapter with a problem related to techniques used in prosthetic applications. Consider how a scheme using stimulating and recording techniques, with the appropriate microelectronics, might be used to overcome some disease or injury state of the nervous system. Further consider the possible drawbacks associated with your scheme. You might want to return to reconsider this question after you have read further in this book.

Chapter 11

Generation of the Membrane Potential

Although knowledge of the existence of bioelectric potentials certainly goes back to the first encounters with electric fish, an understanding of their origin awaited the advances in physical chemistry that occurred near the end of the nineteenth century. The basic elements necessary to establish such a potential were understood then to be mobile charged ions in a solution, a membrane that allows the passage of only one species of these ions, and some means by which a concentration gradient of this species of ions can be established across the membrane. The advances in our understanding since then have provided considerable insight into how excitable cells provide for these necessary elements of potential generation. This chapter will focus on the mechanisms by which fixed potentials are established across cell membranes, and the next chapter will focus on the various means by which these potentials are changed to produce the basis of nervous system signaling.

Excitable cells have a potential difference between their inside and the solution bathing their outside.

As we noted in chapter 10, Luigi Galvani observed that a frog muscle, with its innervation intact, contracted when there was a static electrical discharge in the same room. Galvani was a keen experimenter and surmised that electricity from other sources also should cause contractions. He made many experiments to test this point and used, most spectacularly, atmospheric electrical discharge as one of his electrical sources. His conclusion from these experiments was that there existed "animal electricity" that was intrinsic to the nerve and muscle and that it was through this animal electricity that muscle contraction was initiated.

Large cells or small probes allow direct measurement of intracellular potentials. Both approaches have been used to obtain quantitative measurements of potentials that could only be surmised from the early extracellular measurements. Figure 11.1 is an example of an intracellular recording from the cell body of a

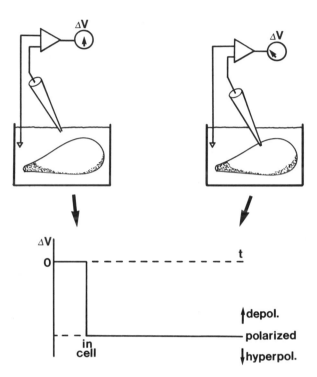

Figure 11.1
Resting membrane potential. A neuron (here schematically shown to be of gigantic size) is placed in a dish of physiological salt solution. The intracellular potential of this neuron is measured with a microelectrode attached to a differential amplifier whose output is the *difference* between the potential at the tip of the microelectrode and an indifferent electrode in the bathing solution. This difference is zero as long as the microelectrode is in the salt solution but registers a negative resting membrane potential when the electrode is advanced into the interior of the cell.

large neuron such as found in some invertebrate ganglia. A fine glass microelectrode can be inserted into the inside of the cell with minimal damage to the cell's integrity. The potential recorded between this electrode and an external reference electrode is amplified with an appropriate amplifier and then recorded on a cathode ray oscilloscope. The measured potential varies from cell to cell but has an average value that is typical for a specific cell type. As we will see below, however, this potential is very dependent on the extracellular potassium concentration. The salient points here are that the inside of the cell is electrically negative with respect to the outside, this *membrane potential* is equal to approximately 1/10 V, and in an unexcited cell, the *resting membrane potential* is stable. Resting membrane potentials are an essential feature of excitable cells but are also commonly found in inexcitable cells such as red blood cells. The membrane potential is a physicochemical property that exists whenever a membrane, with ion-selective channels, separates two solutions with different concentrations of an ion that is capable of passing through the selective channels. Excitable cells are specialized by having the ability to change this potential in response to an appropriate signal.

In 1785 Charles Coulomb described the force between charged particles. The law named for him states that there exists a force that is proportional to the charge, q, on the particles and inversely proportional to the square of the distance between them. When taken to atomic distances, this force is considerable. Thus the force between a proton and an electron at these distances is approximately 10^{40} times as great as gravitational force. We must deal, at this point, with this force in two guises. First we encounter it in the measurement of potential. *Electrical potential* (E) or *voltage* (V) is the work required to bring two charges together. This work is positive if the charges have the same sign and negative if they have opposite signs. A voltage can be measured whenever charges have been separated. Since a voltage is a potential *difference,* voltages must be referenced to another value. The second place we encounter coulombic force is in a *capacitor,* a device that separates and stores charges of opposite sign. Biological membranes in excitable cells maintain a potential difference in the resting state because the membrane is a capacitor. This membrane capacitance is given by

$$C_m = \frac{q}{V_m}$$

where C_m is the capacitance of the cell membrane, q is the charge displaced across the membrane, and V_m is the voltage across the membrane.

11.1.* Problem: How many moles of monovalent cations must a nerve membrane separate to establish a resting potential of 100 mV? The capacitance of biological membranes can be taken to be 1×10^{-6} F/cm^2, and you will remember that Faraday's constant is approximately 10^5 C/mol.

To simplify our discussion of membrane potentials we will use several important terms, which are shown in figure 11.1. When there is a potential across the membrane with a specific polarity, the membrane is said to be *polarized*. By convention, changes in membrane potential are referenced to this polarized condition. Thus, if the potential is made more negative (more polarized) it is said to be *hyperpolarized*. By contrast, when it is made less negative, it is said to be *depolarized*. (In some literature, especially related to cardiac muscle, the term *hypopolarized* is used for this latter condition.) A return to the polarized state following a change of potential is termed *repolarization*.

The Nernst equation describes the relationship between a concentration gradient and a voltage gradient at which a particular ion will diffuse without a directional bias.

As mentioned above, three conditions are necessary for the establishment of potentials across membranes: (1) mobile charged ions, (2) a concentration gradient across the membrane, and (3) the characteristic permeability of the membrane to specific species of these ions. Selective permeability is an extremely important and complex property of the membranes of excitable cells. We will have much more to say about this subject in later sections, but will begin here with a simple statement. Selective permeability is imparted to generally impermeable biological membranes by intrinsic membrane protein molecules that form *channels* through which charged ions can transit the membrane.

Figure 11.2 shows qualitatively how a membrane potential is established. The initial conditions are that there is a concentration gradient across the membrane but electroneutrality on either side. That is, the total number of charged ions on side 2 is greater than on side 1 but there are still the same number of (+) and (−) ions *on each side*. Since there is a concentration gradient across the membrane, there is a greater tendency for ions to move from side 2 to side 1 than in the opposite direction. The selective channels in the membrane will allow, in this example, only the (+) ions actually to move. In the first instant some (+) ions will move from side 2 to side 1, so that there is some reduction in the concen-

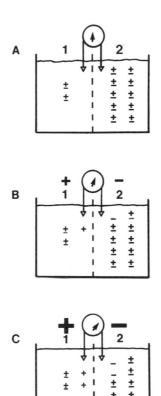

Figure 11.2
Establishment of a diffusion potential. A selectively permeable membrane (permeable only to [+] ions) is used to separate two halves of a container of an ionized salt solution. Initially (A) both sides are neutral but side 2 has a higher concentration of (+) and (−) ions than does side 1. At the first instance (B), some (+) ions move down their concentration gradient from side 2 to side 1 and, in doing so, cause side 1 to have a net (+) charge with respect to side 2. At equilibrium (C) enough (+) ions have moved to side 1 so that the electrical force on an ion from side 1 to side 2 exactly balances the tendency for ions to move from side 2 to side 1 under the influence of their concentration gradient.

tration gradient and side 1 obtains a slight excess of (+) charge with respect to side 2. In the next instant more (+) ions will continue to move from side 2 to side 1, but now they are beginning to experience a repulsive electrical force due to the excess (+) charge on side 1. Eventually an *equilibrium* condition is established where the movement of (+) ions from side 2 to side 1 because of their concentration gradient will be exactly balanced by the movement of (+) ions from side 1 to side 2 because of the electrical repulsive force on them. There is thus an *equilibrium potential* established passively across the membrane because of the concentration gradient. The equation that describes this equilibrium condition is the *Nernst equation*.

The preceding discussion may have left the impression that there is a considerable movement of ions necessary for the establishment of an equilibrium potential. Certainly there must be movement of ions for without the separation of charges there would be no potential. It is important to realize, however, that only a very small and insignificant fraction of the total number of ions that are separated by the membrane actually moves. The effect of the charge of an ion in establishing an electrical force on other ions is much greater than the influence of that one ion in the determination of a concentration gradient. It is a very reasonable approximation that there is no measurable change in the concentration gradient necessary to establish an equilibrium potential.

11.2. Question: Given a cell with (1) a high concentration of KCl on the inside and a low concentration of KCl on the outside and (2) a cell membrane selectively permeable to K^+ ions, will the inside potential at equilibrium be (+) or (−) with respect to the outside? The actual potential established across the membrane at equilibrium is defined by the Nernst equation.

The Nernst equation states that

$$E_1 - E_2 = \frac{RT}{Fz_s} \ln \frac{[S]_2}{[S]_1}$$

Where $E_1 - E_2$ is the potential difference across the membrane, R is the gas constant, T is the absolute temperature, F is Faraday's constant, z_s is the valence of substance s, ln is the natural logarithm, and $[S]_1$ and $[S]_2$ are the concentrations of substance s on sides 1 and 2 of the membrane. (The details of the derivation of the Nernst equation are given in appendix I.)

For our purposes we will write the Nernst equation in a reduced form applicable to excitable mammalian cells. The two sides of the membrane are intracellular (or inside, i) and extracellular (or outside, o). The extracellular potential is usually defined as zero, so the intracellular potential is the potential across the membrane or E_m. More generally, the Nernst equilibrium potential for some substance, s, is given as E_s. We will assign T to be body temperature, give F and R their appropriate values, assume that $z_s = +1$, and, for convenience, convert natural logarithms to common logarithms. This yields

$$E_s = 62 \text{ mV log} \frac{[S]_o}{[S]_i}$$

By considering some properties of logarithmic relationships, we can make some simple approximations to the Nernst equilibrium potentials. Recall that log 10 = 1, log 100 = 2, and so on, and log 1/10 = −1, log 1/100 = −2, and so on. Thus equilibrium potentials increase by 62 mV for every 10 times increase in concentration gradient of the permeant ion between the inside and the outside of the cell. Furthermore, the direction of the concentration gradient of the permeant ion determines the sign of the potential difference. When the inside concentration of a permeant cation is greater than the outside concentration, the potential is negative on the inside and when the outside concentration of a permeant cation is greater than the inside concentration, the potential is positive on the inside.

Exact values for logarithms can be obtained from published log tables, conveniently by a keystroke on most scientific calculators, or by direct comparison of the linear and logarithmic scales on a slide rule. Figure 11.3 presents the same information in graphic form and is of sufficient accuracy for equilibrium potential calculations. On a semilog graph such as this, log(N) is simply the ordinate for points along the diagonal line when N has been located as the abscissa.

We can use the Nernst equation, with the concentration gradients that exist between the inside and outside of mammalian muscle cells, to calculate several equilibrium potentials. These are the membrane potentials that we would expect if the membrane were selectively permeable only to K^+, Na^+, or Cl^- ions, in other words, for a membrane that contained only potassium or only sodium or only chloride channels.

For a membrane with only potassium channels

$$E_K = 62 \text{ mV log} \frac{[K]_o}{[K]_i} = 62 \text{ mV log} \frac{4}{155} = -98.5 \text{ mV}$$

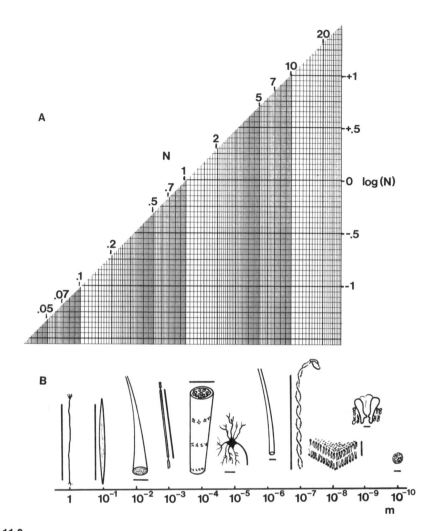

Figure 11.3

Log relationships. (A) This log graph can be used to determine the log of numbers between 0.03 and 30. Numbers on the abscissa, here shown along the diagonal line, have their log value on the ordinate. (B) One important characteristic of a logarithmic graph is that it compresses a range of numbers whose values are many orders of magnitude apart. This diagram shows a logarithmic scale of dimensions of structures discussed in this book. Moving from the left to the right, each scale line represents a length that is progressively 1/10 of the previous one. This log scale shows the length of a long axon, the length of a long muscle fiber, the diameter of a large peripheral nerve, the internodal length of a myelinated axon, the diameter of a muscle fiber, the diameter of a neuron cell body, the diameter of an unmyelinated axon, the length of the light meromyosin molecule, the thickness of a cell membrane, the diameter of the selectivity filter of an ion channel, and the diameter of a sodium ion. Extending this logarithmic scale to the left to 10^{+24} m would bring us to the size of galaxy clusters, and extending it to the right to 10^{-15} m would bring us to the dimensions of the inner structure of the proton.

For a membrane with only sodium channels

$$E_{Na} = 62 \text{ mV} \log \frac{[Na]_o}{[Na]_i} = 62 \text{ mV} \log \frac{145}{12} = +67.1 \text{ mV}$$

For a membrane with only chloride channels

$$E_{Cl} = \frac{62 \text{ mV}}{-1} \log \frac{[Cl]_o}{[Cl]_i} = -62 \text{ mV} \log \frac{120}{4} = -96.6 \text{ mV}$$

(In the last instance we need to include a value of -1 for z since Cl^- ions have a charge of -1.)

11.3. Problem: Check the preceding math for yourself in two ways. (1) Make an approximate check without determining exact log values by setting limits on the exact answer. For example, to estimate E_K, observe that $1/100 < 4/155 < 1/10$ so that $-2 < \log (4/155) < -1$ and $-124 \text{ mV} < E_K < -62 \text{ mV}$. (2) Use the log graph in figure 11.3, the log function on a calculator, a published log table, or a slide rule to calculate accurate values for each of these Nernst equilibrium potentials.

The actual measured resting membrane potential of about 1/10 V, or 100 mV, is close to E_K and E_{Cl} and far away from E_{Na}. A measured membrane potential near a calculated equilibrium potential for some ion implies one of two things: either that this ion is the major contributory ion to the genesis of the membrane potential or that the membrane potential is determined by another factor, and that the ion in question has distributed itself passively across the membrane to be at an equilibrium concentration at that potential. For many excitable cells at rest, K^+ meets the first of these conditions and Cl^- meets the second.

Ion channels provide the means for selected species of ions to cross the hydrophobic cell membrane.

Ion-selective channels in cell membranes probably evolved very early during development of complex cellular functions. As we have seen already, ion-selective channels are the structures necessary for cells to be able to establish membrane potentials by using the ionic gradients that exist across cell membranes.

Metabolism of carbon-containing molecules in cells proceeds, in part, through the flow of electrons in a series of coupled oxidation-reduction reactions, a process known as electron transport. Because of this process, energy-storing ATP molecules are produced. The ATP molecules are eventually used as an energy source in such functions as the establishment of ion gradients by pumps or the contraction of muscles. Ion-selective channels probably evolved at the time of transition from prokaryotic to eukaryotic cells. At that time the H^+ gradient necessary for biochemical electron transport shifted to intracellular structures (mitochondria), and the cell membrane became available for other ionic gradients.

The record of evolution of ion channels is at best an inferential one. One possibility is that rather nonspecific channels, selective for only cations, evolved first. From these probably evolved the more specific K^+- and Ca^{2+}-selective channels and then later Na^+-selective channels. The vast variety of human neural functions are most basically differentiated by the 50 or so types of ion channels found in the membranes of our neurons. These all appear to be large protein molecules for which our genome must carry the coding information. Ion-selective channels differ in several characteristics, and we will return in the next chapter to some of these characteristics. The one channel characteristic of interest here is *selectivity*. By various physicochemical means, ion channels allow some ions to pass while excluding most others.

Ion channels produce what is in effect a water-filled hole through the lipid membrane. Ions that diffuse freely in water move through these holes along with water molecules. Sometimes selectivity is produced in the channel sterically; that is, some ions are just too large to fit through the hole. In other cases, highly charged regions of the ion channel introduce selectivity by favoring the passage of certain ions because of their unique charge densities.

Ion channels can, in a limited sense, be regarded as enzymes that catalyze the movement of ions across a high energy barrier, the lipid membrane. The macroscopic interpretation of this is that channels impart selective permeability to the cell membrane. One additional observation about channels is worth mentioning here. Usually they are rare contaminants of the lipid membrane. One could conceivably pack as many as 30,000 channel-sized proteins into 1 μm^2 of membrane. The actual channel density, however, seldom exceeds about 300 per μm^2.

Energy-requiring pumps are necessary to maintain concentration gradients across membranes.

Membrane potentials are a passive property of any membrane that contains ion-selective channels and that separates solutions of different ionic concentration. The generation and maintenance of a concentration gradient, however, require an ion pump that uses metabolic energy. The most ubiquitous ion pump in biological membranes is the one that pumps Na^+ ions out of the cell and, simultaneously, pumps K^+ ions into the cell. To do this the pump uses the energy stored in a high-energy phosphate bond of ATP.

This pump establishes a K^+ ion gradient that underlies the resting potential and a Na^+ gradient, in the reverse direction, that has several important functions. Again, the resting potential is a passive property, but it depends on a previously established concentration gradient. The sodium-potassium pump moves ions much more slowly than ion channels do. This slow, steady pumping action is perfectly adequate, though, to restore whatever diminution of concentration gradients results from ions moving through open membrane channels down their electrochemical gradients (figure 11.4).

An electroneutral pump, exchanging one Na^+ for one K^+, would be sufficient to establish concentration gradients for Na^+ and K^+. Sodium-potassium pumps have, however, a stochiometry of 3 Na^+ to 2 K^+ for 1 ATP hydrolyzed. The pump is thus *electrogenic,* producing a net outward current across the membrane. Such an outwardly directed, ionic current would be expected to make a contribution to the resting potential. The amount of this contribution is usually small and depends on the resting membrane resistance.

Besides its role in the action potential, which will be discussed in chapter 12, the Na^+ gradient that is established by the sodium-potassium pump has another important role. It is used as an energy storage device. Most cells take advantage of the Na^+ gradient to maintain concentration gradients for other ions or molecules. These specific exchange mechanisms allow Na^+ to move down its concentration gradient in *obligatory exchange* for the other substance moving up its concentration gradient either into or out of the cell. Thus, intracellular Ca^{2+} concentration is kept low in neurons, in part, because of intracellular Ca^{2+} ions being exchanged for extracellular Na^+ ions. A cellular pH gradient is, in some cells, maintained by a similar sodium-hydrogen ion exchange process.

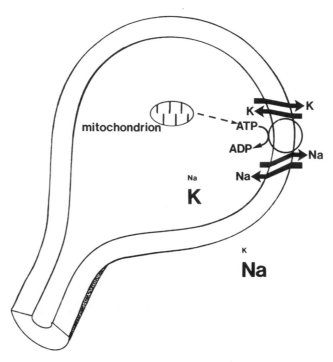

Figure 11.4
Cell concentration gradients. The active sodium-potassium pump maintains the concentration gradients of Na^+ and K^+ across the cell membrane. It compensates for the passive fluxes of these ions down their electrochemical gradients. To move ions up their gradients, the pump uses cellular energy in the form of ATP.

Membranes with permeabilities to several ions maintain a potential difference that is determined by the concentration gradients of and the permeabilities to the various ions for which ion channels exist.

Table 11.1 shows typical values for intracellular and extracellular concentrations of various ions in mammalian muscle. The membranes of excitable cells delineate concentration gradients for several species of ions. These membranes, because of their varied palettes of ion channels, have selective permeabilities to many of these species of ions. The Nernst equation, however, requires monoionic concentrations to be strictly applicable. In dealing with membranes of actual excitable

Table 11.1
Ion Concentrations

S	$[S]_o$	$[S]_i$	$[S]_o/[S]_i$	$E_s(mV)$
Na^+	145	12	12.08	+67.1
K^+	4	155	0.026	−98.5
Cl^-	120	4	30.0	−91.6

cells, we need another method to determine the steady-state potential across the membrane. This is accomplished with a relationship that looks similar to the Nernst equation but includes terms for multiple ion concentration gradients and permeabilities. This relationship, the *Goldman-Hodgkin-Katz equation,* is named after three physiologists who contributed to its derivation. The relationship states that a steady-state potential is established across a membrane with a value determined by the various ionic concentration gradients each to the extent that the membrane is permeable to that ion. The original papers that present the Goldman-Hodgkin-Katz equation are by David Goldman (1943) and Alan Hodgkin and Bernard Katz (1949). These papers are worth reading; they show how biologists have the opportunity to deal in a very quantitative way with the physical principles that underlie biological phenomena.

11.4.* Question: The resting membrane potential is not even approximately equal to the Nernst equilibrium potential for Na^+. The Nernst potential for sodium results from the Na^+ ion gradient that actually exists across the membrane. Can you propose why this might be possible without violating any physical chemical properties?

The Nernst equation for monovalent cations could be interpreted as defining a potential equal to a constant (RT/F) times the natural logarithm (ln) of the ratio of the tendency of substance s to go into the cell (the concentration of s on the outside) to the tendency of substance s to go out of the cell (the concentration of s on the inside). Extending this to a more general case:

$$E = \frac{RT}{F} \ln \frac{\Sigma \text{ monovalent cation influx}}{\Sigma \text{ monovalent cation effux}}$$

For a + ion (e.g., Na^+ or K^+), the tendency of an ion to move across the membrane is simply the product of the membrane permeability and the appropriate concentration. The situation for $(-)$ ions (e.g., Cl^-) is different. We note that an *inwardly* directed electrical current (equivalent to the flow of $(+)$ charges) is produced when $(-)$ ions are allowed to flow out across the cell membrane. Thus, for a $(-)$ ion, the tendencies discussed above become the product of the membrane permeability and the concentration on the opposite side of the membrane.

For Na^+, K^+, and Cl^- ions, the Goldman-Hodgkin-Katz equation is

$$E_m = \frac{RT}{F} \ln \frac{p_{Na}[Na]_o + p_K[K]_o + p_{Cl}[Cl]_i}{p_{Na}[Na]_i + p_K[K]_i + p_{Cl}[Cl]_o}$$

where p_S is the membrane permeability to ion S. It is important to remember that this equation describes a steady-state and not an equilibrium condition. But it is an equation that can be applied to determine E_m whenever the values of concentration and membrane permeabilities are known.

We can now see why the resting membrane potential is approximately, but not exactly, equal to the potassium equilibrium potential. If p_{Na} and p_{Cl} were equal to zero, then

$$E_m = \frac{RT}{F} \ln \frac{p_K[K]_o}{p_K[K]_i} = \frac{RT}{F} \ln \frac{[K]_o}{[K]_i}$$

which is the Nernst equation for potassium. If p_{Na} were to have a small, but nonzero value, E_m would be displaced from E_K by a small amount toward E_{Na}.

11.5.* Problem: How much is the membrane potential displaced from the potassium equilibrium potential if the membrane is 1/100 as permeable to Na^+ as to K^+ (disregarding any Cl^- permeability)? Use the values of concentrations given in table 11.1.

11.6.* Problem: Impaired renal function can lead to hyperkalemia (increased plasma K^+ concentration). This may have dangerous consequences because of the resultant depolarization of cardiac muscle. Assuming that $p_{Na}/p_K = 0.01$, using concentration values from table 11.1, and again disregarding any effect of Cl^- how much depolarization would result if $[K]_o$ were increased to 6.5 mM?

Calcium ions enter the intracellular compartment of cells through selective channels because of their electrochemical gradient. Once in the cytoplasm, these ions regulate many important cellular processes.

The function of the nervous system is to regulate intracellular calcium.

This statement is one of those gross oversimplifications to which there are few exceptions. Intracellular calcium levels control such important functions as *excitation–contraction coupling* in muscle (discussed in chapter 14), *excitation–secretion coupling* in secretory cells and presynaptic terminals (discussed in chapter 13), *excitation–gating coupling* of gated ion channels, and *Ca-dependent regulation* of intracellular enzyme systems. Intracellular Ca^{2+} activity is maintained at an exceedingly low level in most excitable cells through exchange pumping with Na^+ across the cell membrane, or with H^+ across the mitochondrial membrane, and by various intracellular buffering mechanisms. Intracellular Ca^{2+} activity is increased when membrane calcium channels open and thereby allow Ca^{2+} ions to move, down their electrochemical gradient, into the cell. The major consideration of this chapter has been cases in which ionic gradients determine membrane potentials. Here, by contrast, is an important example in which an electrochemical driving force can effectively change an important intracellular ionic concentration.

11.7.* Problem: What is the driving force on Ca^{2+} ions in a resting cell? Assume that extracellular $[Ca^{2+}] = 10^{-2}$ M, intracellular $[Ca^{2+}] = 10^{-8}$ M, and $E_m = -90$ mV.

We have seen in this chapter that when a membrane separates solutions of differing concentrations of a mobile ion and when this membrane contains channels selective for some species of these ions, a transmembrane potential is established. If there is only one ionic species, this is a Nernst equilibrium potential. In multiionic environments with multiple selective ion channels, a membrane potential is established that is a weighted sum of the various Nernst equilibrium potentials. Excitable cells regulate their membrane potentials and some intracellular ionic concentrations by opening and closing ion-selective channels in their membranes. We will return in the next two chapters to the mechanisms by which the opening and closing of ion selective channels are regulated.

Chapter 12

Alterations of Membrane Potential

We began our investigation of cellular electrical properties, in the last chapter, with a look at the resting potential. The resting potential is the ultimate power source for nervous system signaling. We will begin this chapter with a discussion of ways in which the membrane potential is altered so that signaling occurs over short distances (i.e., tens or hundreds of micrometers). In the second part of the chapter, we will again return to signaling based on changes in the membrane potential, but there we will emphasize long-distance signaling (i.e., up to meters).

12.1.* Question: Where, in the nervous system, would local signaling be important, and where would specialized long-distance signaling become necessary?

There are three basic characteristics of electrical current flow: (1) current tends to flow whenever unlike charges have been separated; (2) current always flows in a closed circuit; and (3) current flow can be either resistive or capacitive.

1. Whenever unlike charges have been separated, the electrostatic forces between them tend to bring them back together. Since the movement of electrical charges is an electrical current, separation of unlike charges results in a tendency for an electrical current flow. In the absence of any other forces, the extent of this current flow depends on the *conductance* of the medium separating the charges.

The preceding is simply a statement of *Ohm's law:*

$$I = \frac{\Delta E}{R}$$

It is often more useful to use the inverse of resistance (R), which is conductance (G). Thus Ohm's law can be written:

$$I = G\Delta E$$

2. Our second point is that current always flows in a circuit. This may seem a trivial point, but it has, more than once, led to confusion for an unwary student or researcher who forgot to consider where the return current pathway was. Whenever we follow the movement of a charge from point A to point B, there also must be a return path for the same amount of charge from point B to point A.

3. Current flow in excitable cells can take one of two very different forms. *Resistive current* flows through an electrical conductor and represents continuous movement of electrons or charged ions from one end of the conductor to the other end. The movement of Na^+ or K^+ ions through a membrane channel is a resistive current. *Capacitive current* flows whenever an excess charge on one side of a capacitor displaces another charge on the other side of the capacitor. The net effect is a current through the capacitor, although there is no actual movement of an electron or ion from one side of the capacitor to the other side. Whenever charges are added to one side and a corresponding number removed from the opposite side of the lipid portion of a biological membrane, there is a capacitive current across the membrane.

Ion-permeable channels within the matrix of the ion-impermeable lipid that constitutes the membrane of excitable cells create a parallel combination of a resistive and a capacitive current pathway (figure 12.1). Current flowing across cell membranes always has these two paths as options. Current takes the resistive pathway and flows through ion channels whenever the gates on these channels are open and there is an electrochemical driving force on the ions. If G_m represents the total conductance of open channels in the membrane and ΔE represents the electrochemical driving force on the ions, Ohm's law predicts that

$$I_r = G_m \Delta E$$

Current will, on the other hand, take the capacitive pathway whenever the voltage across the membrane is changing, that is, whenever dE/dt is not zero. If C_m represents the membrane capacitance and dE/dt the rate of change of voltage, then

$$I_c = C_m \frac{dE}{dt}$$

The membrane potential will change characteristically if a small current is applied suddenly to the membrane. Initially, most of the current flows through the ca-

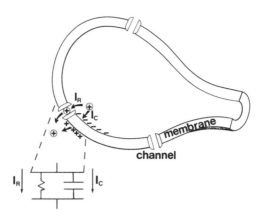

Figure 12.1
Current pathways across a cell membrane. Current can flow across a cell membrane by two different pathways—as a resistive current (I_R) or as a capacitive current (I_C). Ion flux through ion channels is resistive current and obeys Ohm's law, that is, $I_R = G\Delta E$. Current also can flow across the lipid bilayer by adding charge to one side and removing charge from the other side of the membrane. Such current is capacitive and obeys the equation, $I_C = C\, dV/dt$.

pacitance pathway causing the potential to change rapidly toward the maximum value of the applied voltage as charges are deposited on the membrane capacitor. As the charge on and the voltage across the membrane capacitor increase, the rate of potential change decreases. The increasing potential leads to an increased resistive current with the effect that the division of current shifts progressively from the capacitance pathway to the resistance pathway. Eventually, only a steady resistive current will flow through whichever membrane channels are open. The potential change, because of this transition between capacitive and resistive currents, is characteristically exponential.

The total current across the membrane equals the sum of the resistive and capacitive components (figure 12.2):

$$I_m = I_r + I_c = G_m E + C_m \frac{dE}{dt}$$

This differential equation can be solved to yield the potential change that follows a step in membrane current:

$$E_f - E_i = \frac{I}{G_m} (1 - e^{-t/\tau_m})$$

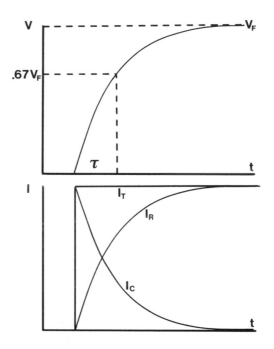

Figure 12.2
Resistive and capacitive components of total current. A step of current applied to a membrane will flow initially as capacitive current. As charge accumulates on the membrane and the potential exponentially approaches a new value, the capacitive component will decrease exponentially and the resistive component will increase exponentially. These exponential processes are described by a time constant, τ, that represents the time necessary for the potential or current change to achieve $1/e$ (≈ 0.67) of its final value. The final voltage (V_F) is determined by the potential drop ($= I/G$ or IR) across the resistor when all the current is flowing through this pathway.

where E_f and E_i are the final and initial voltages, I is the applied current, G_m is the membrane conductance and τ_m is the membrane *time constant*, which is, in turn, equal to C_m/G_m.

12.2.* Problem: A postsynaptic potential occurs whenever a presynaptic cell releases a neurotransmitter that suddenly opens many gated ion channels on the postsynaptic cell. At many synapses, a specific process will then rapidly terminate the neurotransmitter's effect, thereby leading to a rapid closure of the transmitter-gated channels. Thus, with each release of transmitter, the postsynaptic cell is subjected to a short current pulse. Draw the shape and define the final value of the resultant potential change. Assume that the membrane time constant equals the duration of the postsynaptic current pulse. How does the relationship between membrane time constant and duration of transmitter action affect the amplitude and duration of the postsynaptic potential change?

Except under certain experimental conditions, potential changes across the membranes of excitable cells are localized to one region of the membrane and decrease to insignificance at more distant regions of the cell.

We have already seen that whenever there is a difference in potential (separation of unlike charges) there is a current flow in a direction that would eliminate this potential difference. This current flow will, without necessarily affecting any channel gates, change the potential in adjacent regions of the cell. Because of the requisite distribution of the available current between transmembrane current and longitudinal current, the membrane current will diminish exponentially with distance along the cell and the membrane potential difference will likewise diminish exponentially with distance.

As we discussed in chapter 2, passive spread of current along a nerve fiber is described by the *cable theory*. The simplest cable network is derived from a series and parallel combination of resistors. Some rules of these electrical circuits will be reviewed below.

The total *resistance* in a group of resistors connected in series is equal to the sum of the individual resistances (figure 12.3). When a voltage, E, is applied across the series, the voltage drop across each component is proportional to the fraction of the total resistance that is in that component. Ohm's law describes the relationships between current and voltage in a series circuit.

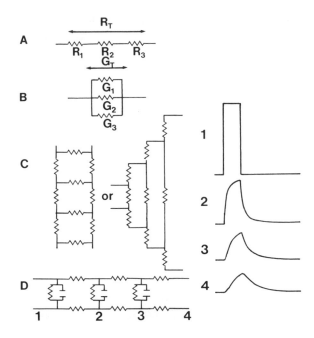

Figure 12.3
Membrane resistive networks. (A) In a series combination, the total resistance is the sum of the individual resistances ($R_T = R_1 + R_2 + R_3$). (B) In a parallel combination the total conductance is the combination of the individual conductances ($G_T = G_1 + G_2 + G_3$). (C) A ladder network, represented here in two forms, approximates some of the passive properties of a nerve membrane. The "rungs" on the ladder represent resistance across the membrane as a result of membrane channels and the "uprights" of the ladder represent the resistance of the intracellular and extracellular solutions. A rearrangement of the ladder components shows it to be a sequence of voltage dividers. The fraction of voltage across each transverse segment of the membrane becomes the source that drives the next segment. (D) A more complete representation of the passive properties of a nerve fiber includes the capacitive component representing the lipid bilayer. At successive points along such a cable, potential change is both progressively slowed and its amplitude is diminished. The inset shows the voltage response, measured at each successive segment, to a step of voltage applied at the left end of the network.

$$I = \frac{\Delta E}{R_1 + R_2 + R_3}$$

or using

$$R_T = R_1 + R_2 + R_3$$

then

$$I = \frac{\Delta E}{R_T}$$

The total *conductance* of a group of resistors connected in parallel is equal to the sum of the individual conductances. In biological systems, an increase in area (e.g., the cross-sectional area of a nerve fiber or the area of a membrane) usually results in increased conductance. Although conductance summation is more intuitively grasped, most readers will be more familiar with the equation for combining resistances.

$$\frac{1}{R_T} = \frac{1}{R_1} + \frac{1}{R_2} + \frac{1}{R_3}$$

which is identical to the equation

$$G_T = G_1 + G_2 + G_3$$

A *ladder network* is a network containing series and parallel resistors. This combination approximates some passive properties of a nerve fiber. In such a network, the voltage at one segment becomes the source of voltage for the next segment. With simple resistors, the voltage will decrease as the distance from the source increases. The spatial course of this decrease depends on the ratio of the longitudinal resistances to the cross-resistances. If the membrane is taken, more realistically, to include capacitors, the slowed voltage change of one segment causes an even more slowed driving of the next segment.

Passive electrical properties of the cell, including the membrane resistance and capacitance and the cytoplasmic resistance, determine its space and time constants.

The voltage drops that occur along a cable conductor originate in the flow of current through the conductive pathways of the core and the external medium.

All the current that flows because of the applied voltage flows through the initial portion of the core. As current, in proportion to the local transmembrane voltage difference, is successively shunted through the membrane conductance along the fiber, the current flowing down the core is reduced. If the core and external conductance pathways are uniform, the decrease of voltage will be the same for equal distances, that is, the voltage drops exponentially with distance.

In a manner analogous to the membrane time constant, we can define a membrane *space constant:*

$$E_x = E_0 e^{-x/\lambda}$$

Where E_x is the final voltage developed at some location, x, E_o is the voltage at the source of the current, x is the distance along a long cell, and λ is the membrane space constant. The space constant is given as the square root of the ratio of the longitudinal conductance to the membrane conductance.

$$\lambda = \sqrt{\frac{G_l}{G_m}}$$

When, as is often the case, the extracellular conductance is high, the longitudinal conductance is almost entirely restricted by the conductance within the cell.

Typically, space constants are between 0.01 to 1.0 cm. Potential will fall to about 37% of its initial value for each space constant; thus, by four space constants the voltage will be but 2% (0.37^4) of what it is at the initial site.

The ladder circuit approximation of a cable conductor is an incomplete representation of the passive nerve fiber. As we have already seen, the membrane also acts as a capacitor. It is thus necessary to include capacitors in parallel with the membrane conductance units (figure 12.3D). The ladder circuit is equivalent to a filter circuit in which each step slows change with a time constant. Just as the potential at the point where current is applied to the membrane changes exponentially with time, so does the potential at an instant of time vary exponentially with distance along a long cell process. The time constant is a membrane characteristic that describes how rapidly potential can be varied in time. The space constant is a characteristic of a cell that describes how the potential will vary in space along a long cell process. Figure 12.4 shows this in graphic form. This graph shows the spatial and temporal changes in voltage in a long cylindrical cell as the result of a sudden step of current applied to point 0. At point 0 the voltage rises exponentially as defined by the membrane time constant; this is

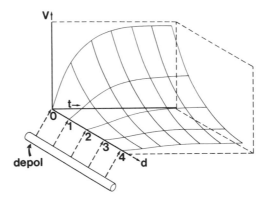

Figure 12.4
Changes in potential in time and distance along an axon when a subthreshold depolarization is applied at one end. At the site where the depolarization current is applied (0), the potential rises exponentially to a final value. At successively greater distances from this point (1–4), the potential rises more slowly (with a sigmoidal time course) to a final value that decreases exponentially with distance.

exactly the situation shown in figure 12.2. At points 1, 2, 3, and 4, however, the voltage is seen to rise progressively more slowly to progressively smaller values. The final value to which these voltages rise decreases exponentially with distance and is defined by the membrane space constant.

12.3. Problem: How might the membrane space constant affect the evolution of cell size? (or vice versa?)

Membrane conductance and capacitance determine how rapidly the membrane potential can be changed at a point where a current is applied to the cell. As we have seen, potential will change as an exponential function of time that is described by the membrane time constant, $\tau = C_m/G_m$. Small electrical events within a neuron will sum during any temporal overlap of each of their exponential responses. This is a basic aspect of neuronal integration. Although the output of a neuron is a sequence of all-or-nothing pulses, the inputs are inevitably small summating positive and negative events. The membrane time constant is thus a crucial determinant in the process of convergence.

12.4.* Problem: Remember that the time constant is the ratio of membrane capacitance to membrane conductance. What effect would the opening of transmitter-gated channels have locally on the membrane time constant? How would this affect the integration of a neuron's inputs?

The space constants that depend on geometric characteristics of various cell types are important in determining the effect of local potential changes in those cells.

Many excitable cells exhibit a rather unique morphology of having very long, but thin processes. Although the membrane time constant is determined by characteristics intrinsic to the membrane, the membrane space constant is dependent largely on the size of the cell. The longitudinal conductance along a long cell process is a crucial determinant. This conductance is greater when the diameter of the cell is larger. As we have already seen, a larger longitudinal conductance yields a longer space constant. Thus, the space constant will vary considerably between long, thick muscle cells and long, thin nerve axons.

The necessity for packing large numbers of individual conducting pathways within a small nerve trunk places constraints on the diameter of individual nerve axons. A single nerve axon may be a meter long but only a micrometer in diameter. Small-diameter axons have shorter space constants, restricting the effectiveness of local electrical events to only short distances from the site of their initiation. This limitation leads to the need for propagated conduction, in which energy is repeatedly added to the information signal. In a fashion similar to that of microwave repeater stations, the exponential decay of a signal dictated by the space constant is overcome by repeatedly regenerating the signal. This process will be discussed at greater length in our discussion of action potential propagation.

Muscle fibers, too, depend on electrical signaling for regulation of their contraction. The interaction of the electrical signal, initiated postsynaptically in the muscle cell, with the contraction is called excitation–contraction coupling. This process involves an electrically initiated release of calcium from internal sites all along the muscle fiber. The rapid dispersement of an electrical signal along a fiber that might be many centimeters long is crucial to the process of excitation–contraction coupling. The diameter of muscle fibers is typically greater than nerve fibers, and, thus, their space constants are proportionally longer. Still, as in nerve fibers, the length of muscle fibers far exceeds even their space constants, making regenerative propagation necessary.

In the regions of dendrites where synaptic inputs converge on central neurons, space constants are complex. This results from the variations in diameter of the dendrites and their complex branching patterns (see, for example, Rall and Rinzel, 1973). These variations in space (and time) constants have important influences on both the relative intensity and timing of inputs arriving at different locations within the dendritic arborization.

As was discussed in chapter 4, the initial stage of sensory transduction involves the generation of locally acting currents. These currents produce local, graded, nonpropagating potentials called *receptor potentials*. Receptor potentials, as is characteristic of local potentials, can summate whenever stimuli come at an interval sufficiently short in comparison to the membrane time constant. Receptor potentials are effective in signaling only at distances that are short compared to the membrane space constant.

12.5.* Problem: If a receptor has a space constant of 0.1 mm, how large could that receptor be without need for signal amplification? Assume that the signal is effective as long as it is greater than 14% of its initial value. What are typical sizes of sensory receptor cells?

The term *safety factor,* introduced in chapter 2, is used to describe the stimulating effectiveness of an electronically spread voltage at a particular site some distance from the electrical source. A response site might be the location where the signal is amplified for a propagated action potential or the location where transmitter is released at the presynaptic terminal of a small neuron or receptor. The site of origin of the electrical signal might be ion channels whose gates are sensitive to the presence of a neurotransmitter at a postsynaptic membrane or it might be ion channels whose gates are sensitive to some form of external energy of a sensory receptor. In any of these cases, the cell has an adequate safety factor when the distance between the two sites is small when measured in units of the membrane space constant.

The junctions between neurons and between neurons and muscles are specialized structures that allow an electrical event in one cell to produce an electrical event in the second cell. We will return to discuss synapses in chapter 13. Synapses typically occur on regions of excitable cells that are not involved in long-distance transmission of information. Thus synapses are found in the endplate region of muscle and on the soma or dendrites of neurons. The potential changes at these specific locations lead to local responses of adjacent areas of the cells. Spatial and temporal summations of these local potential changes are an important means by which excitable cells integrate information.

The ability to generate all-or-nothing action potentials sets excitable cells apart from all other types of cells.

In earlier chapters, we have discussed the origin of what Galvani called "animal electricity." So far in this chapter we have concerned ourselves with small-amplitude electrical events of excitable cells. These local signals follow the constraints of the time and space constants that impose temporal and spatial limitations on the effectiveness of applied potentials. We will extend this discussion to include the *sine qua non* of excitable cells, the *action potential*. The action potential is essential for long-distance signaling whereas the local potentials perform the integrative and information processing functions of the neuron. Consequently, long distance signaling is generally insensitive to small changes in potential that would be very important to the local integrative action of a neuron.

Our understanding of the action potential has advanced rapidly during the last decades. A century ago it was known that action potentials existed, but relatively little was known of the underlying mechanisms of their generation. During an exciting 20-year period in the middle of this century, the underlying ionic currents were described. At present, huge strides are being made toward understanding these phenomena at a molecular level. At each step in this process, old questions have been answered and new ones asked.

Ion channels, protein molecules in the lipid cell membrane, are responsible for both resting and action potentials.

We have already introduced the idea of ion channels. These ion-selective, hydrophilic (Greek: υδωρ = water + φιλειν = loving) pores through the membrane are the underlying basis for membrane potentials. Membrane potentials are a ubiquitous property of living cells. Excitable cells are set apart because of their ability to change this potential in response to an appropriate stimulus. Gated ion channels instill this characteristic of excitability in cells.

A considerable amount is now known about ion channels, and our understanding is advancing rapidly with the work of many biophysicists, molecular biologists, geneticists, and biochemists. In 1991 a Nobel Prize was awarded to Erwin Neher and Bert Sakmann for their introduction and use of the patch clamp technique. This clever technique now makes it possible to measure the flow of ions through a single ion channel, to characterize the conditions and kinetics of channel gates, and to produce state diagrams for the conditions of ion channels. Equally clever techniques of the molecular biologists, geneticists, and biochemists have made it possible to sequence the amino acids making up the channel protein, to make reasonable hypotheses about the tertiary structure of channel proteins, and to manipulate the genetic expression of channels. Figure 12.5 summarizes some of what is known about channel structure. The molecular and electrical information is rapidly converging to a very detailed and consistent picture of exactly what constitutes an ion channel.

The function of ion channels depends on certain highly specialized properties of these protein molecules.

Gated ion channels have four important properties that are best considered to be independent: (1) *selectivity,* or the ability of a channel to distinguish a specific ionic species; (2) *conductance,* or the measure of how well an ion, once selected, travels through the channel (conductance is proportional to the permeability of the channel to a particular ion); (3) *gating,* or the process by which channels are opened or closed to the flow of ions; and (4) *sensing* (voltage, chemical, or mechanical), or the characteristic of a channel that allows it to change its gating state in response to an external stimulus.

We will address, in more detail, these properties of ion channels.

1. *Selectivity:* In the simplest approximation, selectivity is accomplished by steric means; that is, the channel acts like a sieve. This mechanism obviously only works in situations where small ions are to be passed and large ions rejected. Additional means by which channels accomplish selectivity are related to the relative binding strength of the ion to sites within the channel compared to the strength of binding of that ion to water. With some notable exceptions, channels are quite selective, passing preferred ions a hundred or more times better than rejected ions.

2. *Conductance:* Conductance is an electrical measurement relating current flow and driving potential:

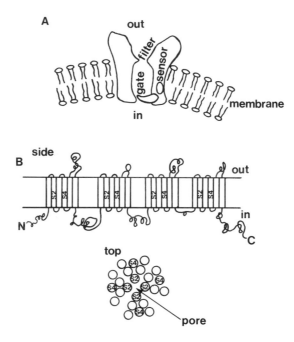

Figure 12.5
The ion channel. Ion channels are intrinsic, membrane-spanning protein molecules. They typically have a sensor that senses the voltage across the membrane or the presence of a chemical substance on either the inside or the outside of the membrane. The sensor activates a gate that can be either open or closed and, only when open, permits ions to pass through the channel. Channels also have some region, the selectivity filter, that allows them to select between those ions that can and those that cannot pass through the channel. (A) A highly schematized ion channel emphasizing the aspects of channel function that have been most extensively studied with electrical measurements. (B) Schematic representation of some details of the sodium channel gleaned from molecular biological investigations. This channel, with striking similarities to several other channels, is thought to have four similar regions, each of which has six membrane-spanning segments. These membrane-spanning segments consist of 20 amino acids and they are all strung together as a protein molecule that is 1820 amino acids long. It is thought that the segments labeled S2 form the walls of the transmembrane pore and that the segments labeled S4 serve as voltage sensors. (A brief review of the current understanding of sodium channel structure can be found in Catterall, 1991.)

$$G = \frac{1}{R} = \frac{I}{\Delta E}$$

where I is current, ΔE is electrical driving force, which for cell membranes with mobile ions is $E_m - E_s$ (E_s is the Nernst equilibrium potential that depends on the concentration gradient of substance s), and R is the electrical resistance to the movement of that ion. In discussions of the conductance of single ion channels, the Greek letter γ is used to represent conductance. Single channels pass picoamperes (10^{-12} A) of current and have conductances of picosemens (10^{-12} Ω^{-1}).

3. *Gating:* To a first approximation, channels have only two states, open or closed. Generally a fraction of the gates on a population of channels moves from the closed to the open state as a function of the effective strength of the stimulus and then return to the closed state with kinetics intrinsic to the channel. When the conductance of the membrane varies in time, we can usually be certain that it is the number of channels open that is varying and not the conductance of each individual channel.

4. *Sensing:* The gating sensors of ion channels in excitable cells respond to the electrical field across the cell membrane, the presence of chemical substances (ligands) at the inside or outside of the membrane, or to other conditions such as mechanical deformation of the membrane. In each instance, the sensor responds by changing the probability of the channel's gates being open. Voltage sensors make essential contributions to the generation of the action potential.

12.6.* Problem: The voltage sensors of sodium channels sense the electrical field change that exists across the membrane during the rising phase of the action potential and, in response to this, open sodium channel gates. Another way of saying this is that the sodium channel protein undergoes a configuration change when the electric field changes. What is this field change across the cell membrane (thickness = 100×10^{-10} m) if the potential changes by 100 mV?

The second broad category of gating sensors is the chemical sensors, which can be further subdivided based on the location of the chemical molecules. First, there are the neurotransmitter receptors, which cause a change in gating when a specific neurotransmitter molecule is present at an external membrane site. The acetylcholine-sensitive channel at the neuromuscular junction is a well-studied example of this type of sensor. Second, there are sensors to various intracellular chemical substances. The study of channels whose gating is sensitive to these *second messengers* has opened vast new insights into the way that neurons function.

For various technical reasons it has been difficult to study mechanically sensitive channels. Although there is still controversy about their exact nature, their long-suspected presence has now been confirmed.

Opening of individual channels is a probabilistic function, with the probability being a function of the state of the sensor. One cannot guarantee that a specific channel will be open at any particular time; however, one can predict with a fair degree of accuracy what will be the percentage of time that a channel will be open given the state of the sensor. Thus, total membrane conductance is a *stochastic* function (i.e., random but predictable) and is described by the probability equation

$$G = pN\gamma$$

where p $(0 \leq p \leq 1)$ is the probability of a channel being open, N is the total number of channels, and γ is the conductance of a single channel. For the sodium channel, G is a function of voltage and time because p is a function of voltage and time.

The action potential shares with various electronically generated time-marking pulses two important and related properties: it has a *threshold,* and once that threshold is exceeded the resultant potential change is *all-or-nothing.*

In 1926 Edgar Adrian and Yngve Zotterman made the important discovery that action potentials are of constant amplitude and that a stronger stimulus elicits more excited units and a higher frequency of action potentials but not larger individual action potentials. Long distance signaling in the nervous system has since been understood to be accomplished by a firing rate code with additional importance placed on the internal patterns of the rate in time. A corollary to this is that the action potential serves as a time marker and thus can be very stereotypic (figure 12.6).

Neurons can be stimulated by passing a current across their membranes. Depending on the direction of this current flow, the membrane potential will be either depolarized or hyperpolarized. One finds, when doing such an experiment,

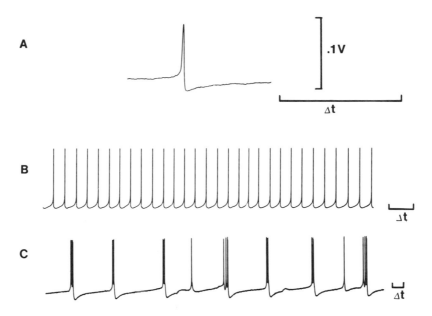

Figure 12.6
Pulse coding. These records show intracellular recordings of (A) a single action potential, (B) a very regular repetition of action potentials, and (C) an irregular grouping of action potentials into bursts. All the records are shown to the same vertical scale but with a successively more compressed time axis.

that the amount of hyperpolarization is approximately proportional to the amount of current passed. This proportionality is also true for depolarizations, but only up to a point. When the amount of depolarization exceeds this critical level, there is a very predictable change in the membrane potential that proceeds without further dependence on the current the experimenter was passing. This critical level is known as the threshold, and the stereotypic change in membrane potential is the all-or-nothing action potential.

Two characteristics of this voltage trajectory are important in understanding what is happening with the gated ion channels that cause the action potential.

1. The action potential is not simply a return of the intracellular potential to zero from a negatively polarized condition. Rather, the action potential carries the membrane potential to a positive value, that is, the action potential *overshoots* zero.

2. The return of the potential from its peak is not a simple decay to resume the resting potential. There can be a period of hyperpolarization, the *afterhyperpolarization* before the resting condition is reattained.

12.7.* Problem: At the beginning of this century, Julius Bernstein (1902) predicted that nervous activity resulted from the loss of selective permeability. Improved measurement instruments by the 1940s allowed Alan Hodgkin and Bernard Katz (1949) to measure an overshooting action potential. How do Hodgkin and Katz's observations disprove Bernstein's hypothesis, and what do these observations predict?

In 1952 Alan Hodgkin and Andrew Huxley tamed the explosive action potential with the *voltage clamp*. This technique makes it possible to switch the independent and dependent variables in electrophysiological experiments. Without the voltage clamp, the experimenter controls the initial current and measures the resultant voltage; with the voltage clamp, the experimenter can control voltage and measure the resultant current. This is an exceedingly important difference since, with constant voltage, current is approximately proportional to membrane conductance and is thus a measure of channel gating. The voltage clamp uses a feedback circuit that measures intracellular potential, compares it with a reference level, and passes a current back into the cell to negate any difference between these two potentials. The current passed by the feedback amplifier is thus equal, but opposite, to the current flowing through membrane channels at any time. Hodgkin and Huxley used their measurements to derive a quantitative description of the ionic basis for the action potential. These descriptions are now understood in terms of the combined effect of ion currents through many single channels.

12.8.* Problem: Would a circuit such as that shown in figure 12.7 be inherently stable? What parameters might affect the stability?

During an action potential, sodium channels open by the process of activation and subsequently close through the process of inactivation. With a somewhat slower time course, potassium channels also open because of their own activation process.

Hodgkin and Huxley found that a step change of the membrane potential, to a sufficiently depolarized value, causes first an inward ionic current followed by a

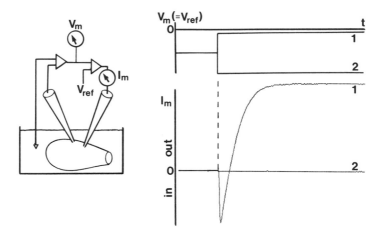

Figure 12.7
Voltage clamp experiment. (A) Voltage clamp circuit. By means of two intracellular electrodes, the intracellular voltage (V_m) is measured and, by means of current feedback through the second electrode, is made to follow changes in the reference voltage (V_{ref}). The time-varying feedback current must then equal the time-varying current across the membrane (I_m) at any voltage. (B) Time graph showing two successive voltage steps that have been superimposed. When the reference voltage is stepped from resting potential to a hyperpolarized value (2), there is very little change in membrane current. However, when the reference voltage is stepped from resting potential to a depolarized value (1), there is first an inward current flow and then an outward current flow.

maintained outward ionic current (figure 12.7). They went on further to show that the inward current is carried by Na^+ ions. The membrane conductance to Na^+ first increases, by a process known as *activation,* and then decreases, by a process known as *inactivation.* The outward current is carried by K^+ ions, as a result of increased membrane conductance to K^+ on depolarization because of an *activation* process. Their further analysis revealed the time and voltage dependencies of sodium activation and inactivation and potassium activation. With this information, they were able to reconstruct the sequence of conductance changes that underlies the action potential.

Sodium channels are a destabilizing membrane element because their gates open when the sensor measures a depolarization and the resultant Na^+ influx discharges the membrane capacitance and leads to more depolarization. Such a *positive feedback cycle* underlies much of the all-or-nothing nature of the action potential. This phenomenon is called the *Hodgkin cycle* (figure 12.8). Sodium

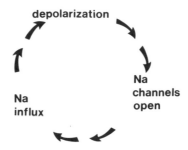

Figure 12.8
The positive feedback Hodgkin cycle. This cycle is initiated by an externally applied depolarization that can come from, for example, an electrical stimulator, local circuit currents from an adjacent excited region of the membrane, or stimulus activated channels in a sensory receptor.

channels have a second voltage sensor that closes another gate when the sensor measures a depolarization. This process is called *sodium inactivation*. The kinetics of this gate are enough slower than those of the activation gate so that the sodium channel first opens and then closes following a depolarization of the membrane.

There is no threshold in the stochastic probability of channel opening. However, when the destabilizing sodium channel activation process predominates over the stabilizing potassium channel process, the positive feedback nature of the array of sodium channels takes over and an action potential is initiated. Threshold is thus a membrane and not a channel phenomenon.

Potassium channel gating is also dependent on a voltage sensor that causes gates to open on depolarization. Potassium gating kinetics are, however, slower than those of sodium channels. Thus, following the depolarizing drive initiated by the opening of sodium channels, there is a repolarizing drive due to potassium channel opening. The increased potassium channel opening also underlies the afterhyperpolarization of the membrane after an action potential.

The period of sodium channel inactivation and potassium channel activation following the peak of an action potential delimits a time of decreased membrane excitability. This time is known as the *refractory period*. The initial preponderance of *inactivated* sodium channels prevents any reexcitation. During this time, the membrane is said to be *absolutely refractory*. There follows a period when most of the sodium channels have recovered from being inactivated but there are still an excess of open potassium channels. During this time, the membrane is excitable, but a larger stimulus is necessary to reach threshold. The membrane is then said to be *relatively refractory.*

12.9.* Problem: The nervous system uses a firing rate code for long-distance transmission. We can calculate the upper limit of the rate available in this code. The action potential is about 1 msec in duration, and this is followed by an absolute refractory period of another millisecond. What is the maximum frequency of action potentials for a stimulus great enough to overcome all the relative refractoriness of the membrane?

The auditory system is sensitive to sound pressure waves over the range of 20 to 20,000 Hz. How much of this frequency range might be encoded directly by a pulse rate signal on an individual fiber? Can the auditory nerve function by a direct transmission of input frequencies? What other means does it employ?

These descriptions of channel characteristics explain, at the single channel level, the model of membrane conductances invoked by Hodgkin and Huxley to explain the action potential. Sodium conductance rises as the result of a depolarizing stimulus until it just exceeds the resting potassium conductance (threshold). The positive feedback nature of the Hodgkin cycle causes the depolarizing drive toward the sodium equilibrium potential (overshoot). A combination of inactivation of the sodium conductance and the rising potassium conductance forces the membrane potential back toward the potassium equilibrium potential and, in fact, can hold it transiently more hyperpolarized than at rest (afterhyperpolarization) (figure 12.9).

We can now explain the process of *accommodation* that was introduced in chapter 2. This form of decreased excitability occurs when a depolarizing stimulus is applied slowly. Since all sodium channels proceed through the sequence of first activation and then inactivation, a slow depolarization will cause inactivation of some sodium channels to occur before enough sodium channels have opened to bring the membrane to threshold. Thus threshold is not a fixed potential, but is dependent on both the level and the rate of change of the stimulus.

Two previously mentioned phenomena combine to show just how efficient this mechanism of excitation is.

1. The effect of the charge of an ion in solution is much more significant than is that ion's effect on concentration. Thus only a small fraction of the ions that are

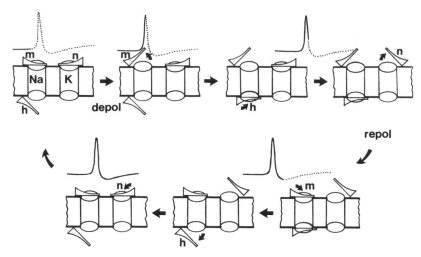

Figure 12.9
Schematic representation of the sequence of channel gating movements during an action potential. The *m* and *h* gates are associated with the sodium channel and the *n* gates with the potassium channel. Depolarization increases the probability that *m* and *n* gates will be open and that *h* gates will be closed, Repolarization increases the probability that *m* and *n* gates will be closed and that *h* gates will be open. *m* gates have the fastest kinetics and will be the first ones to move in response to a potential change; *n* gates have intermediate kinetics, while *n* gates have the slowest kinetics. It is important to realize that this is a very schematic representation of just two representative channels. Movements of the various gates overlap in time and are stochastic, and the gates are much more of an integral part of the channel molecule than is suggested here.

unequally distributed across a cell membrane need move to produce the change in potential that occurs during an action potential.

2. Each channel can process a large number of ions in a short time. Thus only a sparse distribution of channels is necessary, and, even then, they need be open for only a short time in order for an action potential to occur.

12.10.* Problem: If a sodium channel passes 1 pA of current, how many channels per square micrometer are necessary to change the membrane potential by 100 mV in 1 msec?

12.11.* Problem: The extracellular surface of most cell membranes is negatively charged. At normal calcium concentrations, these surface charges are negated by a shielding layer of Ca^{2+} ions. The voltage sensor senses a field that is affected by the net surface charge on the membrane. Hypocalcemia (low extracellular Ca^{2+}) causes an increase in excitability of neurons. Explain the clinical symptoms of hypocalcemia based on the surface charge effect of divalent ions.

Local current flow permits action potentials to propagate along long fibers.

Since action potentials are pulses in a rate code, their function is important in the transmission of information from one place to another in the nervous system. Much of the nervous system's signaling occurs either over very short distances or in a much more diffuse manner and makes use of electrical and chemical phenomena other than an action potential-dependent frequency code. However, for those specifically directed, long-distance, transmission chores such as bringing sensory information from the periphery, sending motor information to the periphery, or communicating over distances greater than a few millimeters within the central nervous system, the transmission of action potentials along nerves is essential.

The propagation of action potentials depends on three basic properties of electricity that have already been introduced.

1. Current always flows between any two regions of unlike charge.

2. Ohm's law ($E = I/G$) dictates that a change of current flowing across the cell membrane always changes the potential across that membrane. If an action potential has occurred at one site on an axon, it will set up *local circuit currents* that flow to other sites where the membrane is in the resting state. When this current flows in the appropriate direction across an unexcited area of membrane, it will depolarize that membrane and initiate an action potential there.

3. Current always flows in a complete circuit. Current flowing between regions of differing charge inside the axon must flow across the membrane and then must flow back through the extracellular solution to the region of initial excitation (figure 12.10).

Neurons conduct action potentials over considerable distances as a continuous propagated wave of excitation. Local currents bring adjacent regions of the membrane to threshold so that each region of the membrane passes successively through excitation, and then refractoriness. There is no degradation of the propagated action potential because each membrane region provides energy, in the

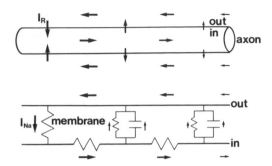

Figure 12.10
Local circuit current flow in an unmyelinated fiber. The top figure shows current flow in a
section of axon that is excited (inward I_R) at its left end. The current flows longitudinally to
the right inside the axon and causes an outward capacitive current that reduces the charge on
the membrane capacitance at adjacent nonexcited regions. The lower figure is the circuit
representation of the membrane of this axon with the inward resistance current as a Na current.
This circuit differs from that in figure 12.3D in that the resistance of the external solution is
considered small enough to be negligible. Why is the external resistance much smaller than the
longitudinal internal resistance?

form of a locally maintained concentration gradient, to the passing action potential. This is a very effective, albeit slower, means of propagation than is obtained
by electrotonic spread of potential.

**Saltatory conduction provides rapid, efficient conduction of action potentials over relatively small
diameter fibers.**

Certain axons are capable of faster and more efficient conduction because of
specialized nonneuronal, glial cells. In the central nervous system these cells are
oligodendrocytes, and in the peripheral nervous system they are Schwann cells.
In both cases they wrap repeatedly around the axon, forming a coating that is
many cell membranes thick. Periodically there is a break in this *myelin sheath*.
These breaks are known as *nodes of Ranvier,* and at them the axon membrane
is, at least electrically, exposed to the extracellular medium (see figures 2.2 and
2.6).

12.12.* Problem: Calculate the voltage as it falls along a frog nerve fiber away
from the source of a constant applied voltage. To estimate the bounds for the

Table 12.1
Nerve Fiber Electrical Properties

	Mechanical values
Core diameter	10 μm
Myelin thickness	2 μm
Distance between nodes	2 mm
Width of node	0.7 μm
Thickness of membrane	8 nm
	Resistance and conductance values
Core resistance	140 MΩ/cm of length
Membrane conductance	290 mS/cm of length
Myelin conductance	3.5 mS/cm of length
Node resistance	50 MΩ per node
	Capacitance values
Membrane capacitance	160 pF/cm of length
Myelin capacitance	12 pF/cm of length
Node capacitance	1 pF per node
	Voltage values
Membrane resting voltage	−70 mV
Applied voltage	+20 mV

answer, calculate values first with no myelin and second with a continuous myelin sheath. Table 12.1 gives some useful values for properties of a frog nerve fiber [from Rall (1977) in the *Handbook of Physiology*].

One can approach this calculation in two manners. A numeric approximation, based on a ladder network, can be calculated using small steps of distance along the fiber (e.g., <0.5 mm). Alternatively one can derive a differential equation for the voltage as a function of distance and source voltage and then solve the equation for the local voltage at any distance. In either case, the external resistance is needed. One can estimate this value by assuming a cross section of external solution of 1 mm^2 with a longitudinal resistance of 0.01% of the internal resistance. A proper calculation of external resistance is complex and depends on the geometry and electrolyte composition of the space surrounding the nerve fiber.

12.13. Problem: One interesting characteristic of an action potential propagated along a myelinated axon can be derived by repeating the calculation from problem 10.5. Assume that the action potential is conducted at 100 m/sec and has a duration of 1 msec. How many nodes of Ranvier participate in this action potential at any instant in time?

The myelin sheath provides a means of directing the current flow from an excited locus to successive nodes of Ranvier that are specialized regions of excitability because they have high densities of sodium channels and only a few potassium channels. The action potential jumps from one node to the next in a discontinuous manner. This type of conduction is called *saltatory conduction* after the Latin word, *saltare,* meaning to dance or to leap. It is important to keep in mind that although the membrane potential change may be spatially discontinuous, there is a continuous flow of current from one node of Ranvier to the next. Saltatory conduction over myelinated fibers has two notable advantages over propagation on unmyelinated fibers: (1) Local circuit currents flow at a greater distance and thus speed conduction of the action potential wave. (2) Since Na^+ influx is limited to specific small regions of the membrane, there is a decrease in Na^+ influx per action potential and thus in the metabolic cost of signaling.

A more accurate description of a myelinated or unmyelinated axon must include the capacitance of the lipid bilayer. The membrane can be approximated as a series of independent, but adjacent patches, each of which supports both resistive and capacitive current flow. The number of open sodium channels at an excited region of an axon determines the current density of the inward ionic current. This current then flows down the axon cylinder and outward across the capacitor of unexcited regions of the membrane. The density of the outward capacitive current determines how large a region of membrane capacitance is discharged and how much depolarization occurs. As the current flows out through ion channels and across the membrane capacitance of each patch, there is less remaining of the initial current for the next patch.

Conduction velocity in unmyelinated axons is limited by the distance ahead of the wave of excitation at which the current is still sufficient to discharge adequately the membrane capacitor (figure 12.11). Myelination increases conduction velocity by decreasing the resistive and capacitive current loss in the patches just ahead of the excitation. The layers of enveloping membrane accomplish this in two ways. Each layer of the membrane has a large, constant resistance (nongated channels) and capacitance (lipid bilayer). The multiple layers of membrane

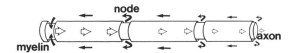

Figure 12.11
Current flow in a myelinated axon. The current flow in a myelinated axon is exactly equivalent to that in the unmyelinated axon in figure 12.10 with the exception that the outward capacitive current occurs almost exclusively at the nodes of Ranvier. Actually the number of nodes of Ranvier that are involved at any instant is considerably greater than that illustrated (see problem 12.13).

produce a series combination of both the resistance and capacitance. Series resistors produce a total resistance greater than any of the individual values, whereas series capacitors produce a total that is less than the smallest of the individual values. Thus myelin causes, in the internodal region, a decrease in resistive current since $I_R = E/R_m$ and a decrease in capacitive current since $I_C = C_m \, dE/dt$. With a decreased current loss to patches in the internodal region, more of the current is left at the appreciable distance of the next node.

12.14.* Problem: Multiple sclerosis and Guillain-Barré syndrome are diseases in which axons become demyelinated. It is observed that some of these patients experience a decrease in function when they are placed in a warm therapy pool. Can you explain this observation based on what you know about saltatory conduction? A possibly useful piece of information is that an increase in temperature decreases the action potential duration.

We have discussed, in this chapter, the stereotypic pulse of excitable cells, the action potential. These pulses are used by the nervous system as time markers in a repetitive rate code. Information is transmitted from point to point by the propagation of groups of action potentials over nerve axons. We are at the exciting juncture of beginning to understand, at a molecular level, how excitable membranes generate action potentials.

Chapter 13

Chemical Effectors

Until the latter half of the nineteenth century, it was assumed that neurons formed a continuous network and that this network was also continuous with muscles. The extensive histological work of Santiago Ramon y Cajal before the turn of this century established that neurons were separate, distinct entities. This debate is summarized in the book *Neuron Theory or Reticular Theory* by Cajal (1908). The existence of separate neurons implies that some specialized communication must occur between cells. Sir Charles Sherrington, in 1897 called this region a *synapse*, deriving the term from the Greek words συν—together and απτειν—to touch. The basis of synaptic communication forms the major topic of this chapter.

Most cell-to-cell communication results when a presynaptic cell releases a neurotransmitter that acts on a postsynaptic cell.

The physiologist Emil Du Bois Reymond set the stage for decades of debate about the nature of intracellular communication with the following statement written in 1875. "Of the presently known natural processes that could mediate excitation, I can only see two that are worth considering. Either there must be an irritating secretion such as ammonium, lactic acid or another violently exciting substance at the boundary of the contractile elements of muscle; or the effect must be electrical." His choice of the chemical substance was wrong, but he was absolutely correct in implying that transmission of information from one cell to another requires either a specialized chemical process or a specialized electrical contact.

The physiological investigations of the late nineteenth and early twentieth centuries were directed mainly toward finding an electrical means by which information could be transferred between cells. As early as 1904, T.R. Elliott suggested that liberation of adrenaline by nerves might serve as a means of communication between cells. The beginnings of the acceptance of chemical transmission are often associated with the work of Otto Loewi in the 1920s. The idea for an experiment using frog hearts came to Loewi in a dream and although he awoke and took some notes on the idea, he could not decipher the notes the next morning. On the following night he again had the dream and this time arose at 3 A.M. and went to the laboratory to do the experiment. His experiments showed that the vagus nerve to the heart released a chemical, *Vagusstoff,* that could affect cardiac muscle cells by slowing their firing. Sir Henry Dale identified *Vagusstoff* as the neurotransmitter acetylcholine. He went on to identify some nerves, which he named *cholinergic,* that were capable of releasing acetylcholine; and other nerves, which he named *adrenergic,* that were capable of releasing adrenaline. Even by 1936, when Loewi and Dale received the Nobel Prize for their work on chemical transmission, considerable debate continued. Some physiologists, including R. Beutner, R. Gesell, B. Katz, and D. Nachmanshon, accepted the existence of chemical mediators of information transfer between neurons and between nerves and muscles, whereas many others did not. Sir John Eccles was one of those who did not accept the idea of chemical transmission and he continued for about 10 years to explain his results based on electrical interactions between neurons. Eventually the evidence for chemical transmission became overwhelming and as Eccles wrote, "around 1945 it became clear to me (although I did not want to admit this in public) that my hypothesis was in bad shape" (Kodahl and Issekutz, 1966, p. 446). Eccles' subsequent work on chemical transmission led to a Nobel Prize for him in 1963.

It is now apparent that sometimes there is also electrical communication between cells. Many neurons in invertebrates communicate through direct electrical connections, as do certain cells in the retina of vertebrates, and as do cardiac and smooth muscle cells. A very important means of communication between cells is, however, by a chemical that is released by an initial *presynaptic* neuron and whose presence is sensed by a second *postsynaptic* cell. Because of the size and accessibility of the neuromuscular synapse, many details of chemical synaptic transmission were determined at this specialized structure. We will begin our discussion of chemical effectors with a discussion of the neuromuscular synapse and then go on to discuss other types of synaptic action.

The neuromuscular junction is a highly specialized region of contact between a motor nerve and a muscle fiber.

The neuromuscular synapse, or *neuromuscular junction,* is a specialized region of contact between a single nerve fiber and a muscle fiber. We need to point out some notable features of this region before discussing its function. First, the postsynaptic muscle cell is considerably larger than the presynaptic nerve ending. Typically, the muscle will have a diameter 100 times as great as that of the nerve fiber. Second, although the pre- and postsynaptic cells do not have cytoplasmic continuity, they are so closely juxtaposed that the actual *synaptic cleft* is only about 500 Å. Third, the postsynaptic membrane forms a relatively large area of contact because it exhibits extensive folding into the muscle cell. Finally, the presynaptic terminal is specialized in that it contains many *synaptic vesicles* that are congregated in *active zones* adjacent to the folds of the postsynaptic membrane; and it contains many mitochondria, organelles associated with metabolic activity (figure 13.1).

In vertebrates, decisions regarding muscle contraction are made in the central nervous system and not in the periphery. That is, whenever a motoneuron in the spinal cord fires an action potential, the muscle fibers on which it has synaptic contact invariably fire action potentials and subsequently contract. The problem of neuromuscular transmission is then reliably to bring the postsynaptic membrane to threshold each time an action potential arrives at the presynaptic terminal. Electrical propagation to the presynaptic ending occurs, as we saw in chapter 12, when an excited region of membrane provides adequate local current to excite an adjacent region of membrane. The size differential between nerve fibers and muscle fibers is not conducive to such local current excitation of the postsynaptic muscle. The small nerve fiber can produce only a small current density, whereas the large muscle fiber requires a large amount of current to depolarize it to threshold level.

13.1.* Problem: Calculate the current that a presynaptic nerve can supply and the current required to bring a muscle fiber to threshold. Values of the current supplied by the nerve can be calculated since an action potential will produce about 1 mA/cm^2 of current and the typical area of a neuromuscular junction is around 2×10^{-5} cm^2. The necessary current in the muscle fiber can be calculated from Ohm's law taking the total resistance to current supplied at a point to be 40 kΩ and the requisite depolarization as 40 mV (assuming $E_m = -90$ mV and $E_{thresh} = -50$ mV).

Some means are required at the neuromuscular junction to amplify the energy of the presynaptic current to an amount adequate for postsynaptic excitation. Chemical transmission provides this necessary amplification.

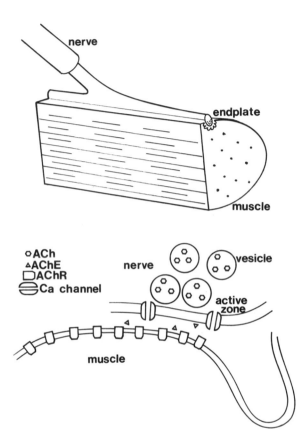

Figure 13.1
The neuromuscular junction. This schematic figure shows the junction of a nerve fiber with a muscle fiber and a detailed view of the opposing pre- and postsynaptic membranes. There are several morphological features of this motor endplate that are important to its function. (1) The cross sectional area of the nerve is considerably smaller than that of the muscle. (2) The actual synaptic cleft between pre- and postsynaptic cells is only about 500 Å. (3) The postsynaptic membrane has a relatively large surface area and contains acetylcholine-gated channels where it opposes the active zone of the nerve. (4) The presynaptic terminal has many synaptic vesicles and has voltage-gated calcium channels in its membrane. ACh, acetylcholine; AChE, acetylcholinesterase, the enzyme that hydrolyzes acetylcholine; AChR, acetylcholine-gated channel (receptor), a ligand-gated channel.)

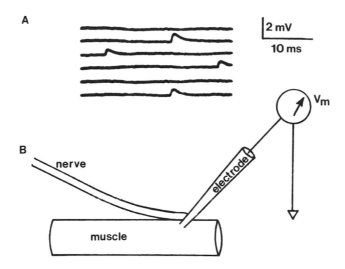

Figure 13.2
Miniature endplate potentials (mepps). Small spontaneous depolarizations (A) are recorded in the endplate region of muscle fiber (B). These potential fluctuations occur randomly and are always in multiples of a quantal unit of about 1 mV. (Records from a mammalian motor endplate recorded by Liley, 1956.)

Even when it is not conducting action potentials, the presynaptic nerve releases quanta of neurotransmitter that produce small depolarizations of the postsynaptic cell.

In the early 1950s, Paul Fatt and Sir Bernard Katz (1951, 1952) made several important observations about the mechanisms of synaptic transmission from their experiments using the neuromuscular junction of the frog. The first of these observations was that the postsynaptic membrane undergoes rapid, small depolarizations even when the presynaptic nerve is not being stimulated. The small, spontaneous depolarizations of the postsynaptic membrane were consistently about 1 mV in amplitude and lasted a few milliseconds. They were observed only when the recording was made near the neuromuscular junction. These small fluctuations are called *miniature endplate potentials,* or *mepps*. Mepps were found to be the result of the spontaneous release of *quanta* of neurotransmitter from the presynaptic terminal and are a common feature of a multitude of types of neuromuscular junctions (figure 13.2).

Mepps may represent simply an inadequate control of the neurotransmitter release mechanisms so that occasionally neurotransmitter is released without a presynaptic action potential. However, the presynaptic nerve has important effects on the muscle fiber other than just excitation. If the presynaptic nerve is cut, that is, the muscle fiber is *denervated,* two important consequences follow. First, the neurotransmitter receptors that are generally localized strictly on the postsynaptic membrane immediately opposite to the presynaptic terminal become dispersed over the whole surface of the muscle fiber. Second, the muscle fiber will eventually atrophy. The mepps may play a role in preventing these two consequences of denervation from occurring.

In the presence of Ca^{2+}, presynaptic action potentials initiate the release of a large number of quanta of neurotransmitter.

A second important observation made by Fatt and Katz was that Ca^{2+} is crucial for successful neuromuscular transmission. If the Ca^{2+} concentration in the solution bathing the neuromuscular junction is reduced, the size of the postsynaptic response to a presynaptic action potential is similarly diminished. At low concentrations of Ca^{2+}, the size of the postsynaptic response falls to small number multiples of the amplitude of the mepp. Thus the quantum that constitutes the spontaneous miniature endplate potential is also the quantum unit underlying the normal postsynaptic response, the *endplate potential* or *epp* (figure 13.3).

Of particular interest is that at low Ca^{2+} concentrations, the amplitudes of the now drastically reduced endplate potentials can be predicted by a Poisson distribution. The Poisson distribution, which is a special case of a binomial distribution, states that

$$\frac{n_x}{N} = e^{-m} \frac{m^x}{x!}$$

where n_x is the number of responses containing x quanta, N is the total number of observed responses, and m is the average number of quanta per response, the *mean quantal content*.

J. del Castillo and Bernard Katz (1954) showed that two, independent measurements, in low Ca^{2+}, give the same value for the mean quantal content. One way to determine m is simply to divide the mean amplitude of an epp by the mean amplitude of a mepp. A second way to determine m is to count the number

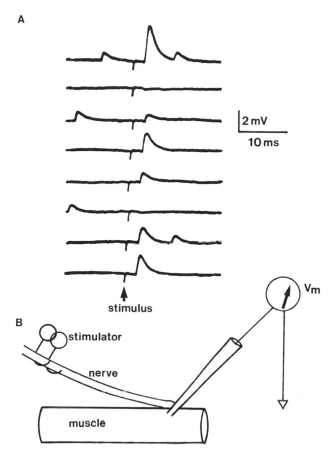

Figure 13.3
Distribution of endplate potentials. As in figure 13.2, small quantal potential fluctuations are recorded independent of any stimulation to the presynaptic nerve (B). Responses in quantal increments of amplitude (A) are observed when the nerve fiber is stimulated (↑) while the neuromuscular junction is made less responsive by being bathed in a low Ca^{2+} solution. (Records from a mammalian motor endplate recorded by Liley, 1956.)

of times that presynaptic stimulation causes no postsynaptic response. The Poisson distribution predicts a certain number of failures, i.e., those cases of $x = 0$. For this condition, the Poisson distribution simplifies to

$$\frac{n_o}{N} = e^{-m}$$

or

$$m = \ln \frac{N}{n_0}$$

Under a variety of conditions, m calculated by these two independent techniques agrees well, thereby supporting the Poisson nature of neurotransmitter release. The implications of the Poisson nature of neurotransmitter release are that the release of any one quantum occurs with low probability and is independent of the release of any other quantum. A single presynaptic action potential, at a neuromuscular junction bathed in a normal Ca^{2+} concentration, causes the simultaneous release of about 300 quanta out of a large reserve supply.

The coupling between depolarization of the membrane of the presynaptic terminal and the release of synaptic vesicles is accomplished by a rise in intracellular Ca^{2+} concentration.

We saw, in chapter 11, the importance of Ca^{2+} in regulating the effector functions of the nervous system. An important example is *excitation-secretion coupling* in which an electrical signal causes a neuron to release some chemical substance. For the neuromuscular junction, the chemical substance is the neurotransmitter acetylcholine. We will discuss other types of excitation-secretion coupling later in this chapter and we will see that they all depend on Ca^{2+} influx into the secretory neuron. This *calcium hypothesis* originated in the work of Katz and his colleagues. Although it is generally accepted today, several aspects of the underlying mechanisms are not entirely understood.

The Ca^{2+} concentration within the presynaptic terminal is normally maintained at the low level of 10^{-8} to 10^{-7} M. Voltage-dependent calcium channels are present in the presynaptic terminal with a density of around 10 channels/μm^2. These channels are most likely concentrated near the active zone where the synaptic vesicles lie. Because of the slow kinetics of both activation and inactivation gating, the calcium channel remains open for a relatively long time. Thus a single presynaptic action potential may permit an increase of the intracellular Ca^{2+} concentration, at least locally, by around 20-fold.

Excitation–secretion coupling consists of the following three steps (figure 13.4):

1. Voltage-dependent presynaptic calcium channels open in response to a presynaptic action potential.

2. Consequently, there is a rise in intracellular Ca^{2+} concentration that is probably greatest in the region of the active zone.

3. Ca^{2+} activates intracellular processes that promote movement of synaptic vesicles to the presynaptic membrane and their fusion with that membrane followed by release of the vesicular contents into the synaptic cleft.

Ca^{2+} plays a role in two processes that are necessary for the release of neurotransmitter from the presynaptic terminal. First, vesicles are made available to their active site by a Ca^{2+}-dependent protein called synapsin. Second, the available vesicles fuse with the presynaptic membrane through the action of other Ca^{2+}-dependent proteins. When the vesicles fuse with the membrane, their contents are released by *exocytosis* into the synaptic cleft.

13.2.* Clinical Problem: Lambert-Eaton myasthenic syndrome is an autoimmune disease where the target of the immune attack is calcium channels in the presynaptic membrane. Patients with this disorder have a significant reduction in functional calcium channels. What would you expect the symptoms of this disease to be? What types of treatment might you propose?

While the nature of the presynaptic intracellular sites of Ca^{2+} action is not entirely understood, considerable research is currently addressing this question and some interesting possibilities are being investigated. Ca^{2+} might interact directly with certain phospholipid molecules in the membrane of the synaptic vesicles or Ca^{2+} might activate specific ion channels in the vesicular membrane. Ca^{2+} might act through a specific receptor site on a molecule such as calmodulin or troponin C. Ca^{2+} might activate a protein kinase and have its effect through the resultant phosphorylation of some protein molecule. Whatever the intermediate step, it can amplify significantly the presynaptic electrical signal. In experiments in which the extracellular Ca^{2+} concentration has been varied, there can be as much as a fourth power relationship between Ca^{2+} concentration and neurotransmitter release.

A

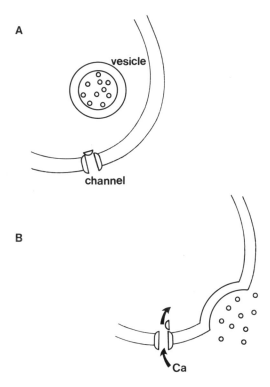

Figure 13.4
Excitation-secretion coupling. Voltage-gated calcium channels in the presynaptic membrane (A) increase their probability of being open when the presynaptic terminal is depolarized by an action potential. These open calcium channels allow a transient Ca^{2+} influx (B) that promotes fusion of the synaptic vesicles with the presynaptic membrane and subsequent exocytosis of neurotransmitter into the synaptic cleft.

Although counterarguments need still be taken seriously, the synaptic quanta probably can be associated with synaptic vesicles. Such a conclusion is certainly parsimonious with several experimental observations. Acetylcholine can be supplied directly to the neuromuscular junction from a dilute solution contained in a micropipette. If the application time is short and if the solution is sufficiently dilute, a postsynaptic depolarization resembling a mepp can be produced. Since in these experiments the concentration of acetylcholine is known, one can calculate the amount required to produce a depolarization equivalent to a mepp. Such calculations yield a quantum content of about 10^4 molecules of acetylcholine. This amount of acetylcholine is consistent with the amount that is thought to be contained within a single synaptic vesicle.

13.3.* Problem: Calculate the number of molecules of acetylcholine (ACh) present in a synaptic vesicle if the diameter of the vesicle is 500 Å (500×10^{-10} m) and the concentration within the vesicle is 150 mM. Can you think of any means by which to estimate the concentration of acetylcholine within a synaptic vesicle?

Another piece of evidence supporting the vesicular hypothesis of quantum release is that when synaptic vesicles are separated from the other subcellular organelles of neurons, the vesicles are found to contain a high concentration of acetylcholine. Finally, the venom of the black widow spider is known to release neurotransmitter from the presynaptic terminal. When black widow spider venom-treated terminals are studied under the electron microscope, they are found to have fewer synaptic vesicles.

Neurotransmitter is released from the presynaptic terminal in quantum units. It is most probable that these quantum units represent the contents of single vesicles containing neurotransmitter. A miniature endplate potential represents the spontaneous release of a single vesicle, whereas the endplate potential represents the approximately simultaneous release of many vesicles in response to a presynaptic action potential.

Acetylcholine initiates electrical events in skeletal muscle cells by binding to ligand-gated channels in the postsynaptic membrane.

Once the acetylcholine diffuses the short distance across the synaptic cleft it binds to specific molecular receptors on the postsynaptic membrane. These receptors make up part of a complex protein molecule that also forms an ion channel. These nicotinic acetylcholine-gated channels represent a vast and important class of *ligand-gated channels* (or *receptors*). These channels are distinct from the voltage-gated channels discussed in chapter 12 in that they are not influenced by the voltage gradient across the membrane but only by the presence of a specific ligand molecule.

The acetylcholine-gated channel molecules are very densely concentrated in the postsynaptic membrane of the neuromuscular junction. Some estimates place the number of these molecules as high as 10^4 μm^2. (Compare this with the density of sodium channels in nerve membrane or the density of calcium channels in the presynaptic membrane.) This high density of channels provides many receptor sites for the acetylcholine molecules that are released into the synaptic cleft and it also makes possible the large ionic current flow into the postsynaptic cell when the channel gates open.

13.4.* Problem: What is the gain of the neuromuscular junction? The postsynaptic current that flows following the release of a single quantum carries about 5×10^{-12} C of charge. If a quantum contains 10^4 monovalent acetylcholine molecules, what is the maximum "gain" of charge transfer resulting from chemical transmission at the neuromuscular junction? What did you assume about the stoichiometry of acetylcholine's postsynaptic action?

Molecular genetic techniques have provided considerable information about the structure of the nicotinic acetylcholine-gated channel at the neuromuscular junction. This molecule is a pentapeptide with four distinct subunits, one being repeated twice. Each subunit is capable of spanning the cell membrane and at least four of them do so. The space between the membrane-spanning subunits forms an aqueous pore through the membrane when acetylcholine is bound to specific receptor regions of the molecule. The amino acid sequence of each subunit has been determined using cDNA cloning techniques. When comparison is made of the amino acid sequence of the acetylcholine-gated channel derived from several species, it is seen to be a highly conserved molecule.

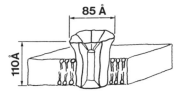

Figure 13.5
Dimensions of the nicotinic acetylcholine-gated channel. Molecular biological techniques have provided considerable information about the structure of the nicotinic acetylcholine-gated channel. The channel is a pentapeptide with units, $\alpha_2\beta\gamma\delta$. The α units are the part of the molecule that acts as receptors for two acetylcholine molecules. When acetylcholine is present the molecule forms a membrane-spanning water-filled pore that is nonselective among many monovalent cations.

Nicotinic acetylcholine-gated channels open following the binding of two acetylcholine molecules to binding sites that are part of the channel molecule.

The ability to record the current through single channels has made it possible to elucidate many details about the kinetics of acetylcholine-gated channels at the neuromuscular junctions of skeletal muscles (figure 13.5). (These acetylcholine-gated channels are called *nicotinic* acetylcholine-gated channels because of their sensitivity to nicotine and are distinguished from a second quite different group of acetylcholine-gated channels that are sensitive to muscarine and are therefore called *muscarinic* acetylcholine-gated channels.) It is now known that the nicotinic acetylcholine-gated channel's gate opens when two acetylcholine molecules are present on the receptor sites of the molecule. The gate subsequently closes, dependent on kinetics intrinsic to the protein molecule, that is, it is not the result of simple diffusion of the acetylcholine molecules away from their receptor sites.

Figure 13.6 shows the kinetic scheme for acetylcholine-gated channel opening. When two acetylcholine molecules have bound to their receptor sites, the channel is in a permissive state for opening. This initial binding reaction is extremely rapid so that free acetylcholine comes rapidly into equilibrium with channels in the permissive channel state. Channels make the transition from the permissive state to the open state with a rate that is dependent on structural changes in the channel protein. Similarly, channels close to the permissive state based on the kinetics inherent in the structural change of the channel protein. Since the concentration of acetylcholine in the synaptic cleft has meanwhile rapidly fallen, the

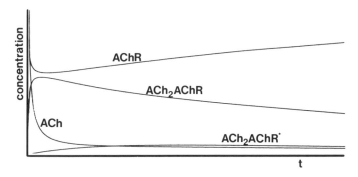

Figure 13.6
Nicotinic acetylcholine-gated channel kinetics. The interaction of acetylcholine with its receptor follows the following kinetic scheme:

$$2\ ACh + AChR \rightleftharpoons ACh_2AChR \rightleftharpoons ACh_2AChR*$$
$$\downarrow (AChE)$$
$$2\ A + 2\ Ch$$

The following abbreviations are used in this scheme: ACh, acetylcholine; AChR, nicotinic acetylcholine receptor (acetylcholine-gated channel); AChE, acetylcholinesterase; A, acetate; Ch, choline; ACh_2AChR and ACh_2AChR*, the closed and open form of the acetylcholine-gated channel, respectively. The graph above shows the calculated time course for concentrations of the various molecules in this scheme for one set of kinetic rate constants.

equilibrium condition dictates a rapid removal of the acetylcholine from their receptor sites. The limiting step in this process is the kinetics inherent in the channel protein molecule and thus the decay of the postsynaptic response depends more on channel kinetics and than on acetylcholine concentration.

Nicotinic acetylcholine-gated channels are nonselective among many small cations.

An important factor in characterizing nicotinic acetylcholine-gated channels is a determination of their ionic selectivity. Since we know that the endplate potential is excitatory (depolarizing), one would anticipate that the potential predicted by the Goldman-Hodgkin-Katz equation for the open channels would be more depolarized than the resting potential. In fact this potential is approximately -15 mV.

13.5.* Problem: Use the Goldman-Hodgkin-Katz equation discussed in chapter 11 to calculate the maximum depolarization of an epp. We will assume that the membrane is impermeable to Cl^- and that the open acetylcholine-gated channels have a $P_K = P_{Na}$. Use the concentration values that are given in table 11.1.

Determination of acetylcholine-gated channel selectivity is based on measurements of the potential at which the current through a single open channel reverses direction. This potential (the *reversal potential*) is the point at which there is no driving force on the ions that flow through the channel (figure 13.7). The current through open acetylcholine-gated channels has been found to reverse at a potential around -15 mV. This finding is, on first thought, curious since none of the ions listed in table 11.1 would be expected to have a Nernst equilibrium potential in this range. It would be possible to obtain such a reversal potential if the channel allowed several different ions to pass through it. Apparently the acetylcholine-gated channel is rather nonselective among small cations. Various lines of evidence have led to the conclusion that the acetylcholine-gated channel is a relatively large pore through the membrane. Judging from the diameters of the ions that can pass through it, its most narrow point must be at least a 6.5×6.5 Å. Perhaps this represents a surviving member of an ancient category of nonselective channels from which the more selective Na, K, and Ca channels evolved.

The enzyme acetylcholinesterase is responsible for the rapid degradation of acetylcholine.

The neuromuscular junction contains an enzyme that rapidly depletes the supply of acetylcholine in the synaptic cleft by breaking an acetylcholine molecule down into molecules of acetate and choline. Because this enzyme, *acetylcholinesterase,* acts rapidly, the postsynaptic effect of released acetylcholine is transient.

Acetylcholinesterase, found in very significant concentration in the extracellular matrix of the synaptic cleft, begins enzymatic degradation of acetylcholine immediately on its release. As a result, lateral spread of an individual vesicle's contents is minimized and the highest concentration of acetylcholine is localized on the postsynaptic membrane. The 300 or so quanta released during an epp probably act independently of each other producing punctate chemical stimuli to the postsynaptic receptors. On their release from the postsynaptic receptors, acetylcholine molecules are rapidly degraded and have only a negligible probability of interacting again with another receptor.

Acetylcholine is synthesized in the presynaptic terminal from acetate and choline, and acetylcholinesterase hydrolyzes acetylcholine again into these two

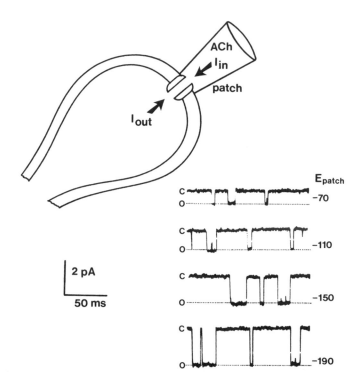

Figure 13.7
The patch clamp technique can be effectively used to measure the current through a single acetylcholine-gated channel. The channel opens and closes in the presence of acetylcholine in a probabilistic manner so that current is suddenly turned on and off. The amplitude of the current through the open channel depends on the potential across the patch of membrane: $I_{channel} = \gamma_{channel} \Delta E_{patch}$ where $I_{channel}$ is the current through a single channel, $\gamma_{channel}$ is the single channel conductance, and ΔE_{patch} is the driving force across the patch for the ions that flow through the channel. As is shown in this record, as the potential is made less hyperpolarized, current amplitude decreases. Although not shown, the current *reverses* at approximately -15 mV. (Records from Hamil et al., 1981.)

molecules. Acetate is a common molecule in the body and is a product of intermediary metabolism; choline, on the other hand, is important in fat metabolism and its level is dependent on dietary input. Choline, at the neuromuscular junction, is conserved by being transported back into the presynaptic terminal where it is subsequently resynthesized into more acetylcholine.

Myasthenia gravis is a disease in which the patients suffer muscle weakness. It has been shown that the cause of the disease is an autoimmune reaction to the acetylcholine-gated channels at the neuromuscular junction. Myasthenia patients have fewer functioning acetylcholine-gated channel molecules. One treatment for the disease is to give the patients antiacetylcholinesterase drugs. Why would these drugs be effective in treating the symptoms of this disease?

Many drugs and toxins are known to have their effects through specific actions at the neuromuscular junction. Some examples from the extensive compendium are *black widow spider venom* that causes release of acetylcholine from its presynaptic stores, *botulinum toxin* (produced by *Clostridium botulinum* in improperly canned food) that blocks the release of acetylcholine, *insecticides* and *nerve gas* that block the action of acetylcholinesterase, and *curare* that binds to the nicotinic acetylcholine-gated channel and prevents acetylcholine from having its effect.

13.6. Problem: Describe the effect that you would expect to observe in an individual who had been poisoned with each of these substances. Might any of these drugs or toxins be useful in the treatment of some pathological condition?

Neuron-to-neuron synaptic transmission uses a multitude of different neurotransmitters whose postsynaptic effects can be excitatory, inhibitory, or modulatory.

Thus far we have considered only the neuromuscular junction in our discussion of synaptic transmission. Although this is perhaps warranted since many details are known about this synapse, synapses between neurons are becoming better and better understood. Acetylcholine is only one of perhaps 50 neurotransmitters that are chemical effectors of the various neurons of the body. Four rather specific requirements have been established to identify a chemical as a neurotransmitter.

1. It must be synthesized by the presynaptic neuron.
2. It must be present in the presynaptic terminals of the neuron.

3. Its application to the postsynaptic neuron must mimic the natural response of transmission at that synapse.

4. There must be a mechanism to remove it from the synapse.

Although all these requirements have been successfully applied to only a few neurotransmitters, many different chemicals have satisfied at least some of the criteria at specific synapses. Strictly speaking, chemicals should be called *putative neurotransmitters* until all the criteria have been established.

There are three general categories of neurotransmitters that fall into a natural hierarchy. The first category includes amino acids, the secondary category includes biogenic amines (e.g., acetylcholine), and the third category includes peptides.

The first category of neurotransmitters includes amino acids. Amino acids, the building blocks of all proteins, are very common in the nervous system. Some amino acids have been shown to function as neurotransmitters and these generally have effects throughout the brain. Most neurons have specific receptors for some of these neurotransmitters and when they respond they do so rapidly. A very common amino acid neurotransmitter is γ-*aminobutyric acid* or *GABA*. This neurotransmitter is found in 25% to 40% of all synapses and its effect is universally one of inhibition of the postsynaptic neuron. Another amino acid, *glutamic acid,* is probably the dominant excitatory neurotransmitter of the brain. One of the receptors for glutamic acid, the *NMDA receptor,* plays an important role in such diverse phenomena as learning and epilepsy.

The second category of neurotransmitters includes biogenic amines. This category includes neurotransmitters that are relatively small molecules containing an amino group. These neurotransmitters are found in lower concentrations than those in the first category and their actions are usually localized to specific regions of the brain. It is these neurotransmitters that are most often associated with specific neurological or psychological states of the individual. *Acetylcholine* is a member of this category that we have already discussed. Another neurotransmitter that was identified early, *norepinephrine,* is also a member of this category. Norepinephrine, among other things, is the neurotransmitter that plays a prominent role in the response to emergency situations.

The third category of neurotransmitters includes many neurally active peptides. The significance of this category of neurotransmitters, the *neuropeptides,* has only recently been appreciated. These neurotransmitters are found in the smallest quantities in the brain and their role is generally one of modulation of synaptic efficacy. The *enkephalins* are prominent examples of this category. These peptides bind to the specific receptors to which the opiate drugs also can bind.

Evidence has recently been accumulating that a gas, nitric oxide, may act as a neurotransmitter. Nitric oxide is not contained in vesicles, it is not released by exocytosis, and it has no specific postsynaptic receptor molecules. It may, however, play an important role in the transmission of information between cells in the brain (see Snyder and Bredt, 1991).

Dale's principle, important in shaping the thinking of neurophysiologists over the last quarter century, was delineated by Eccles et al. (1956) and attributed to the earlier work of Dale. In its simplest form, the principle states that a neuron secretes only one type of neurotransmitter. There is considerable recent evidence that this principle is not valid. Certainly, developing neurons can produce and secrete several different neurotransmitters and they may change neurotransmitter types during development. Mature neurons probably can change the type of neurotransmitter that they release and there is some evidence that neurons can secrete simultaneously more than one type of neurotransmitter.

We saw, in the first part of this chapter, that acetylcholine has a rapid action partly because the enzyme acetylcholinesterase rapidly degrades the available neurotransmitter in the synaptic cleft. Not all synaptic action is terminated by enzymatic degradation of the neurotransmitter. In all synapses, simple diffusion of the neurotransmitter away from the receptor sites is one mechanism of neurotransmitter removal. In some synapses, diffusion appears to be the only mechanism, and, as expected, this results in a slower termination of the synaptic event. In other synapses, a third mechanism of neurotransmitter removal exists, namely specific membrane transport mechanisms pump the neurotransmitter back into the presynaptic terminal or into other adjacent cells.

Chemical synapses are sites of amplification, susceptibility to drugs and toxins, unidirectionality of transmission, and integration of information.

In our discussion of transmission at the neuromuscular junction, we covered three properties of synapses; we now add to this list the fact that synapses are the sites where information is integrated. The skeletal neuromuscular junction is an *obligatory synapse,* that is, each presynaptic action potential initiates enough current through neurotransmitter-gated channels in the postsynaptic cell to guarantee a postsynaptic potential that exceeds threshold. Except for a few special cases, neurons do not behave in this manner. Normally thousands of distinct presynaptic endings synapse on a single postsynaptic neuron each with its own characteristic effectiveness (figure 13.8). Each postsynaptic potential, by itself, is not sufficient to initiate an action potential. Temporal and spatial summation is required at a specialized low threshold region of the neuron called the *axon hillock* for an action potential to be initiated. Sometimes the summed potential can lead not just to a single action potential but to a rapid burst or long train of action potentials. Furthermore, the postsynaptic responses need not always be excitatory.

Excitatory postsynaptic potentials or *EPSPs* result from the action of neurotransmitters that open gated channels for ions whose reversal potential is more depolarized than the resting potential. In fact, this response is similar to the epp that we have already discussed. These channels are frequently nonselective among small cations and the current through these nonselective channels reverses direction when the potential across the membrane is approximately -15 mV. Most EPSPs decay within 10 to 15 msec as do epps, but EPSP amplitude depends on the number and effectiveness of simultaneously activated presynaptic terminals.

Inhibitory postsynaptic potentials or *IPSPs* result from the action of neurotransmitters that open gated channels for ions whose equilibrium potential is near to or more hyperpolarized than the resting potential (figure 13.9). A quick review of table 11.1 will show that the two best candidates for this process are K^+ and Cl^- (although other ions such as HCO_3^- also may be involved).

There are two, somewhat different, mechanisms of generation of inhibitory responses. A neurotransmitter-induced increase in permeability to K^+ will generally cause a hyperpolarization of the membrane potential since the potassium equilibrium potential is invariably more hyperpolarized than the resting potential. The resulting negative-going potential will subtract from the positive-going potentials generated by excitatory synaptic inputs into the neuron. On the other hand, a neurotransmitter-induced increase in permeability to Cl^- will often cause minimal change in the membrane potential since the chloride equilibrium potential is generally very close to the resting potential. The effect of increased Cl^- permeability is also inhibitory in that it increases the tendency for the membrane potential to remain near rest and decreases the effectiveness of excitatory postsynaptic potentials.

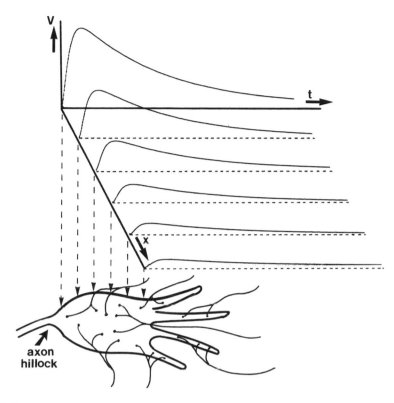

Figure 13.8
Spatial effects of synaptic inputs. This figure shows the time course, *at the axon hillock,* of constant amplitude EPSPs applied at more and more distant locations over the surface of the cell. Note the similarities and differences between this figure and figure 12.4.

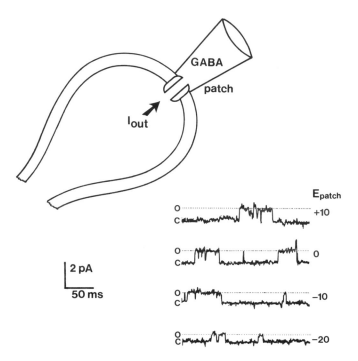

Figure 13.9
This figure is similar to figure 13.7 except that the patch clamp electrode is over a GABA receptor (channel) and the electrode contains GABA instead of acetylcholine. All currents in this record are outward and the current would not reverse until the patch was polarized to about −75 mV. (Records from Bormann et al., 1987.)

Just as is true for neurotransmitter release at the neuromuscular junction, neurotransmitter is released in quantal units at synapses in the central nervous system. Elegant experiments using the patch clamp technique have permitted the direct measurement of quantal effects at both excitatory and inhibitory synapses on neurons. These measurements show that one quantum opens 10–250 postsynaptic ligand-gated channels.

The amino acid γ-aminobutyric acid or GABA is the most prevalent inhibitory neurotransmitter in the brain. Its response is mediated by two types of postsynaptic receptors, GABA$_A$ and GABA$_B$ receptors. GABA$_A$ receptors respond to the presence of the neurotransmitter by opening gates on chloride channels and GABA$_B$ receptors respond by opening gates on potassium channels. The drug Valium has its effect by potentiating the effect of GABA at GABA$_A$ receptors.

13.7.* Problem: Demonstrate the effectiveness of Cl⁻ permeability in preventing the depolarizing effect of an EPSP. Calculate the membrane potential with the Goldman-Hodgkin-Katz equation using the concentrations of Na^+, K^+, and Cl^- given in table 11.1 under the following conditions:

1. At rest with $P_{Na} = P_{Cl} = 0.001 \times P_K$,
2. During an IPSP alone with $P_K = P_{Cl} = 100 \times P_{Na}$,
3. During an EPSP alone with $P_{Na} = P_K = 100 \times P_{Cl}$,
4. During a simultaneous IPSP and EPSP with $P_K = P_{Na} = P_{Cl}$.

Compare especially the effectiveness of the Cl⁻ permeability in altering membrane potential during an IPSP with its effectiveness in altering the amplitude of an EPSP.

The importance of inhibitory postsynaptic effects in the nervous system is dramatically demonstrated by the effects of the drug strychnine. Strychnine causes convulsions with sustained muscle contraction as the result of a general excitation of neurons in the central nervous system. The synaptic effect of strychnine is to block the action of the *inhibitory* neurotransmitter glycine. An important idea demonstrated here is that tonic inhibition is essential in the nervous system to prevent runaway excitation.

Not all synaptic effects are the result of a direct action of a neurotransmitter on a postsynaptic receptor–channel molecule. A very important aspect of the operation of synapses in the function of the nervous system stems from the modulation of synaptic and electrical properties by neurotransmitters.

Recent study has greatly expanded the understanding of those areas of neuronal function that can be modulated by neurotransmitters. We will simply list some examples here with the understanding that they probably represent only a fraction of the realm of neuromodulatory effects in the nervous system. These three are examples of the modulation of firing pattern, the modulation of action potential shape, and the modulation of synaptic efficacy.

1. The simple encoding of stimulus intensity by the repetition rate of action potentials has a limited capability to transfer information. Certainly, temporal patterns of firing are important in encoding within the nervous system. Synaptic

inputs to neurons play an important role in determining temporal firing patterns. One dramatic example of such an effect is the production of bursts of action potentials in a neuron when excitatory and inhibitory inputs alternate. Bursts of action potentials can be more effective in causing neurotransmitter release to the next neuron than would the same number of action potentials fired regularly over the same period.

2. Action potentials have long been considered as time marking pulses in a frequency code but recent evidence has shown that their amplitude and duration can change and that these changes can also have important functional significance. In some important instances, action potential duration is determined by a synaptic input that modulates the intracellular concentration of Ca^{2+}.

13.8.* Questions: Why would a long duration action potential in a presynaptic neuron cause an increased synaptic efficacy? Is a varying duration action potential consistent with the supposition that a neuron can carry only one dimension of information?

3. We have just mentioned one instance where one synapse could affect the efficacy of synaptic transmission at another synapse and there are many other examples. This kind of modulation often occurs when one neuron makes a synaptic contact on the *pre*synaptic terminal of a second neuron where it, in turn, synapses onto a third neuron. The neuron making the presynaptic contact often uses a peptide neurotransmitter to regulate neurotransmitter release by the second neuron.

Presynaptic inhibition occurs because of a reduction of the amount of excitatory neurotransmitter released by the presynaptic neuron.

One of the first examples of neuromodulation that was discovered was *presynaptic inhibition* where a modulatory neuron depresses the amount of excitatory neurotransmitter released by a second neuron. Presynaptic inhibition has some different characteristics from postsynaptic inhibition. It is very selective; that is, it can affect only one of the multitude of excitatory inputs onto a neuron and even then it can only have its effect when the excitatory neuron is active. Presynaptic inhibition lacks any direct effect on the final postsynaptic neuron. Presynaptic inhibition is of longer duration than postsynaptic inhibition, lasting for 100 to 150 msec, and thus can be effective on excitatory inputs that occur over a considerable period (figure 13.10).

Presynaptic inhibition appears to operate through one of two mechanisms. In both cases, the result is a reduction of the release of an *excitatory* neurotransmitter from a second neuron. In some neurons, the presynaptic inhibitory neurotransmitter decreases the amplitude of the depolarization of the presynaptic terminals of the excitatory neuron with a consequent diminution in the number of voltage-gated calcium channels that are opened. In other neurons, the presynaptic inhibitory neurotransmitter has its effect by directly blocking presynaptic calcium channels in the terminal of the excitatory neuron.

Synaptic events can have two different effects in postsynaptic cells.

1. When the membrane potential is significantly different from the equilibrium potential of the postsynaptic conductance change, the EPSP or IPSP produces a potential change that is *additive* with other postsynaptic potential changes.

2a. When the membrane potential is close to the equilibrium potential for the postsynaptic conductance change (generally only possible for IPSPs), the predominant effect is *multiplicitive*, changing the amplitude of other postsynaptic potentials.

2b. In addition, the process of presynaptic inhibition is also a multiplicitive rather than an additive process.

When P is the summed postsynaptic potential, E is the amplitude of an EPSP, I is the amplitude of an IPSP when the membrane potential is different from the equilibrium potential, and i is the multiplicitive effect of an IPSP near its equilibrium potential or of presynaptic inhibition, the three cases above become

$$P = E_1 + E_2 - I_1 - I_2 \tag{1}$$

$$P = i(E_1 + E_2 + E_3) \tag{2a}$$

$$P = iE_1 + E_2 + E_3 \tag{2b}$$

The *gate theory of pain* proposed in 1965 by Ronald Melzack and Patrick Wall invokes presynaptic inhibition for its operation. Here, cutaneous sensory information entering the central nervous system traverses, at its first synapse, a possible locus of presynaptic inhibition. Rubbing or vibration of the skin around a source of pain, or electrical stimulation with a transcutaneous nerve stimulation, TNS, unit selectively stimulates those fibers that produce the presynaptic inhi-

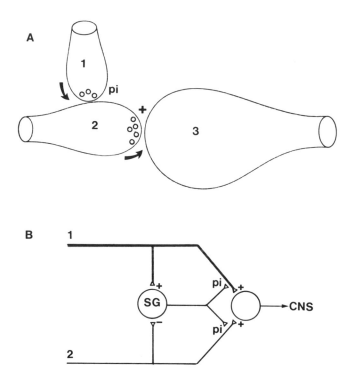

Figure 13.10
Presynaptic inhibition. (A) A generalized scheme for presynaptic inhibition. Neuron 2, when stimulated, releases neurotransmitter that causes an EPSP in postsynaptic neuron 3. The terminal of neuron 2 is, however, itself postsynaptic to neuron 1. If neuron 1 is stimulated slightly before neuron 2, its synaptic action on 2 will cause neuron 2 to release less neurotransmitter with a consequent depression of EPSP amplitude in neuron 3. (B) A classic example of the application of presynaptic inhibition in the gate theory of pain. The cell labeled SG produces presynaptic inhibition of the terminals of afferent fibers 1 (large diameter) and 2 (small diameter) at their first relay neuron to the CNS. A painful stimulus will cause a predominant activity on fiber 2 thereby inhibiting the SG cell and preventing any presynaptic inhibition from occurring. Selective activation of fiber 1 by electrical stimulation or rubbing of the skin will excite the SG cell and lead to presynaptic inhibition of all afferent input to the CNS relay neuron.

bition. Thus, afferent input from nociceptors can be selectively blocked before it can have an excitatory effect in the central nervous system. Some effects of acupuncture may be related to this action.

Second messengers act intracellularly in postsynaptic cells.

Our discussion thus far has centered mainly on instances where the receptor molecule for the neurotransmitter is also an ion channel. These are sometimes called *ionotropic* receptors. In many synapses, the postsynaptic receptor has its effect indirectly through intracellular processes in the postsynaptic cell. Intracellular substances act as another neurotransmitter or *second messenger* to initiate the postsynaptic response. Second messengers introduce the possibility for much greater complexity of synaptic response. One presynaptic neurotransmitter can bind to receptors that affect different second messenger systems and can thereby regulate several postsynaptic ion channels (or other cellular processes). Alternatively, one ion channel can be regulated by the action of any one of several neurotransmitter-receptor systems if the ion channel is sensitive to the effects of several second messengers. One class of indirect effects utilizes *metabotropic receptors* that accomplish intracellular signaling without necessarily involving ion channels. The fine tuning that is possible with indirect synaptic action is a dramatic contrast to the obligatory neuromuscular synapse (figure 13.11).

The patch clamp technique has provided conclusive evidence for the separation of receptor and channel functions at some synapses. The seal formed by the patch clamp pipette onto the surface of the cell is sufficiently tight that neurotransmitter molecules cannot cross it. Sometimes it is found that only if the neurotransmitter is actually included within the pipette is a current measured through ion channels under the tip of the pipette. This type of experiment argues strongly for the existence of a direct synaptic action where the ion channel protein and the neurotransmitter receptor protein are either the same or very closely associated. In other instances, it is found that only when the neurotransmitter is applied outside the pipette is a current measured through ion channels under the tip of the pipette. These experiments argue for an indirect synaptic action where the ion channel protein and the neurotransmitter receptor protein are clearly separated and are coupled intracellularly through second messengers.

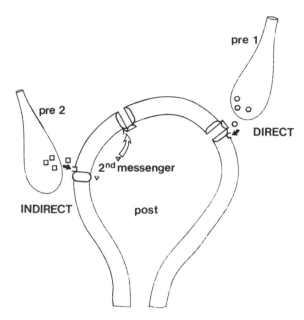

Figure 13.11
Direct and indirect synaptic action. Presynaptic neuron 1 produces a direct action at a post-synaptic channel as in the classic case of the nicotinic acetylcholine-gated channel at the neuromuscular junction. Presynaptic neuron 2, however, has an indirect action on channels in the postsynaptic neuron. Neurotransmitter released from the terminal of 2 binds to a post-synaptic receptor that causes a second messenger to be released or produced in the postsynaptic neuron. It is this second messenger that is responsible for the indirect activation of the post-synaptic channels.

There are many different second messenger systems and we will mention only two of them here: Ca^{2+} and cAMP. We have discussed, on several occasions, the importance of intracellular Ca^{2+} in regulating cellular functions. Most recently we considered its role in excitation-secretion coupling. Ca^{2+} also plays an important role in gating of ion channels or *excitation-gating coupling*. Notably, Ca^{2+} has been shown to affect the gating of certain potassium channels, certain calcium channels, certain chloride channels, and a class of nonspecific cation channels. Several examples now exist where the effect of a neurotransmitter at its receptor is to control the release of intracellular Ca^{2+} and thereby regulate flux through Ca^{2+}-activated ion channels. A second, very important, second messenger system involves the production of the molecule cyclic adenosine monophosphate, cAMP. This molecule is synthesized from the body's paramount energy storage molecule, ATP, by an enzyme that can be either activated or inhibited by the effects of a neurotransmitter. Cyclic nucleotides (cAMP and cGMP) act as second messengers to affect the gating of important ion channels in retinal rods and certain other cells. In addition, the levels of cAMP regulate many cellular functions, one in particular being the phosphorylation of proteins. (See chapter 9 for a short review of protein phosphorylation.) The phosphorylation of ion channel protein molecules can have important modulatory effects on channel function.

In addition to the effects of postsynaptic potentials, neurotransmitters can have a variety of other effects in postsynaptic cells.

We began this chapter with an extensive discussion of the best studied, classic synapse, the neuromuscular junction. We will end the chapter with a consideration of some more diverse actions that chemical effectors can have. As examples we will mention the control of electrical synapses, gene expression, and exocrine cell secretion.

The receptive fields in the retina of the eye have complex forms due, in part, to the interaction, through electrical connections, of adjacent neurons in the retina. These cells also have postsynaptic receptors for the neurotransmitter dopamine. When dopamine is present on its receptors, it acts through a cAMP second messenger system to uncouple the electrical synapses and thus decrease the size of the receptive fields.

The genetic material present in any cell contains the code for all the proteins that are made by the whole organism. Cell specialization arises through the selective expression of only parts of the genetic code contained within the cell. Several examples now exist to show the ability of a neurotransmitter, acting through a postsynaptic receptor, to regulate the level of production of messenger RNA and therefore specific proteins in a cell. In one specific example, the neurotransmitter norepinephrine regulates synthesis of the peptide neurotransmitter, substance P.

The secretory cells of the pancreas have receptors for acetylcholine, norepinephrine, and peptide neurotransmitters. One function regulated by the action of these receptors is the control of intracellular Ca^{2+} levels. The Ca^{2+}, in turn, is capable of controlling the release by the cell of both small ions and secretory proteins.

The comment has been made that we secrete our thoughts. Certainly the release of chemical effectors by neurons and the subsequent action of these chemicals on other cells is a primary action of the nervous system. The diversity of these chemical effectors, and the even greater diversity of their actions, warrants the digression that we have made in this chapter from electricity to chemistry.

Chapter 14

Mechanical Effectors

A major aspect of nervous system function is its physical expression through muscle activity.

Muscle activity results in effects as diverse as the locomotion of the body and the internal movement of substances in the cardiovascular and gastrointestinal systems. Muscle also plays an important role in the control of body heat—as a heat generator, as a regulator of heat loss by controlling skin blood vessels, and, in fur-bearing animals, as a regulator of heat conservation through the movement of individual hairs. If muscle acted only as a simple transducer of nerve signals, it would not be such an important topic of nervous system function. However, muscle is also very much an active processor of neural signals. Mechanical response is certainly strongly dependent on neural drive over an appreciable period of past time, but muscle activity depends almost as much on the mechanical interactions with its load. Much of the processing and combination of signals that determine the motor output of the nervous system occur in the muscle and a study of the functions of the nervous system is incomplete unless the role of muscle is included. Since the modification of information by muscle is closely tied to the mechanism of muscle function, the modification itself becomes part of the functional system. The kinesiological role of muscle was discussed in chapter 7 and this chapter will deal with muscle only as manifest in a free muscle system.

Much of what is known about muscle function was derived from experiments using electrical stimulation. As early as 1791, Galvani discussed muscle as an electrically excitable tissue. He stated: "Now from the experiments performed, this fact emerges without difficulty, that there is a swift and violent excursion of neuro-electric fluid through the muscle to that nerve whereby chiefly muscular contractions and motions are excited." Both Helmholtz and du Bois Reymond, two central figures in nineteenth-century physiology, made extensive quantitative studies of the electrical properties of muscle. However, it was Weber's treatise *Muskelbewegung* (1846) that laid the foundation of most of our current knowledge of muscle as the motor of neural control.

Today muscle is variously studied as an excitable cell with electrotonic properties and ion channels, as a Ca^{2+}-regulated effector that uses chemical energy to produce work and heat, and as a biological machine that operates in thermal-length-velocity-force-impedance space. The other mechanical effectors of the nervous system, cardiac and smooth muscle, react to their neural signals in a way that is distinctly different from that of skeletal muscle. The varieties of both structure and function of smooth and cardiac muscle are more diverse than those of skeletal muscle. Although we concentrate on skeletal muscle in this book, this should not be taken to show a lack of study of cardiac and smooth muscle.

For those with a special interest in muscle and its control, there is a very large ($>10^5$ item) literature base. It is advisable to start with a study of secondary sources such as the *Handbook of Physiology*. One whole volume, *Skeletal Muscle,* in this series has 20 chapters devoted to excitation, the contractile process, and its anatomical substrate. The volume *Motor Control* contains one chapter (Partridge and Benton, 1981) on the motor function of skeletal muscle. Cardiac muscle is treated in some detail in the *Cardiovascular* section and the smooth muscle of the respiratory tract is discussed in the *Respiratory* section. The *Gastrointestinal* section has one whole volume of 31 chapters devoted to structure, excitation, and mechanical function of smooth muscle in different parts of the gastrointestinal system. Other sections of this series treat the smooth muscle of blood vessels, bladder, and uterus. An example of the many specialized monographs on muscle is that by Squire (1990).

The motor unit is the effector unit of neural control in skeletal muscle.

Each individual skeletal muscle contains between 10 and 10^3 independent *motor units* with the individual units composed of one motoneuron and its innervated muscle fibers. The tens to hundreds of fibers of one motor unit are intermixed with those of other motor units within one restricted region of a gross muscle. The fibers of a motor unit may be arranged in a variety of geometric patterns with different directions of action, but the individual fibers of a muscle generally act in a qualitatively similar manner. Muscle fibers fall into different classes based either on their chemical composition or on the resulting differences in speed, force, or fatigue resistance. Individual motor units are generally made up of all the same type of fiber. Gross muscles have characteristic distributions of fiber types that range from purely slow, fatigue-resistant fibers, to purely fast, rapidly fatiguing fibers.

The neurons of a motoneuron pool that drive a particular muscle commonly receive overlapping inputs although impulse firing is separately determined in each neuron. The average firing rate of different motor units fluctuates in a generally parallel manner, although the individual motor units are not synchronized. At high firing rates, the greater probability of an impulse occurring within any period may yield the false impression of synchronized firing.

In contrast to skeletal muscle, neither cardiac nor smooth muscle fibers have individual connections with specific nerve fibers. These classes of muscles often receive two types of innervation, sympathetic and parasympathetic, that rely on different neurotransmitter systems. Cardiac muscle cells and some smooth muscle cells are electrically interconnected whereas other smooth muscle cells operate independently.

The nerve signals that drive skeletal muscles regulate the intensity of response in two ways: by changes in the firing rate of individual motor units and by variation in the number of motor units that are active simultaneously.

A skeletal muscle unit, innervated by only excitatory cholinergic nerve fibers, can be "inhibited" only when its motoneuron is inhibited so that a lower frequency of impulses arrives at the innervated muscle fibers. The whole muscle, with a response dependent on the number of motor units recruited at a given time, also can show "inhibition" with a reduced number of active units (figure 14.1).

Activities such as quiet walking require perhaps only 5% of the motor units of a primary muscle to be excited, and these motor units need only fire at a low rate. During a step, there is an abrupt jump in firing rate from 0 to about 5 pulses/sec as those nerve fibers that innervate slow, fatigue-resistant muscle fibers are recruited. Strenuous activity ordinarily involves very strong contraction of the slow muscle units with the addition of very brief periods of activation of the fast, rapidly fatiguing fibers that make up the remainder of the muscle. The firing rate of individual motor units peaks at about 50 pulses/sec. The *recruitment order* of slow and then fast fibers has been shown in most studies, although there are instances where there is isolated recruitment of fast fibers.

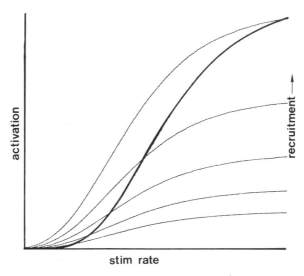

Figure 14.1
Schematic representation of effect of stimulus rate and recruitment on muscle force and stiffness. Activation of a motoneuron pool results in changes in both firing rate of units and in the number of units active. Small units are activated first and then produce increasing firing rate before larger units are recruited and exhibit their increasing firing. The individual curves show a nonlinear relationship between the firing rate of an activated group of motor units and the total muscle activity. Different curves correspond to different levels of recruitment. The heavy curve results from a combination of recruitment and firing rate of motor units as total activation increases.

The neural control of cardiac and smooth muscle is generally modulatory and a particular nerve fiber can be either excitatory or inhibitory.

Cardiac and smooth muscle contraction differs from that of skeletal muscle in that it can be driven by local processes with nerves providing only modulatory control. A further difference is that both excitatory and inhibitory neural control of an individual organ is possible because of the frequent occurrence of dual innervation.

The cholinergic parasympathetic fibers to the heart generally reduce cardiac muscle activity. Some of these nerve fibers end at a group of specialized muscle cells that are responsible for the normal rhythm of cardiac muscle contraction. This parasympathetic inhibition can actually stop the heart for a period long enough to be detrimental to an already compromised heart. Parasympathetic fibers also end in other regions of the heart where they may depress conduction of excitation over other specialized muscle fibers or where they can depress the speed and intensity of contraction of ordinary cardiac muscle. Adrenergic sympathetic fibers generally have the opposite effect on these different types of cardiac muscle fibers.

14.1. Problem: Application of a parasympathetic blocking agent presumably blocks all inhibitory nerve input to the heart. It is noted that the patient still experiences a *reduction* in heart rate following a reduction in emotional stress. How is this possible?

14.2. Question: What significance is there to the difference between nerve function in the heart and in skeletal muscle with respect to heart transplantation operations? If reinnervation is not possible, what restrictions on physiological function would be expected in a person with a transplanted heart?

Electrical excitation of a muscle fiber occurs when an action potential propagates over the sarcolemma.

Forty to fifty percent of the mass of the human body is composed of the muscles that move joints of the skeleton. These *striated* or *skeletal muscles* can propagate action potentials over their cell membranes. The action potentials of muscle cells, as those of nerve cells, result from the action of voltage-gated sodium and potassium channels.

The prefix *sarco* is derived from the Greek word σαρξ for flesh and is used in the various words describing the morphology of skeletal muscle. The cell membrane of a single muscle cell, over which the action potential is propagated, is the *sarcolemma* (from flesh + husk). The contractile unit of a skeletal muscle cell is a *sarcomere* (from flesh + part), and the cytoplasm of a muscle cell is the *sarcoplasm* (figure 14.2).

Individual muscle cells, or fibers, are relatively large cells with diameters from 10 to 100 μm and lengths up to many centimeters. We saw in chapter 12 that the space constant that defines the spatial distribution of potentials in a cell is

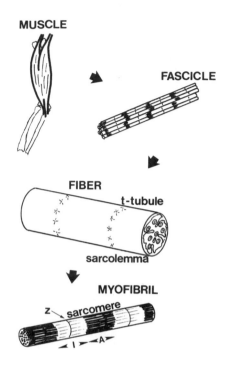

Figure 14.2
Gross organization of muscle. A skeletal muscle can be conveniently subdivided into three smaller units. The fiber bundles (or fascicles) may be arranged in various orientations, are surrounded by blood vessels and connective tissue, and are attached, at their ends, to tendons or other tissues. The muscle fiber is a cell so its boundary, the sarcolemma, is the cell membrane. Muscle fibers receive postsynaptic activation from motor nerve fibers and propagate action potentials over their cell membrane. The myofibrils are the actual contractile filaments made up of interdigitating thin and thick filaments. The basic contractile unit is the sarcomere measured from z-line to z-line along parallel myofibrils.

$$\lambda = \sqrt{\frac{g_\mathrm{l}}{g_\mathrm{m}}}$$

The longitudinal conductance, g_l increases with increasing cell diameter so muscle cells, with a large diameter, should have a long space constant. Measured space constants for skeletal muscle fibers are typically around 2 mm. A potential change at a point on the muscle cell (e.g., at the neuromuscular junction) will change the potential some distance away. Muscle cells are, however, long—too long to allow electrotonic potential changes to produce an effective electrical signal over the whole of the cell surface.

The study of electrotonic properties of skeletal muscle is complicated because the sarcolemma does not form a smooth cylindrical sheet over a muscle fiber. It has many invaginations (*transverse tubules* or *T-tubules*) that plunge deeply into the interior of the fiber. The surface area of a muscle fiber is probably increased by 3 to 10 times by the inclusion of the additional area of the transverse tubules. The exact details of the potential change in these T-tubules is not known, but they provide a means by which the signaling action potential that is propagated over the sarcolemma can have an effect deep within the large diameter muscle fiber. The cell membrane of muscle cells contains voltage-gated sodium and potassium channels. The sodium channels are found in approximately the same density as those on the surface of the squid axon and have a very similar voltage dependence of their gating. The T-tubules also contain sodium channels, but these are only at one-half the density.

Muscle fibers have resting potentials near the upper limits of those recorded in any excitable cells—in many cells they approach 100 mV. Depolarization of these cells to their threshold causes the initiation of robust, overshooting action potentials with durations of a few milliseconds. Local current flow causes these action potentials to propagate away from their site of origin resulting in a rapid, transient depolarization of the whole surface of the muscle fiber (figure 14.3A).

Individual motor units are activated independently, thus the extracellular potentials from these different units can occur independently or overlap in time or they can cancel each other. The resultant electromyogram (EMG) develops a complex *interference pattern* with increasing contraction strength. The EMG does not increase in proportion to the sum of the underlying unit activity because of variable summation and cancellation. The EMG resulting from a *single motor unit,* however, involves an almost synchronous activity that does sum to a noticeably longer and larger recorded spike than is found in a single muscle fiber.

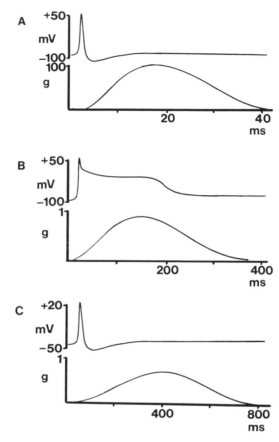

Figure 14.3
Electrical and mechanical events in various muscle types. Muscle action potentials propagate over the membrane of a muscle cell and initiate the events of contraction that result, after a delay, in a transient increase in tension—the twitch. This figure shows schematic action potentials and twitches in (A) skeletal muscle, (B) cardiac muscle, and (C) one type of smooth muscle. (Note different scales used.)

Muscle fibers that have been denervated by trauma or motoneuron disease tend to generate spontaneous and independent impulses that can be recorded in an EMG. The electrical manifestation of this is a *fibrillation potential*. Over a long period, the remaining motor axons to a partially denervated muscle develop sprouts that make synaptic connections and assume control of nearby denervated muscle fibers, resulting in enlarged motor units. Simultaneously some damaged nerve fibers may regrow and recover control of originally denervated fibers.

14.3.* Problem: Describe the sequence of changes that you would expect to find in the EMG of a muscle at various times following crushing of the motor nerve. Include a description of the EMG at rest and during attempted contraction. What variability of recovery might you expect in both ability to contract and in the EMG? How might these variations be used diagnostically?

Excitation of cardiac and smooth muscle fibers can originate in muscle cells themselves.

Although the bulk of the muscle fibers in the body function to move the skeleton, many important functions are accomplished by contraction of muscle fibers in the heart, blood vessels, and viscera. The smooth muscle fibers of the viscera differ in many ways from skeletal muscle fibers both in morphology and function. Cardiac muscle fibers are intermediary between these extremes, in some ways being more like smooth muscle and in other ways being more like skeletal muscle.

Both cardiac and smooth muscle fibers have a negative intracellular potential, although calling it a resting membrane potential is somewhat of a misnomer since the potential is rarely at rest. Mammalian cardiac cells have a potential near -80 to -95 mV and smooth muscle cells typically have a potential near -50 to -60 mV. Both cell types have voltage-gated sodium, calcium, and potassium channels and produce action potentials upon excitation.

14.4.* Questions: Just as a review, what effect on membrane potential would you expect when a calcium channel opens to allow a Ca^{2+} flux? Why might a flux of Ca^{2+} ions have a different effect than a similar flux of Na^{+} ions?

The patterns of conductance changes that underlie action potentials in cardiac and smooth muscle are even more complex than the dual conductance mechanism of skeletal muscle. Muscle, from the ventricle of the heart, has a rapid, transient sodium conductance increase followed by a *decrease* and subsequent increase in potassium conductance and a simultaneous slow rise and fall of calcium conductance. The resultant cardiac action potential has an initial peak followed by a plateau that lasts about 200 msec (figure 14.3B).

The refractory period of ventricular muscle fibers barely extends beyond the long cardiac action potential, but, because of the length of the action potential, a second action potential cannot occur for about 300 msec after an initial action potential. This then sets an upper limit on ventricular muscle firing rate. Since the rise and fall of tension in a single twitch also last about 300 msec, twitches in ventricular muscle cannot sum as twitches in skeletal muscle can. Clearly in small animals, such as birds, with very high heart rates the cardiac muscle fibers must have correspondingly shorter refractory periods.

Because of its large surface areas and synchronous depolarization, cardiac muscle generates relatively large electrical fields that can be recorded at a distance. The electrocardiogram (EKG or ECG) deflection is shorter than would be expected from the prolonged depolarization of the cardiac action potential. This is the result of the cancellation of fields when oppositely oriented regions follow each other rapidly in depolarization. Tissue damage that blocks normal conduction of excitation can leave part of the initial depolarization uncancelled.

The action potentials of smooth muscle cells (figure 14.3C) are only now being extensively investigated and they appear to have a depolarizing phase that results from an increased sodium and/or calcium conductance and a falling phase that results from an increase in potassium conductance.

Both cardiac and smooth muscle fibers can produce *pacemaker potentials,* that is, spontaneous oscillations of their membrane potentials that lead to the rhythmic generation of action potentials. This characteristic is especially pronounced in special *nodal cells* of the heart where a relatively high continuous depolarizing drive from sodium channels interacts with a delayed hyperpolarization from potassium channels to produce an oscillation that determines the heart rate. Many smooth muscle cells can produce similar spontaneous oscillations. These cells are subject to an additional feedback in their electrical properties because they have stretch-activated depolarizing channels.

Cardiac and smooth muscle cells, rarely exceeding 200 μm in length, are small in comparison with skeletal muscle cells. In both of the former tissues, however, low-resistance electrical pathways are found between adjacent cells. Thus current from one cell can easily pass into adjacent cells. Consequently, the space constants of cardiac and smooth muscle cells may be 1 to 2 mm, or about 10 times the size of an individual cell. The large area that is affected electrically from a site of excitation allows effective spread of propagated action potentials and subsequent coordination of fiber contraction.

The coupling of electrical excitation with mechanical contraction is accomplished through the action of Ca^{2+} ions.

Thus far we have discussed only the excitation of muscle cells, represented by the potential change on their surface membrane. We will soon turn our attention to the generation of force that results from this excitation and comes about by the interaction of protein molecules within the muscle fiber. One might well ask how the electrical event at the cell membrane can produce this generalized cellular response. Part of the answer lies in the somewhat cryptic statement, made in chapter 11, that the role of the nervous system is to regulate intracellular Ca^{2+}. The coupling of electrical excitation to mechanical contraction (*excitation-contraction coupling*) requires Ca^{2+} ions. We might still ask, though, about the source of this Ca^{2+} and how it acts as rapidly as it does.

The rate at which excitation is propagated radially into the center of a skeletal muscle fiber is about 700 times as great as one would expect for the diffusion of Ca^{2+} ions over this distance. Slower, smooth muscle fibers exhibit a much slower spread of excitation because they depend on Ca^{2+} diffusion from the surface. Skeletal muscle fibers attain their speed of contraction because the *T-tubules* and *sarcoplasmic reticulum* provide a means by which Ca^{2+} can be released from many sites *within* the muscle fiber (figure 14.4).

We have already mentioned that the T-tubules are a network of invaginations of the surface membrane into the depths of a skeletal muscle fiber. Although the density of sodium channels is less in the T-tubules, there is probably a sufficient number for action potential propagation. Thus the surface excitatory event is rapidly transmitted into the interior regions of the muscle fiber. At specialized regions called *cisternae,* the T-tubular membranes juxtapose the membrane of the sarcoplasmic reticulum with a gap of only about 300 Å.

14.5.* Questions: How big is 300 Å? How does this distance compare with two distances that we have already discussed, the thickness of a cell membrane and the width of the synaptic cleft?

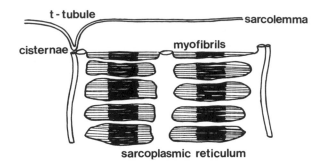

Figure 14.4
The triad. At the point where the sarcolemma invaginates to form the T-tubule, it forms a close apposition with the expanded cisternae of two sections of sarcoplasmic reticulum. At this point, the depolarization of the sarcolemma interacts with the intracellular sarcoplasmic reticulum causing calcium channels in the sarcoplasmic reticulum to open with a resultant efflux of Ca^{2+} into the sarcoplasm.

The sarcoplasmic reticulum can be thought of as a bag filled with a Ca^{2+}-sequestering protein (appropriately named calsequesterin) whose membrane contains calcium channels and calcium pumps. In the resting state, the pumps use metabolic energy, in ATP, to pump Ca^{2+} from the sarcoplasm into the sarcoplasmic reticulum where the Ca^{2+} is captured by the sequestering protein. Because of this action, sarcoplasmic Ca^{2+} concentration is maintained at less than 10^{-7} M. When the sarcoplasmic reticulum responds to electrical excitation of the T-tubules, calcium channels open and this stored Ca^{2+} is rapidly dumped out into the sarcoplasm. This surge of Ca^{2+} can transiently raise the sarcoplasmic Ca^{2+} to as much as 10^{-5} M. Following excitation, the sarcoplasmic Ca^{2+} is again recycled into the sarcoplasmic reticulum by the calcium pumps.

Recent evidence is beginning to elucidate the mechanism of coupling between the T-tubule and the sarcoplasmic reticulum. This evidence suggests that there are two modified calcium channels involved, one in the T-tubule membrane and the other in the sarcoplasmic reticulum membrane. The structure in the T-tubule acts mainly as the voltage sensor and senses the potential across the T-tubule membrane. The structure in the sarcoplasmic reticulum acts as the Ca^{2+} permeant pore. These two macromolecules are connected by a "foot protein" that couples the sensor in the T-tubule membrane to the gate on the pore in the sarcoplasmic reticulum membrane. Because of this two part calcium channel, a depolarization of the T-tubule membrane increases the probability that the gates will be open on Ca^{2+}-permeant pores in the sarcoplasmic reticulum, which results in a flux of Ca^{2+} from the pool in the sarcoplasmic reticulum into the sarcoplasm.

Excitation-contraction coupling of cardiac and smooth muscle differs somewhat from that of skeletal muscle. Cardiac muscle has a less well-developed sarcoplasmic reticulum but has, on the other hand, a significant Ca^{2+} influx across the sarcolemma during the action potential. This Ca^{2+} influx across the cell membrane may provide some of the Ca^{2+} necessary for contraction and it probably triggers the release of additional Ca^{2+} stored in the sarcoplasmic reticulum. Most smooth muscle has much less extensive sarcoplasmic reticulum. It must depend on the Ca^{2+} influx across its cell membrane during the propagated action potential. This mechanism, although effective, produces a much slower excitation-contraction coupling than that found in skeletal muscle.

In summary, skeletal muscle cells are electrically excitable and, when stimulated, propagate action potentials over their cell membranes. These action potentials invade the transverse tubular system and trigger release of stored Ca^{2+} from the sarcoplasmic reticulum. This Ca^{2+} transiently perfuses the contractile proteins in the bulk of the muscle fiber and initiates the events of contraction. Following excitation, the continued Ca^{2+} pumping capability of the sarcoplasmic reticulum membrane causes the sarcoplasmic Ca^{2+} to be pumped back into the sarcoplasmic reticulum thereby terminating the contraction. Cardiac and smooth muscle cells deviate from this scheme somewhat in that some or all of their Ca^{2+} comes from a flux across the cell membrane.

Movement is a common feature to many living cells, including those of animals, plants, and microorganisms.

Movement of living cells includes cytoplasmic streaming, ciliary beating, and muscular contraction. Many molecules responsible for these forms of movement appear to have similar evolutionary origins. The first demonstration of nonmuscle contractile proteins was made in 1952 by A.G. Loewy. This discovery was made in the unassuming, but fascinating organism the slime mold. Further similarities between nonmuscle contractile mechanisms and those of muscle are seen in the previously discussed example of *Paramecium* ciliary beating. Cilia use filamentous contractile proteins, require ATP as an energy source, and use intracellular Ca^{2+} as a regulator.

One form of subcellular movement that is vital to the nervous system is *axoplasmic flow*. By this means various substances are moved from the cell body as much as a meter to axon terminals and other substances are moved from the periphery back to the cell body. There are two distinct types of axoplasmic flow, fast and slow. Slow axoplasmic flow moves substances at rates of 1–2 mm/24 hr and fast axoplasmic flow can be as rapid as 250–400 mm/24 hr. An example of fast axoplasmic flow already considered in chapter 9, the movement of synaptic vesicles, may be part of a mechanism of long-term memory.

An important nonmuscle contractile protein is *tubulin*. This protein forms long structures called microtubules. Microtubules are important in many examples of subcellular movement from the movement of chromosomes during cell division, to the beating of cilia and flagella, to fast axoplasmic flow.

The primary contractile proteins of muscle are actin and myosin. In skeletal muscle contraction is regulated by troponin and tropomyosin.

A mammalian muscle cell contains a number of intracellular structures. About 2% of the cell volume is filled with the sarcoplasmic reticulum and an additional 0.3% with the T-tubular network. Not surprisingly, for such a metabolically active tissue as muscle, about 5% of the cell volume is composed of mitochondria. The major part though, as much as 80% of the cell volume, is made up of the protein molecules involved directly in contraction. These include *actin, myosin,* and the complex of *tropomyosin* and *troponin*. We will consider briefly each of these protein components (figure 14.5).

Actin

G-actin, the simplest form of the molecule, is a globular protein. Under the proper conditions the globules combine in long strings and two of these strings form a double helical filament of *F-actin*. The filaments of F-actin are 80 Å in diameter, 1 μm long, and make one rotation of their spiral every 770 Å. In skeletal muscle, the parallel filaments of actin, called *thin filaments,* are attached at one end to the material that forms a structure called the *Z-line* of the muscle cell. The actin molecules form an array that has a hexagonal cross section. Under the appropriate conditions, myosin will bind to specific binding sites on the actin molecule.

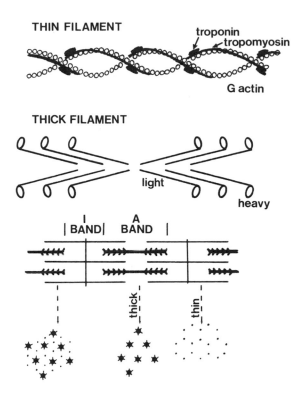

Figure 14.5
Muscle proteins. Thin filaments are made up of a double helix of globular, G-actin, units with two strands of filamentous tropomyosin lying in the two grooves along the helix. At intervals of approximately one-half revolution of the thin filament, globular troponin molecules are attached to the tropomyosin. Thick filaments consist of a regular arrangement of myosin molecules arranged so that the rod-like light meromyosin molecules form a central shaft from which the globular heavy meromyosin heads bristle. Thin and thick filaments interdigitate so that the thin filaments form a hexagonal array around the regularly arrayed thick filaments.

Tropomyosin and Troponin

Tropomyosin is another long filamentous protein molecule. Two tropomyosin molecules lie in the grooves that are formed on either side between two actin molecules. At every one/half revolution of the actin helix, a complex of *troponin* molecules is associated with the tropomyosin. When Ca^{2+} binds to a specific binding site on the troponin molecule, there is a change of configuration of the troponin-tropomyosin complex. Because of this change, the tropomyosin molecule is moved away from myosin-binding sites on the actin filament.

Myosin

The myosin molecule has two components, a globular *heavy meromyosin* and a long tail component called *light meromyosin*. Myosin molecules polymerize into a molecule that is 120 Å in diameter and 1.8 μm long. The light meromyosin tails lie together to form the backbone of this polymer. The globular heavy meromyosin heads project from the backbone approximately every 140 Å and rotate around the backbone 60° with each successive projection. The myosin heads have two very important properties: first, they can use the energy stored in a phosphate bond of ATP to rotate with respect to their tail region, and second, they can bind to binding sites on the actin molecule.

Skeletal muscle has been investigated under the light microscope for many years. Its very regular structure, especially when viewed with polarized light, has led to some important morphological nomenclature. Muscle fibers have light bands (*isotropic* or *I bands*) that alternate with dark (*anisotropic* or *A bands*) along the length of the fiber. The I bands are bisected by a dark line, the *Z-line,* and the distance from one Z-line to another is called a *sarcomere* (see figure 14.2). The A bands consist of a hexagonal array of thick filaments or myosin polymers and the I bands are the nonoverlapping parts of another hexagonal array of thin filaments or actin-tropomyosin-troponin complexes. The actual interdigitation is such that the thin and thick filaments overlap over varying amounts of the A band with each thick filament surrounded by a hexagonal array of thin filaments.

Cardiac muscle has a similar arrangement to skeletal muscle with A and I bands made up of myosin and actin-tropomyosin-troponin filaments. Obviously cardiac muscle fibers are not attached by tendons to bones but contract to apply pressure to the enclosed hollow chambers of the heart. Smooth muscle is different from skeletal or cardiac muscle. Although it contains similar contractile proteins, it does not have the same regular array of bands. The arrangement of the thin

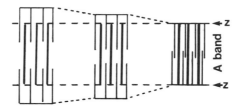

Figure 14.6
Sliding filament theory. Muscle shortening occurs by the increasing overlap of interdigitating thick and thin filaments. The A band representing the thick filaments remains constant in length during shortening while the I band representing the non-overlapping region is compressed and may even disappear during shortening.

and thick filaments is also different in that it is not in a strict hexagonal array. Although skeletal and cardiac muscles are "actin regulated" in that interaction between actin and myosin is regulated by the troponin associated with actin, smooth muscle is "myosin regulated" via an additional protein associated with myosin.

Muscle shortening results from the sliding of interdigitating thin and thick filaments.

Although it has been known since the work of Blix (1893) that the force developed by muscle varies with the length at which it was operating (figure 14.10A), the significance of this to the contractile process was not understood until much later. A considerable amount of work in the laboratories of both A.F. Huxley and of H.E. Huxley, from 1950 onward, has contributed much to our understanding of the mechanism of muscle contraction. This is still very much an area of active research so the explanations, especially the simplifications shown in figure 14.7 should be thought of as working approximations. Three important points are well established.

1. The thin and thick filaments interdigitate and slide together relative to each other during muscle shortening. This is known as the sliding filament theory of muscle contraction and its most obvious evidence is that the thick filaments that make up the A band do not change in length during muscle contraction. Figure 14.6 shows that the length of a sarcomere can range from where there is little if any overlap of thin and thick filaments to where the thick filaments go from one Z-line to the next Z-line.

2. The immediate source of energy for muscle contraction is the hydrolysis of high-energy phosphate bonds in ATP molecules. This is a multistep process that is enzymatically catalyzed by an ATPase associated with the myosin molecule.

3. The source of the force of muscle contraction is the movement of the myosin heads that make up the cross-bridges when these cross-bridges are attached to their binding sites on the actin molecule. The details of cross-bridge interactions are not completely understood at this time.

Figure 14.7 provides one interpretation of the events of the contractile cycle of muscle.

1. The process of excitation-contraction coupling discussed above brings about the release of Ca^{2+} through gated channels in the sarcoplasmic reticulum in response to a depolarization of the T tubules (C).

2. This Ca^{2+} interacts with troponin to allow the myosin head to form an initial association with the binding site on the actin molecule (D). At this point the ATPase on the myosin molecule is activated.

3. The myosin head moves to another binding configuration and, because of this movement, the thin and thick filaments move past each other (E).

4. In the maintained presence of Ca^{2+} and if ATP can be resynthesized, a continued ratcheting movement of the myosin heads along the actin binding sites occurs (F→C).

5. Contraction ends after excitation stops and the sarcoplasmic Ca^{2+} is actively pumped back into the sarcoplasmic reticulum (F→A).

14.6.* Problem: We encourage the interested student to test this simple scheme against the very complex literature on muscle contraction. More complex, and probably more accurate, schemes can be devised.

It is important to remember that the contraction occurs in a three-dimensional structure so that each myosin molecule makes and breaks cross-bridges with six different actin molecules at each end. Force is continually being generated even when some cross-bridges are not bound.

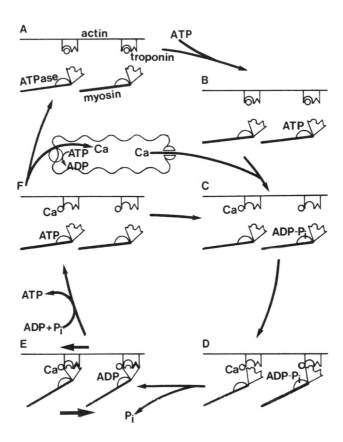

Figure 14.7
Contractile cycle of muscle. Resting muscle (A) has the myosin-binding site on actin blocked by tropomyosin and lacks high-energy ATP molecules on the myosin ATPase. In the presence of ATP (B) and when Ca^{2+} is released from the sarcoplasmic reticulum (C) the binding site is unmasked and a high energy ADP-P_i molecule is available on the myosin molecule. The myosin heads bind to their binding site on actin (D) and, with the release of energy from a high-energy phosphate bond (E), rotate to a second binding position thereby moving the thick and thin filaments with respect to each other. Continued availability of energy (F) and continued release of Ca^{2+} allows the muscle to continue the contraction cycle (F→C→D→E→F→) while removal of Ca^{2+} returns the muscle to its resting state (A).

A single adequate stimulus to a muscle nerve or directly to a muscle will produce a single, rapid contraction of the muscle followed by a relaxation back to its resting condition.

The unitary contraction of a muscle fiber is called a muscle *twitch* (figure 14.8A). Only in the artificial conditions of electrical nerve or muscle stimulation do we find simultaneous twitches in all the constituent fibers of a muscle. Detailed study of the time course of a twitch in a muscle is complicated by the effects of muscle fiber orientation and by the asynchronous activation of different fibers. Selection of thin, parallel-fibered muscles reduces the problems associated with fiber orientation. Simultaneous activation of fibers can be achieved by placing the muscle in an electrolyte bath between two plate electrodes. Further refinement involves the isolation of single fibers to study isolated twitches.

A typical muscle action potential lasts 5 to 10 msec. This is followed by a slight relaxation of muscle tension and then by the muscle twitch. A skeletal muscle twitch lasts from 10 to 100 msec, depending upon the type of muscle fiber and the temperature. If a second twitch is initiated before the end of a first twitch, the tension from the two can sum (figure 14.8B). The increments of tension resulting from the summation of twitches are not linear since the ability to add additional tension decreases as the muscle contracts. If the twitch rate is fast enough, *fusion* of the individual twitches occurs to produce a smooth maintained tension called *tetanus*. (This type of contraction is distinct from the disease called tetanus.) The stimulus rate necessary to produce a fused tetanus depends on the duration of the twitch in an individual fiber. *Fast muscle fibers* (usually white muscle) require a high rate of stimulation to produce a smooth contraction. These muscle fibers can often produce measurable force fluctuation when following up to 60 to 100 stimuli/sec. *Slow muscle fibers* (usually red muscle), as their name implies, have slower twitches that reach smooth tetanus at rates below 20 stimuli/sec. Cardiac muscle fibers, because of the firing rate limitations imposed by their long action potentials and associated refractory period, cannot undergo summation or fusion of individual twitches.

14.7.* Question: Why do the muscle action potential and the twitch have different time courses?

Tetanic stimulation is a convenient means of producing maintained contraction in a muscle that is stimulated in a laboratory experiment but normal contractions

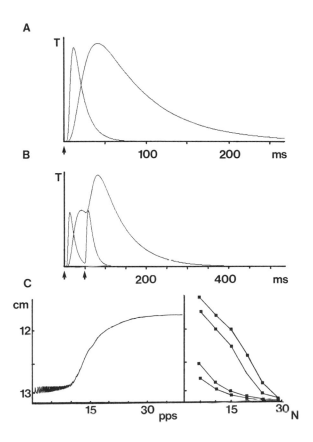

Figure 14.8

Muscle twitches. (A) Simulated muscle twitches following the neural activation and a brief latent period show rapid rise and subsequent fall in tension. The time course of this event varies as is shown between slow and fast fibers. (B) Simulation of the effect of a second action potential arriving before the tension from the first has relaxed. Depending on the particular muscle involved and current conditions the second stimulus may add the same, more, or less to the response than did the first stimulus. (C) Experimental data showing the effect of stimulus rate in pulses per second (pps) on the response of an isotonically loaded muscle. The graph on the left shows changes in muscle length resulting from a continuously increasing stimulus rate from near zero to 40 pps (stimulus rate was changed at 1 pulse/sec/sec). The inflection at about 15 pps probably results from saturation of the slow fibers before there is appreciable summation of fast fibers. The graph on the right shows the interaction of load and muscle length at four different stimulus rates. Each line represents a different stimulus rate. This graph includes four points taken (arranged vertically) from the graph on the left and other points taken from the responses of the same muscle with five other loads.

are seldom tetanic. As we have seen, groups of fibers are under the control of different motoneurons in the spinal cord so that many different neurons need to fire to activate all the fibers in a muscle. Smooth contraction of muscles under physiological conditions involves asynchronous firing of these different motor nerves. Because of the effects of mechanical interactions within the muscle, the actual smoothing is appreciably better than might be expected by simple summation of randomly related unit twitches.

In a resting mammal, it is commonly observed that the muscles are not entirely relaxed. (Simple palpation of a normal limb muscle feels different from a completely flaccid muscle.) This low level of contractile activity is called *tonus*. Tonus occurs in both skeletal and smooth muscle but is generated in different ways in the two cases. In smooth muscle, tonus occurs in the absence of external driving impulses as a result of intrinsically generated muscle action potentials. In skeletal muscle, tonus results from a low level of nerve impulse activity shifting among a few small motor units. The flaccid muscle seen in the absence of tonus is often diagnostic of abnormal function in the central nervous system.

The efficacy of muscle for a given change in enthalpy depends on how the output of that muscle is measured.

It is instructive to consider the efficiency of muscle as a motor. When doing external work over a short period, some energy stored in muscle (enthalpy) is delivered to the load as mechanical energy. Various attempts have been made to estimate the ratio of external work to the decrease of enthalpy of the muscle. When these calculations are based on the assumption that the sum of the mechanical energy and the heat make up the total energy leaving the muscle and should equal the decrease in enthalpy, muscles have been found to have a mechanical efficiency of 50% to 70% for a twitch. During an isometric contraction there is no shortening and thus no work, so there is 0% efficiency in work production. Likewise, after an initial movement, a load-moving contraction that is followed by a holding period has a continued energy expenditure, although the lack of continued work means that the efficiency over the whole period continually decreases. When muscle is stretched during contraction, it absorbs energy and a calculation of mechanical efficiency becomes meaningless. Calculations of muscle efficiency are thus relevant only to specified conditions. Furthermore, 0% efficiency in delivery of mechanical work corresponds to 100% efficiency in delivery of heat.

The heat generated by contracting skeletal muscle was studied extensively by A.V. Hill and his collaborators during the first half of this century. Several general categories of heat can be measured. *Activation heat* can be measured early in a twitch or tetanus and is probably associated with Ca^{2+} movements and the initial interaction of actin and myosin. *Maintenance heat* is measured during continued isometric contraction and is generated by the continued interaction of actin and myosin. Maintenance heat is proportional to the force generated by muscle and is a function of muscle length. Additional heat is created when shortening occurs and work is done. Finally, *recovery heat* can be measured over a period of minutes following the contraction. Recovery heat is approximately equal to the heat generated during contraction and represents the chemical work of replenishing stored energy.

It is now possible to evaluate some parts of muscle function on a micro scale. Because of the regularity of the sarcomere structure, one can examine crossbridge arrangement by using x-ray diffraction. Free Ca^{2+} ion activity within the sarcoplasm can be evaluated with Ca^{2+}-sensitive dyes and spectrographic measurements. Optical measurements make it possible to measure the movement of a single sarcomere. Special isolation techniques have made possible mechanical studies of isolated fractions of the contractile system from muscle fibers. The few milliseconds between excitation and the beginning of the twitch are called the latent period. Several events occur within this time. Immediately following excitation of a muscle fiber there is an increase in free Ca^{2+} in the sarcoplasm. This is followed by a rapid rise in the resistance of the fiber to passive stretch (increased stiffness) and a simultaneous release of activation heat and a small decrease in force. The rise in stiffness probably reflects the formation of crossbridges but there is no currently accepted basis for the activation heat or the decrease in force. The increase in stiffness is sometimes called *active state* and was originally thought to represent an internal force development. It is now thought that a later process in the cross-bridge cycle develops stress and represents the first appearance of mechanical energy.

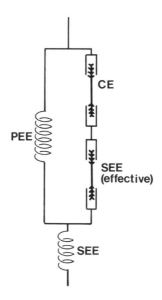

Figure 14.9
Elastic elements. Tension, developed by the contractile element (CE), is delivered to bones through series elastic elements (SEE) consisting of tendons and connective tissue and parts of the actin–myosin system. The sarcolemma and other connective tissue acts as a parallel elastic element (PEE) that gives the stiffness observed in stretch of the passive muscle. The elastic properties of series connected fibers and even sarcomeres within the same fiber provide series elastic contributions to the load on an individual sarcomere. Those parts of the elastic elements that are associated with the contractile system are variable with the level of excitation.

The contractile proteins are contained within a bag that has complex viscous and elastic properties.

Since the tendons that attach muscles to bones can stretch, they provide elastic elements between the force-generating element and the site where this force is applied to the external world (figure 14.9). One commonly used simplification is to lump the elastic elements associated with muscle into two components. In parallel with the contractile elements are the *parallel elastic components;* in series with the contractile elements are the *series elastic components*.

In a gross muscle, with its attachments, energy can be distributed in several parts of the tissue. Contractile elements are attached to their load by series elastic tissue that, when subjected to force, is stretched with a consequent storage of mechanical energy. The contractile proteins that lie in series with the cross-bridges contribute an appreciable series elastic action. When the tensile force changes, the stretch of the series elastic elements changes and the amount of elastic energy stored there also changes. Thus, in a twitch contractile energy is first stored in series elastic elements and then, as the contractile process decreases, this energy still can be delivered to the load. Elastic structures in parallel with the contractile elements, such as the sarcolemma, are also stretched within the functioning range of muscle lengths and can deliver energy during muscle shortening. These tissues are typical of elastic tissue and do not obey Hooke's law. That is, their elastic stiffness increases nonlinearly as the coiled elastic filaments become straightened. *Stiffness* is quantitatively just what we would expect it to be from our everyday experience, that is, the amount of force necessary to effect a given change in length. The stiffness of muscle is further complicated by the contribution of cross-bridges to stiffness. This stiffness varies with the level of excitation of a muscle.

14.8. Problem: Describe the direction of transfer of mechanical energy into and out of the various structures in a pair of muscles, one a plantar flexor of the ankle and the other its antagonist. Consider a simple vertical jump starting before an initial crouch that stretches the plantar flexor, then the rise as the muscle shortens, and then the ballistic movement to peak height. During this sequence, are there any periods in which some nonelastic source or sink of energy must be assumed for an energy balance? Can you identify appropriate candidates for these sources or sinks? Next continue the jump through falling and decelerating phases and return to a flat footed stance. Divide the time to include all the necessary changes in energy transfer. Again account for energy balance. Incidentally, it has been shown that the series elastic element of the long Achilles tendon of the kangaroo contributes to energy conservation by storing energy from one landing and delivering it into the next jump.

14.9.* Questions: How would the force exerted by the elastic elements change with length if this component obeyed Hooke's law? How would the stiffness of muscle vary with length if it obeyed Hooke's law?

The force that a muscle fiber can deliver at any one time depends on a very nonlinear interaction of the muscle length and velocity, its temperature, the level of excitation, and the recent history of the muscle's actions.

The nerve impulses that control muscle are indeed delivered to a very complex motor. To simplify the description of muscle, restraining assumptions of constant length (*isometric*) or constant force (*isotonic*) are often made. We will first describe these reduced conditions and then introduce the more complex condition in which length, velocity, and tension vary.

Weber (1846) showed that muscle response varies with stimulus frequency and Blix (1893) studied the effect of length on the response. The results of these pioneering studies have been confirmed, refined, and extended by many subsequent investigators and students. Levine and Wyman (1927) measured work to study the effect of velocity on force. The extension of this study, and mathematical modeling of the behavior of muscle during shortening, is largely associated with Hill's studies. Although many studies of muscle have concentrated on contraction with shortening, Fenn (1945) brought attention to the effects of "contraction" in lengthening.

The relationship of length and force is generally investigated under isometric conditions.

Although "isometric" means constant length, it does not mean that the length cannot be changed. Length is the independent variable (X axis) in the isometric length-tension relationship. The dependent variable (Y axis) in this plot represents the resultant force generated at those lengths of the muscle that the experimenter has previously fixed. An *isometric length-tension curve* is produced from two sets of experimental measurements. The first or *passive* (F_P) curve is generated by measuring the steady resistive force that results from stretching the muscle to various lengths. This nonlinear relationship, shown in figure 14.10, represents the elastic characteristics of the parallel and series elastic elements. If the muscle is stimulated, while being held at various lengths, a twitch tension can be measured. This tension varies characteristically with muscle length. This is the *total* (F_T) tension curve and it includes both the tension resulting from the passive elastic properties of the muscle and the *active* (F_A) tension resulting from excitation of the contractile elements.

If the force that opposes stretch is given a positive sign, passive stiffness ($\partial F_P/\partial L$), as measured in the length-tension curve, is positive for all lengths (figure 14.10). With a weak contraction, and in some muscles at all strengths of contraction, the total stiffness ($\partial F_T/\partial L$) is also positive at all lengths. Since the active length-tension curve for strong contractions has a maximum within the functional range of lengths, some total length-tension curves have a local maximum followed by a region of negative stiffness within the functional range.

14.10. Problems:

1. Why is the active length-tension curve that is calculated as $F_T - F_P = F_A$ only approximate when determined in whole muscle but better defined when determined from measurements in a single sarcomere?

2. What relationship between $\partial F_A/\partial L$ and $\partial F_P/\partial L$ is implied by a $\partial F_T/\partial L$ curve with a local maximum?

Gordon et al. (1966) measured the active length-tension curve of a single sarcomere. This curve has the same shape as that for the whole muscle (figure 14.10A), and indeed underlies the whole muscle's active length-tension curve. As is represented in figure 14.10B, the single sarcomere length-tension curve can be interpreted as interactions of the thin and thick filaments. When the sarcomere is at its shortest, about 1.65 μm, the thick filaments are butted against the adjacent Z-lines and the thin filaments overlap. In this condition the muscle is incapable of generating force. At the extreme of stretch, about 3.65 μm, there is no overlap of thin and thick filaments and again the contractile elements cannot generate force. Between these extremes, force is generated through cross-bridge interaction. This force has a maximum at a sarcomere length of about 2.2 μm, which is approximately the sarcomere length in resting muscle.

The relationship between force and length in an active muscle, (Partridge, 1966, 1967; Feldman, 1966; Bizzi et al., 1982) within its working range of lengths, can be compared with the relationship between force and displacement in a negative feedback position control system. This relationship also can be compared with that of an adjustable spring. In either case, the force delivered by a constantly excited muscle will be in equilibrium with a particular load at a specific length. As can be seen in a length-tension curve where stiffness is positive at short or long lengths, the force difference will be in a direction that leads to movement toward the equilibrium point. One can consider that the overlap of the filaments

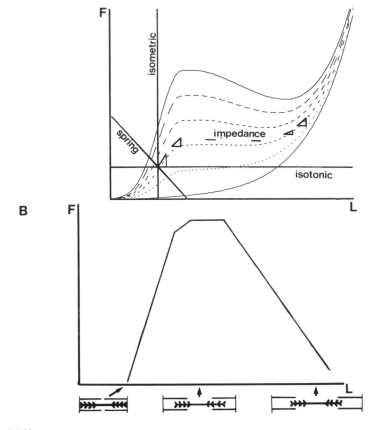

Figure 14.10
(A) Effect of excitation on the interaction between muscle and four types of load: isometric, isotonic, elastic, and one that forces the muscle to move. The six curves of force vs. length represent this relationship with different levels of activation from passive to maximally activated. Interrupted curves represent intermediate levels of excitation; longer dashes indicate higher stimulus rates. An isometric load restricts the control by stimulation to changes in *force* at the prechosen length (vertical line). The effect of stimulus rate on force at one length is shown by the intersections of the isometric line with the different stimulus lines. By definition, isotonic loads restrict the response to changes in *length* at a prechosen force (horizontal line). With most loads, both length and force change (auxotonic). For a purely elastic or spring load, the possible combinations of force and length fall along a diagonal line with a slope determined by the stiffness of the spring. If the load is an external force that moves the muscle, the muscle properties of interest are its mechanical impedance represented here by the stiffness component that changes with length and stimulus rate. The stiffness, $\partial F/\partial L$, is indicated by the slope of a line tangent to the length–force curve at any point. Six slope lines are shown along the curve at one excitation level. This stiffness is shown to vary with the length of the muscle and the stimulus rate. Actual measurements of stiffness by small forced movements will differ with the details of the test conditions (e.g., small stretches vs. small releases). (B) The active contribution to muscle force measured in a single sarcomere is related to the amount of overlapping of thick and thin filaments within the sarcomere. The curve's shape can be explained by the ability of myosin cross-bridges to interact with actin-binding sites. This graphic description has been important to the acceptance of the sliding filament theory of muscle contraction.

senses the actual length and that the contractile process is the effector of the feedback system. This feedback makes the conversion of nerve signals into muscle position much less sensitive to, but not independent of, load than would be the case with a force control.

Cardiac muscle has a similar length-tension effect that leads to the relationship known as *Starling's law* (1918). When the heart is filled more, the subsequent contraction force is increased and can compensate with increased blood output. This is especially important because the effectiveness of tension in the wall of a hollow elastic structure decreases as the diameter increases. Without the increasing muscle force, any increased filling would produce a decreasing ejection force and accumulation of residual blood in the ventricle.

The relationship between force and velocity can be investigated under several conditions of movement.

The *force-velocity curve* can be measured continuously by either stretching or allowing muscle to shorten while recording its force and length. The area under the recorded curve can be the work done on, or by, the muscle at a given constant velocity. In a *passive* (unstimulated) muscle, as was shown by Blix (1893), the work done on stretching is slightly greater than that returned on release, but the conditions of recording the two curves differ only in the sign of the velocity. The area between these two curves represents the amount of energy that is lost in one cycle. In a purely elastic element, even a nonlinear one, the release curve would have exactly retraced the stretching curve. The difference in work in a *passive* muscle is largely a consequence of energy dissipated into the viscosity of the muscle. In an active muscle, the energy loss is much greater and involves energy from chemical and mechanical processes.

A traditional way to measure the force-velocity effect is to measure the maximum velocity of shortening during twitches with different loads. At the peak of velocity there is no acceleration so that the inertial force is zero and at this point the weight equals the force on the muscle. Using this method, Hill showed that the force-velocity relationship during shortening could be fit with a hyperbolic curve (figure 14.11). The equation that he gave for this curve is

$$(P + a)V = (P - P_0)b$$

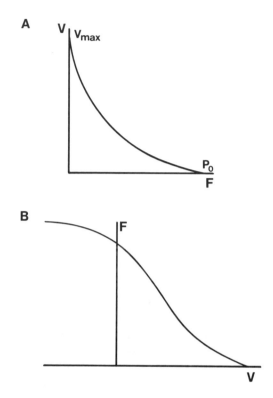

Figure 14.11
Force-velocity relationship. (A) For many years force-velocity effects were determined from the maximum velocity of twitches under conditions of different isotonic loads. Under these conditions, the velocity of shortening is inversely related to the load on the muscle. At zero external load, the muscle has its maximum velocity of shortening, V_{max}, whereas a maximum force, P_o can be developed when no shortening occurs. (B) Recent measurements of the force–velocity effect have used tetanically excited muscle that was driven to shortening or lengthening at a constant rate. These measurements are each made at the same length but at different velocities. Except for the exchange of coordinates of the graphs, the shortening parts of the two types of graph are similar, although one was made at constant length and with tetanic stimulus and the other at different lengths, during twitch responses.

where P = tension (poids), P_0 = tension at zero velocity (isometric tension), V = velocity of shortening, and a and b are constants for a specific muscle.

At the force maximum, force is constant and thus series elastic elements are momentarily at a constant length so that the load velocity is presumed to be equal to the velocity of the contractile element. It is difficult to make measurements during lengthening in experiments using muscle twitches because the length-velocity-force relationship is affected by the length of the interval between application of the stimulus and the load. Force-velocity measurements have been made recently under conditions of servo-control of muscle length using a constant velocity over an appreciable time with measurements made as the muscle passes through a predetermined length. This makes it possible to obtain measurements at both lengthening and shortening velocities and during tetanic excitation. The observed velocity-dependent differences between the stretching and releasing curves are due to changes in the conversion between chemical energy and mechanical energy and between mechanical energy and thermal energy during the cycling of active muscle. This velocity-dependent effect provides the energy absorption that prevents the length-tension effect from interacting with the load to produce an oscillation of length.

In normal activity, length, velocity, and force all change. This is a condition called *auxotonic contraction.*

At any moment, the state of a muscle involves a particular length, velocity, force, and degree of excitation. Each possible combination of length and velocity can be represented as a point on a phase plane graph and all movement trajectories can be shown on the phase plane. At any point on the phase plane, different forces can be generated by adjustment of the excitation. These values are conveniently shown as heights above the phase plane. A point in this length-velocity-force space represents the force at that velocity on the force-velocity curve for the relevant length that is the same as the force on the length-tension curve (figure 14.12). A family of length-tension curves and, at right angles to these curves, a family of force velocity curves can be constructed over the phase plane forming a surface for a particular level of excitation. Projecting a particular movement trajectory up onto this surface leads to the prediction that movement of a constantly excited muscle can be expected to generate a varying force. Different levels of excitation define different theoretical surfaces.

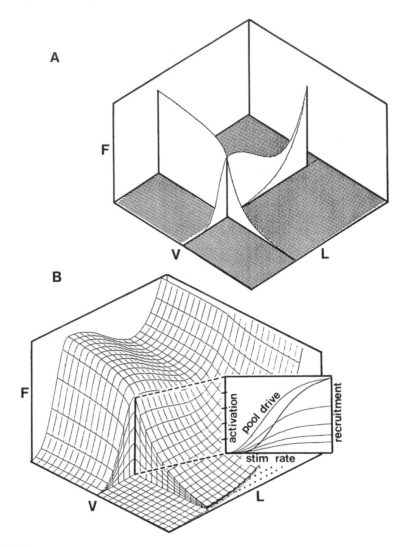

Figure 14.12
(A) An instantaneous measurement of muscle force occurs at some specific point on the length-tension graph (see figure 14.10A) for the velocity and excitation level at the time. Likewise that force also falls at a particular point on the force-velocity curve (see figure 14.11B) for the length and activation at that time. Plotting these two graphs at right angles in a pseudo-three-dimensional graph results in the intersection of the two graphs at the point on the base plane (phase plane graph) representing the length and velocity at the test moment. (B) Interaction of stimulus rate, recruitment, length, and velocity in determining muscle force. The small inset graph duplicates figure 14.1 to show the interaction of stimulus rate and recruitment in determining the activation of a muscle. The surface of the pseudo-three-dimensional graph shows the many combinations of length and velocity that determine force at maximum activation as in (A). The window cut in the lower corner of this surface shows the edges of other surfaces that would result at lower levels of activation. The effects of stimulus and movement history are not represented in this diagram.

The theoretical force surfaces provide a basis for understanding the general relationships of muscle as an effector that operates in an auxotonic world with neural control. The theoretical surface is based on individual tests in which the excitation and mechanical histories were carefully restricted to standard patterns. The differences that occur in normal function introduce appreciable deviations from these theoretical surfaces and we do not yet understand the rules of these complications well enough to make good predictions of expected responses.

In summary, the state of the simplest single muscle determines how that muscle will behave in the immediate future. This state depends on current values of length, velocity, load, excitation, and the history of past excitation and movement. These states could be further subdivided based on energy storage in various elastic elements. Despite the nonlinear complexity of the rules that govern muscle response, the nervous system has developed an adequate means of control. We need a much better understanding of auxotonic signal-following dynamics before we can develop a successful prosthetic substitute for even a single muscle.

Chapter 15

Temporal Modifications

Since the value of the nervous system lies in its contribution to the individual's response to changes, an understanding of dynamic processes is critical to an understanding of neural function.

By the time information has reached the nervous system, it deals with past states of both the individual and the environment. A similar delay exists between the time when a controlling signal is generated in the nervous system and the time when that signal can modify relationships in the world. Since neural control is needed neither to deal with things that do not change nor to send messages to structures that are static, certainly a major factor governing the evolution of the nervous system is its success in dealing with temporal events. Those functions that are tried and proven to be successful in predicting and controlling future states of the individual and environment are those whose genetic basis is most likely to survive. All of those processes that have been preserved through evolution may not have had a direct value. Thus simple delay may have evolved as the by-product of some unrelated process or it may have had its primary role in another function.

That we understand only a few predictive processes of the nervous system results from the difficulty in identifying them and should not be construed as a lack of their importance. This chapter will deal with some processes that alter temporal relationships in neural signals as these signals are produced by receptors, as they are processed in central pathways, and as they exercise control over effectors. The nervous system has four simple actions that change the time relationships of signals: (1) *conduction delay,* (2) *memory,* (3) *summation,* and (4) *adaptation.*

Time-consuming processes of the nervous system delay responses with respect to the stimulus; the first three actions listed above, conduction delay, memory, and summation have just such an effect. We have already considered, in chapters 2 and 12, signal delay in transmission along nerves. Memory processes, discussed in chapter 9, provide long delays before stimuli have their effects. Summating effects at junctions and effectors, as are discussed in chapters 13 and 14, produce *lags* in responses that have temporal effects intermediate between conduction delays and the delays of memory. The existence of a process that could make a response *lead* the stimulus that caused it may not be immediately apparent. Adaptation has just such an ability to produce lead in signals that originate with smoothly changing stimuli. Two other examples of temporal modifications of neural signals have been discussed in previous chapters. In chapter 4 we considered the mechanical tuning of the auditory system that selects the responsiveness of individual nerve fibers based on temporal properties of the stimulus. In chapter 2 we discussed the pulse code of nerve fibers that imposes a limitation on the transmission of high-frequency information. In chapter 16 we will examine the temporal properties introduced by nerve networks. In this chapter, we will first consider delaying temporal effects and then adaptation.

15.1.* Question: What process might contribute to the delays seen between the stimulus and the response in the knee jerk reflex (figure 15.1)?

15.2. Question: Can you propose a situation in which processes, such as those that delay the knee jerk, might contribute to lead of the response to another stimulus?

The time consumed in conduction of nerve impulses along fibers is functionally significant, particularly in dealing with rapidly changing signals.

The magnitude of conduction delays depends on two independently variable factors, conduction velocity and conduction distance. The longest delays are on long, slowly conducting fibers such as the efferent (autonomic) fibers to blood vessels in the foot or equally long, slowly conducting afferent fibers from thermal receptors. The delays over these pathways can approach 1 sec. Conversely, the shortest delays occur in short, rapidly conducting fibers in which the delay may be only a few hundredths of a millisecond.

15.3. Question: Have you checked these statements of conduction times with your calculations? Doing these calculations gives you a chance to learn whether you understand what assumptions are behind the author's claims. Furthermore, textbooks contain errors!

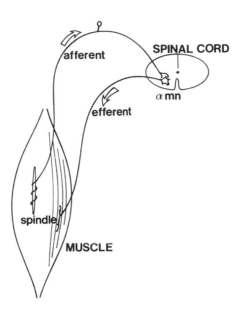

Figure 15.1
The knee jerk reflex. The knee jerk (or stretch or myotatic) reflex is an example of the simplest form of reflex consisting of only a single afferent element, one central synapse, and a single efferent element. The afferent element is from a spindle receptor that senses relative muscle length and rate of change of length. The central synapse is onto an α motoneuron (α mn) in the spinal cord. The efferent element is a motor nerve that innervates (extrafusal) muscle fibers in the muscle containing the spindle receptor. The stretch reflex in a whole muscle has many of these simple pathways in parallel.

The longest nerve fibers in the body carry signals from muscles in the foot uninterrupted to the lower part of the brain, but, because they belong to the most rapidly conducting class of fiber, they have delays of only about 50 msec. The longest conduction delays are over thin, unmyelinated C fibers from nociceptors and some thermoceptors. All other delays in single nerve fibers fall between these extremes because the fibers are of intermediate length or conduction velocity. (Table 10.1 summarizes the conduction velocities of the different fiber types.)

15.4.* Problem: If an object started to fall under the influence of gravity, how fast would it be falling after 100 msec? (This is equivalent to twice the shortest conduction time between the foot and the brain.) How far would it have fallen in this time? How far would you travel at a speed of 50 km/hr (30 miles/hr) during the duration of the conduction delay of the fastest fibers over the distance from mid-biceps to the spinal cord and back? What would this value be if the conduction distance were from the muscle to the cortex and back? (An actual neural response also would include time for central processing and a lag in the muscle's response.)

Conduction delays are nearly constant on a particular fiber over short periods of time; thus, impulse patterns arrive unaltered except for a delay. Over longer periods of time, the delays may be altered by changes of body temperature, although even this does not alter the short-term patterns transmitted. Over a range of temperatures, within the functional range from hypothermia to fever, the variation in delay between impulses conducted on any pathway can span a ratio of at least 1:3.

Correlations exist between function and fiber types so that functions involving rapid changes are generally signaled along the most rapidly conducting fibers.

Much afferent information, such as body temperature, and efferent information, such as the control blood vessel diameter, does not involve changes that are important in much less than a second. These functions are some of those that are subject to the longest conduction delays (figure 15.2). On the other hand, some entire motor actions can be completed in appreciably less than a second. Both the sensory and motor nerves involved with information about these movements are of the most rapidly conducting A class. Since rapid conduction involves large, metabolically extravagant cells, an important factor in evolution has certainly been the compromise between the need for current information and the cost of rapid nerve conduction. The shortness of the pathways for auditory and visual information is probably significant.

The shortest conduction delays are found in the very short connections using large-diameter fibers between adjacent central neurons. Presumably, small delays are important in those networks that involve a sequence of connections to control urgent operations. The advantage of short connections, in accomplishing complex operations quickly, could be a factor in the evolution of localized vs. spatially distributed functions in the nervous system (e.g., Nelson and Bower, 1990).

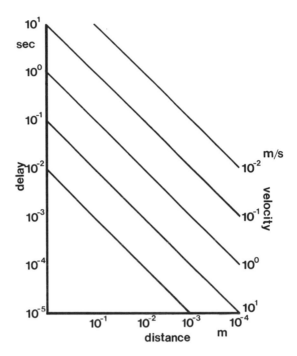

Figure 15.2
Conduction delays. Relationship between conduction distance, conduction velocity, and conduction delay for the ranges of these values found in normal nervous system function.

Memory yields the longest delays between events and the neural consequences of those events.

You will recall from chapter 9 that different types of memory serve the nervous system in different ranges of time. These may occur at different anatomical locations and most certainly represent different biochemical processes. Short-term memory spans a period of awareness and is terminated by sleep or unconsciousness. Long-term memory results from the consolidation of short-term memory, overlaps it in time, and lasts for as long as a lifetime. Genetic determinants of structure of the nervous system store "memories" concerning connections and functions that have proven valuable to the species over many generations. Each of these types of memory provides a way in which inputs can alter responses at a time later than that resulting from simple conduction delays.

Memory is the storage of information. This stored information provides a means of delaying the effect of inputs to the nervous system. Memory allows the past to influence the future over reasonably long periods of time. The action of the past on the future may simply involve the storage of information and later retrieval —a delay. Another application of memory is the modification of the manner in which the nervous system processes the information contained in a particular type of input. This later effect can be accomplished by modifying the parameters of the processing, or by associating a new response with a particular stimulus. Both delays and the modification of parameters are forms by which memory of preceding events affects later behavior. Parameter adjustment, however, is functionally rather different from the various mechanisms that simply process or delay the original signal.

An important result of summation is the smoothing (low pass filtering) of discontinuous signals.

Wave summation was first described with regard to muscle contraction, and, later, *temporal summation* was described in reflex experiments. In both cases, the observation was that when successive input pulses from the same source arrived at a responding system with a short interpulse interval, the effect of each pulse was added to the residual effect of the preceding pulses. The response to a series of pulses rises to a greater value than is produced by a single pulse. The summation reaches a maximal level that varies with the repetition rate of the stimulus and with certain properties of the response system. Summation of inhibition also can occur in reflexes to produce a decreased or zero output.

Information is carried on a single nerve or muscle fiber by a series of brief, discrete events. Even the combination of all the impulses on functionally similar fibers of a whole nerve produces a very discontinuous pattern. The physiological responses, however, to such signals are ordinarily smooth, continuous functions partly because of the lagging effect of temporal summation (figure 15.3).

15.5.* Experiment: Design an experiment to determine whether summation in a particular muscle is a mathematical summation of identical unit responses with each response simply superimposed on the residual response from previous pulses. What results do you expect? Can you explain the results that you obtain in carrying out this experiment?

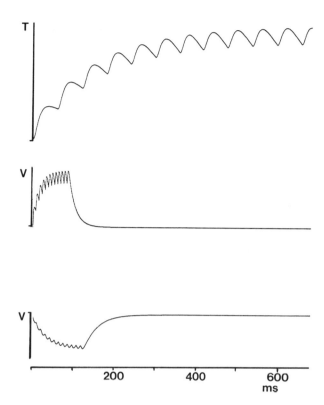

Figure 15.3
Schematic records comparing the time course of summation. Summation of tension in a muscle in response to repetitive stimulation of its motor nerve (top), intracellular potential in a neuron following stimulation of an excitatory presynaptic nerve (middle), and intracellular potential in a neuron following stimulation of an inhibitory presynaptic nerve (bottom).

Frequently substances are delivered to the blood stream over a period while simultaneously excretion by the kidney removes the substance at a rate proportional to the blood concentration. As the accumulated quantity increases, the removal rate also will increase, reaching a steady pattern where the removal during an interval is equal to the delivery during that interval. This balance establishes a steady-state level that depends on the rates of delivery and removal. Similar processes occur in the accumulation of transmitters at a synapse, elastic stored energy in a muscle, or electrical charges on membranes.

15.6.* Problem: Write equations or a program that represent the intuitive model just described. Use this formal model to examine the effect of pulsatile delivery at different rates, different quantities per pulse, and different removal rates on the time course of accumulation. Extend the model to the additional assumption that the accumulation of a first agent determines the rate of addition of a second agent. Now model the accumulation and removal of the second agent. By suitable adjustment, this model can be made to provide an elementary model of endplate potentials, synaptic potentials, and muscle contractions. What has been omitted in this model?

A postsynaptic response, and, even more, the mechanical response of a muscle to a single impulse is much longer in duration than a single action potential. When the driving impulses arrive at a moderate to high rate, the individual responses sum to give a steady response with superimposed fluctuations. These fluctuations make up only a fraction of the total response amplitude. This smoothing action makes it impossible to drive a very fast change in the output. Response smoothing occurs in muscle as *tetanic fusion* when the stimulus rate is sufficiently high that the individual impulses are obscured in the smooth mechanical response. This smoothing and its rejection of high frequency signals is a *low-pass filter* action.

While sensory systems frequently are tested with pulse inputs, in normal function, such isolated impulse stimuli occur only rarely. Inputs that change slowly and continuously are much more common in nature. Important characteristics of the response to continuously changing signals are not easily recognizable in the responses to impulses. A useful alternative is the study of responses to sinusoidal inputs at a series of different frequencies. Such signals better represent the diversity of the continuous waveforms experienced in normal function. Summating systems, and, as we will discuss later in this chapter, adapting systems are both cases in which impulse tests tend to minimize important effects that are easily identified in sinusoidal tests. The rich repertoire of analytic, synthetic, extrapolating, and descriptive tools associated with sinusoidal testing in some engineering fields cannot be fully invoked because of the nonlinearity of neural systems so extensions of the frequency response data beyond a qualitative description should be carried out with careful attention to the validity of superposition of signals.

A stimulus, S, varying sinusoidally over time, t, with an amplitude of $2A$, and a frequency of oscillation, ω, can be described as

$$S = A \sin \omega t$$

This representation describes a signal varying from $-A$ to $+A$ (figure 15.4A). For some stimuli such as rate of drug administration, light intensity, or blood pressure, negative values have no meaning. For such inputs it is necessary to add a bias, B, to the input with $B \geq 1$ (figure 15.4B):

$$S = A(\sin\omega t + B)$$

S cannot be used in a continuous form as an input to a nerve or a muscle but rather a pulse rate that is proportional to the instantaneous value of S is required. A continuous sinusoidal signal can be approximated by a pulse rate that is proportional to the average of the continuous signal during each interpulse interval. Such approximations have been useful for tests of dynamic behavior of neural systems (figure 15.4C).

Two different forms of stimulus modulation are used for functional electrical stimulation. Pulse rate modulation, with constant amplitude pulses, grades muscle responses relatively smoothly. Alternatively, modulation of the intensity of the stimulus can be used to grade the recruitment of motor units. Normal neuronal activity involves both types of modulation, although the physiological recruitment order is different from that attained by a graded stimulus intensity. An electrical stimulus excites large units first, while physiological recruitment starts first with the small units.

15.7.* Problem: The response of a muscle to a sinusoidally modulated rate of nerve action potentials, as shown in a frequency response curve, is one way of describing the dynamic response of the system. The impulse response to a single action potential is an EPSP. With repeated inputs to a motoneuron, these poten-

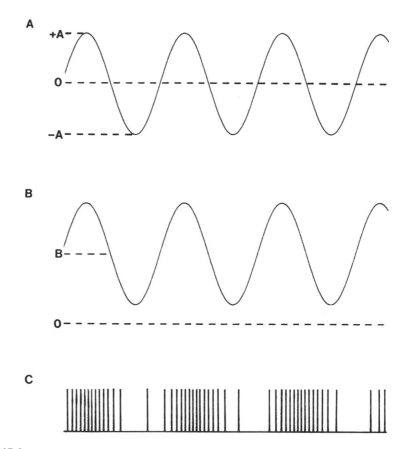

Figure 15.4
Sinusoidal stimulation. (A) Sinusoidal stimulus with an amplitude $2A$ ($S = A \sin \omega t$). (B) Many types of stimuli do not have values corresponding the negative half cycle of a sine wave. Sinusoidal stimulus with an added bias ($S = A \sin \omega t + B$). (C) One pulse rate representation of the sinusoidal stimulus in (B).

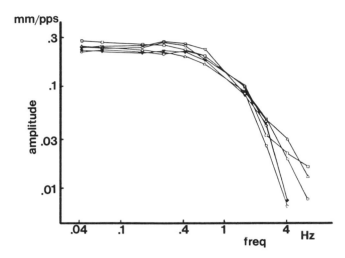

Figure 15.5
Frequency response curve for muscle. The muscle response (amplitude) to different frequencies of sinusoidally modulated pulse rates of nerve action potentials (similar to that in figure 15.4C). Separate lines represent different load inertias over a range of 1:28 (From Partridge, 1966).

tials summate and decay more rapidly than does the tension in the muscle fiber innervated by that motoneuron. Compare the impulse response of an EPSP to that of a muscle. Sketch your estimate of what the frequency response of post-synaptic excitation would look like. Compare this with figure 15.5.

Lags are produced by the temporal effects of summation on periodic inputs.

The relationship between input and output that is classically described as sum-mation is also called *lag* and is distinguished from simple delay by the nature of the modification of the time course of the signal. This process not only delays responses but changes the internal time relationships and in this way provides the nervous system with a computational capability to modify signal dynamics.

At the beginning of a tetanic train, stimulus rate rises abruptly but muscle response does not reach its maximum until several stimuli have been delivered. That is, the change in the response lags behind the instantaneous increase of the stimulus rate. If the rate of firing of the motor nerve changes cyclically, the response always lags a fraction of a cycle behind the excitation. In skeletal muscle, this lag can amount to one second or more (figure 15.5). (At 0.1 Hz, the period of one cycle is 10 sec. Thus a 36° lag = 36°/360° × 10 sec = 1 sec.) The mechanical response of a muscle, especially during a slow movement, is retarded with respect to its neural drive by many times the delay introduced by conduction time in the motor nerve. Both lags and conduction delays in autonomic responses are even larger. Although the lags within central synapses are small, when a signal traverses a series of synapses, the cumulative lag and pattern alteration may be appreciable.

When a light is flashed at a low rate, the visual sensation is one of individual flashes. With an increase of frequency, the sensation is of flicker. At some point above 20 flashes/sec, the perception approaches one of a fused, continuous light although the individual light pulses are still well separated. As flash intensity is increased, this *flicker fusion frequency* increases to a limit of about 50 flashes/ sec. Thus, at some point in the visual system, which could be simply the pulse rate encoding, a low-pass filtering occurs.

In a single nerve cell a single presynaptic nerve impulse or brief stimulus can be below the threshold necessary for a postsynaptic response, but, if the input is repeated, postsynaptic summation can yield a suprathreshold response. This type of summation causes spurious and trivial signals to be rejected without rejecting signals that are confirmed by continuation. In chapter 8 we discussed Sherrington's experiment in which a dog was stimulated with an "artificial flea." In this experiment, summation periods of several seconds were required before the stimulus reached a level that would initiate the scratch reflex.

As signals pass through the nervous system and generate external responses, several different processes introduce delay. These delaying processes have important differences. Lag, pulse encoding, and tuning of receptors modify the information in signals, whereas memory modifies how new signals are processed. Those processes that also modify signal pattern, as opposed to conduction delay, are the ones that have the largest temporal effects.

Adaptation has the remarkable and important effect of causing the output of the adapting system to lead in time any smoothly changing signals on which it operates.

Adaptation, like lag, alters the timing of the dynamic signals that are processed by the nervous system. Unlike lag, however, the change is in the opposite direction, causing the output to *lead* the input. This perhaps surprising action of

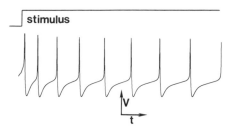

Figure 15.6
Adapting spike train. Computer simulation of an adapting spike train in response to a step in stimulus as shown above.

adaptation is a general characteristic of receptor activities with temporal details and mechanisms that vary appreciably from one receptor to another.

The term *adaptation* refers to a phenomenon common to both sensory experience and experimental study of neural signals. Adaptation is a decrease, over time, of the response to a stimulus that has remained constant following a step increase. Although adaptation is most often studied with a constant stimulus (figure 15.6), the process underlying adaptation also will modify the time course of the response to a changing stimulus. We will consider the effects of adaptation that act during, and after, both increases and decreases of stimulus intensity and include both smooth and abrupt changes. The term *accommodation* is often improperly used interchangeably with adaptation. Accommodation properly refers to one of two processes. As we have seen in chapter 10, accommodation refers to the gradual increase in action potential threshold when the stimulus is increased slowly. In the visual system, accommodation refers to the adjustment of the optical system to varying image distances.

The result of adaptation is a familiar experience in everyday life. For example, after being in a dark room, one has an initial sensation of excess brightness when normal room lights are switched on. If the new light level is maintained, this glare rapidly wanes as the visual system adapts. Similar adaptation, observed in subjective sensation, also occurs on first exposure to diverse sensory stimuli such as a cold swimming pool, a hot shower, loud music, body rotation, a nonirritating odor, firm skin contact, or even a breeze. A socially notorious case in which adaptation causes the loss of appreciation of the intensity of a stimulus involves the sense of smell. A person exposed to a particular perfume, body odor, deodorant substance, or food odor adapts to the stimulus and becomes unaware of how strongly the stimulus is perceived by others who have not adapted. This sensory adaptation has both central and peripheral components and occurs over a time course of seconds to minutes.

15.8.* Demonstration: Set up three containers of water, one with water that feels quite hot, one with water that feels quite cold, and one with water at a temperature roughly midway between the other two. Place one hand in the hot water and the other hand in the cold water and keep them there for 3 min. Does the sensation change with time? Is the time course and amount of adaptation the same or different for the two hands? Now transfer both hands to the container with water of moderate temperature. What is the resulting sensation? Do your hands give a good measure of absolute temperature? What kind of errors might be expected in judging the temperature of milk for a baby or lotion for a massage by using a manual test? Can you tell from this demonstration whether the adaptation observed is a central or a peripheral process?

Most sensory receptors show some form of adaptation to their adequate stimulus.

One can place electrodes on nerve fibers that come from individual receptors. When this is done, adaptation is commonly observed in the output of those receptors. After a step increase in a stimulus, the initial rapid firing rate of the receptor decreases toward a steady level. Some receptors adapt to a zero rate of firing (figure 15.7A1) and others adapt to a level that is related to the maintained level of the stimulus (figure 15.7A2). These two cases are called, respectively, *complete* and *partial adaptation*. In some receptors, the resting, unstimulated state is characterized by a steady firing rate. In these receptors, when the firing returns to that base level while the stimulus continues, it is reasonable to call this complete adaptation. When receptors, which exhibit steady firing under resting conditions, are adapted to an increased stimulus and then returned to a zero stimulus, the response falls to below the resting level. This has an obvious limit at zero firing rate but provides signals below the resting level (figure 15.7A3).

Individual receptors differ in how fast they adapt to a change of stimulus. The speed of adaptation is sometimes described by a time constant although the process of adaptation is generally only approximately exponential. In this first approximation, responses of adapting receptors are composed of the sum of two parts. Initially both parts depend on the magnitude of the step of stimulus. One

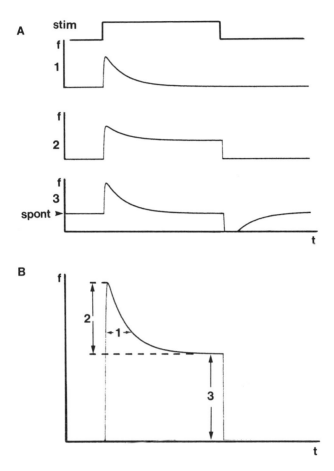

Figure 15.7
Schematic representation of the time course of adaptation. (A) Spike frequency vs. time for a neuron that exhibits complete adaptation (1), partial adaptation (2), and complete adaptation with a spontaneous level of activity (3). (B) Measures that describe adaptation: decay time constant (1), an adapting or phasic portion (2), and a nonadapting portion, part of which can include the spontaneous activity of the neuron (3).

part decays after a step input and the other part continues to represent the magnitude of the step. A variety of responses can be approximated by specifying only three parameters: (1) time constant, (2) relative magnitude of the adapting portion, and (3) relative magnitude of the nonadapting portion (see figure 15.7B). The time constants of different receptors vary widely and, even within one receptor, variations can occur with temperature, pH, stimulus magnitude, and recent stimulus history.

Receptors that adapt completely can produce signals to represent a changing stimulus but not a steady stimulus.

The response of a receptor that adapts completely reflects only the *change* in the stimulus. Thus, a receptor that adapts completely will soon return to its resting output when the stimulus does not change in time but will respond again when the stimulus changes again. The faster the stimulus changes, the more the effect of the change will exceed the loss of response due to adaptation.

15.9. Question: Name at least two different factors in your environment for which a measurement of the absolute value is of less importance to your welfare than a measurement of changes of that value. Might change, in these cases, in some way warn about, or predict, a future state that will be important to you?

While a receptor is responding, a decrease in the stimulus will produce a decrease in the response. In the presence of adaptation, the more rapidly the stimulus decreases, the more the response will decrease. Here the decreased response signals a negative rate of change of the stimulus. Events in the real world (that is, outside the laboratory) tend not to change instantaneously. When they do change, the rate of change usually remains relatively constant over short time periods. Although changes occurring over periods of years are recognized using long-term memory, most of the changes recognized by the nervous system occur in the range of tens of milliseconds to hours. In this important intermediate period, adaptation plays a major role as a predictor of future states. It is possible to use a receptor's combined information about the current value of a stimulus and the rate of change of that value as a predictor of what that value will be at some time in the near future. The output of a partially adapting receptor can signal the predicted magnitude of the stimulus in the near future.

We use predictions of the near future in a variety of everyday activities. While driving, we can estimate how far we will have gone by some future time by adding our current distance to the product of our current speed and the remaining interval. The sources of error in such predictions are obvious but for short time periods, the amount of error is usually small. The mathematical equivalent of this predictive process is the use of a truncated Taylor's series. This series allows extrapolation of values of a function from known values of that function and its derivatives.

Muscle spindles are examples of adapting receptors. Adaptation provides rate of change information that can be used to make predictions about future states of the muscle. The differences in time constants of adaptation and of the ratios of adapting to nonadapting parts of the responses seen among muscle spindles affect how far in advance these predictions are valid. Further combinations of signals from quantitatively different receptors might be used to make predictions over intermediate time intervals. Although such information is available to the nervous system, it is not known how much use is made of it.

15.10.* Problem: A muscle spindle was found to respond to static stretch with an increase of 100 impulses/sec/mm of static stretch. The same spindle responds to the rate of stretch with 3 impulses/sec/mm/sec. When this receptor is stretched at 10 mm/sec, how much faster would it fire than it would if held at the initial stationary length? What additional length would the receptor appear to have because of the additional firing added by the stretching? How long would it take for the receptor to be stretched the additional length that is predicted by its rate sensitivity? How does this lead interval compare with the conduction delays in the stretch reflex? After some interval of stationary length, the receptor's adapting firing rate will be approximately equal to the firing rate that it would reach by a given time if it were responding only to the current position. Try the same calculations using a different rate of stretch but with the same receptor characteristics. Now consider velocities of negative stretch (shortening).

15.11.* Questions: What kind of information would you seek to support the hypothesis that neural control of motor activity takes advantage of a combination of information from receptors with different adaptive properties? Would this same information be available to the nervous system from another source if it did not use adapting receptors?

15.12.* Problem: Write a program that either accepts as an input or generates internally a series of values representing successive samples from a smoothly varying stimulus. Have the program then operate on this stimulus as a simple adapting receptor would. Now have the program either draw a graph or provide a table for hand graphing of both the time series of input values and the corresponding values of the adapting generator potential response. The program should be written so that it is easy to change (1) the input pattern, (2) the adaptation time constant, (3) the adaptation ratio, and (4) the output bias to a zero input. Using this program, simulate enough different combinations of stimuli and receptor characteristics so that you develop the ability to predict the effects of changes in the various parameters before you demonstrate them. To be more realistic, include a procedure that generates a train of impulses at a rate proportional to the response (generator potential) of the adapting model. Putting the output of these pulses through an audio system will give you some experience in interpreting the sounds commonly heard in a neurophysiology research laboratory.

You may have wondered about the fact that the modeling suggestions do not include any consideration for nonlinearity of the receptor's response. In fact, they specifically ignore it in describing the response as proportional to the stimulus magnitude. Congratulations if you noticed this omission; it is more than an isolated case. All models are incomplete and can be misleading when used beyond their appropriate range. The worst examples are verbal models that often have errors of omission that are hard to recognize. On the other hand, a mathematical or other formal model must be specified completely; anything that is not included is specifically omitted and thus limitations are well defined. Since we do not know everything about real neural systems, we always think about them only in terms of our model representations based on some properties. Thus, an important skill in dealing with real systems lies in the ability to recognize how far each of our conceptual models can be used and what its limits are. Whereas excessive extrapolation leads to absurd conclusions, excessive restriction limits thinking. The computer model of pulse coding and adaptation simplifies the actual understanding of the properties of many receptors. The model becomes increasingly incorrect as it is used to represent larger amplitudes of stimulus change where the nonlinearities become more significant. We suggest that you make formal models whenever you can but then subject them to careful criticism!

For receptors that operate over a large range of stimulus intensities, adaptation adjusts function into the current range of intensities.

Adaptation allows the limited range of a pulse rate code to be used at different times for widely varying stimulus intensities. Simultaneously, complete adaptation removes from a neural signal all the information reporting the absolute magnitude of the stimulus.

As we have seen in chapter 2, the pulse rate code used by nerve fibers is limited in its ability to transmit information about the magnitude of a signal. Just as it is not practical to use a truck scale to weigh a letter because the scale lacks sufficient resolution, axons in the optic nerve that report on the light levels on a sunny beach do not have enough resolution to report immediately the differences in light level in a photo darkroom. That the optic nerve, unlike the truck scale, can, at different times, deal with both signals is explained by the effect of adaptation. The ranges spanned by this means can be quite impressive.

The difference in light level between a sunlit snow field and a rural location on an overcast night is $10^{12}:1$ and yet vision operates over the whole range. The functional range of hearing spans a range of $1:10^6$ of sound pressures with a resolution difference as small as $1:1.2$. The ear also has to deal with atmospheric pressure changes superimposed on the sound pressures. The atmospheric pressure variation between sea level and a 6-km mountain is 10^{10} times as large as the pressure variation that produces a threshold sound. The compensation for steady pressure here not only suppresses the near constant offset, but is an essential protection for the delicate receptor structures.

15.13. Questions: Would you expect that hearing threshold would be affected by altitude? Why?

Although adaptation has qualitatively similar effects in many receptors, the mechanisms of its production vary widely from one case to another.

Adaptation, in its broadest sense, includes a multitude of mechanisms. Some of these operate in sensory accessory structures, some in the transduction process, some in transmission, and some in central processing. Visual adaptation, although perhaps the most thoroughly studied, is not yet entirely understood. Increased light level produces pupillary constriction, decreased sensitivity of the receptor cells, a shift from rod vision to less sensitive cone vision, changes in signal processing within the retinal neurons, and probably changes in central processing of optic nerve signals. An important consequence is that the visual system automatically adjusts to operate in an immediate range of variation of perhaps only 1:100 of brightness differences out of a long-term operating range in brightness of $1:10^{12}$.

15.14.* Demonstration: Obtain an assortment of sheets of nonreflecting construction paper including black, several shades of gray, white, and an assortment of saturated colors (red, yellow, green, blue). After adapting for at least 10 min to the light of a single candle at 3–5 m, sort and arrange all the papers in order of your judgment of brightness. Using a very sensitive photometer, measure and record the light reflected from the different papers under the same illumination. (You will need an assistant to read the scale without exposing your eyes to brighter light.) Briefly light the papers with a strong reading light and note any differences in the perceived sequence of brightness immediately after returning to the original test conditions. Has your dark adaptation been decreased by the exposure to the bright light? Illuminate the papers with room light and repeat the sorting and measurements of brightness. Repeat the procedure again in bright sunlight. Compare your judgment of the relative brightness of the colored and gray papers with the luminance readings from the meter.

Do your different judgments of brightness agree across the range of lighting conditions and do they agree with the meter? (Most photometers are designed to have a sensitivity that varies with wavelength roughly corresponding to that of normal human vision.) As judged by meter readings, what information did you have to distinguish among white and black and gray that could be applied across the range of different lighting conditions? Did you note any differences in the appearance of relative brightness of the colored papers? Is the ratio of luminance between papers, or the absolute differences between luminance, the most nearly constant across different conditions of lighting?

The diameter of the human pupil varies from about 1 to 8 mm with changes in light level (and with several drugs). The light admitted varies with the area of the pupil, thus, the pupil provides an adapting adjustment of about 1:64 in the fraction of the incident light that is admitted to the eye. This is a difference comparable to 6 f-stops on a camera. Additional adaptation is achieved through the differing

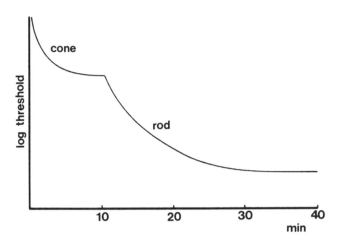

Figure 15.8
Dark adaptation. The dark adaptation curve is measured by taking a subject from a brightly lighted environment to a dark location and measuring his or her visual threshold at various times after the initiation of total darkness. This curve has two components, the first representing the adaptation of the cones, and the second representing the adaptation of the rods.

sensitivities of the rod and cone systems and through the variability of the sensitivity of individual photoreceptors. The sensitivity of the eye, at any state of adaptation, can be determined by measuring the intensity increment of a flash of light that is just noticeable. The required increment of brightness changes in a manner that is roughly proportional to the level to which the eye is adapted. This approximation holds over a range of intensities of $1:10^7$.

The increase in sensitivity that occurs after a time in the dark is called *dark adaptation*. This is one of the slowest forms of adaptation in humans. The time course is, in addition, complex. During the first few seconds, a 50-fold increase of sensitivity occurs with further change continuing over a period of more than 30 additional minutes. When the initial light level is high enough to excite cones, the adaptation is divided into two segments with different time courses. First the cone vision adapts and then, after some delay, the rod vision becomes effective and then it adapts further with a time constant of roughly 6 min. Thus, the whole adaptation curve cannot be reasonably approximated by a single time constant process (figure 15.8). Dark adaptation, necessary for discrimination in a very low light level, can be maintained during activity in moderate light by wearing goggles with lenses that pass only red light. This is effective because the rod system is not sensitive to red light and can adapt even while the red-sensitive cones are being used at the higher light level. (See figure 4.3.)

The Pacinian corpuscle, in responding to mechanical displacement, is probably the most rapidly adapting receptor in humans. This response to a step displacement terminates after only a few milliseconds during which time only one or two impulses are generated. These receptors recover rapidly from adaptation and thus can respond to a succession of displacements (vibration) occurring at as much as 300 Hz. If we define the input to these receptors as *vibration* instead of *displacement,* they do not then adapt. Although it is conventional to define these receptors as rapidly adapting, that definition is dependent on the defined stimulus.

Adaptation, in the Pacinian corpuscle, is a mechanical process. The experimental evidence for this observation was obtained by isolating single Pacinian corpuscles and recording generator potentials from them while they were subjected to external pressure. It was found that the receptor potential showed its normal very rapid adaptation. After the capsule was dissected away, and steps of external pressure were applied, it was found that the generator potential adapted only very slowly (see figure 5.2).

15.15. Problem: If the stimulus to a Pacinian corpuscle is vibration, how would you define adaptation so that you could decide whether these receptors adapt?

Let us consider the combined response of two mechanoreceptors to the same stimulus. The Pacinian corpuscle adapts rapidly and completely whereas the muscle spindle adapts only slowly and, even then, incompletely. A combination of these responses provides distinctive patterns to various inputs that the individual receptors would be unable to differentiate. Low-level step inputs and somewhat larger vibratory inputs would produce the same response from a slowly adapting receptor whereas a brief pulse input and a step input would produce indistinguishable responses in the rapidly adapting receptor. Together, however, the two receptors provide a distinctive output pair for each of these inputs.

We have been stressing the point that the dimensions of sensory receptors are not necessarily those of the physicist. To some extent, the arrangement of the semicircular canals provides a contrast to this observation. Each vestibular apparatus contains three semicircular canals that are in almost orthogonal planes. They can thus resolve complex rotary movement into the three Cartesian coordinates but not in Newtonian units.

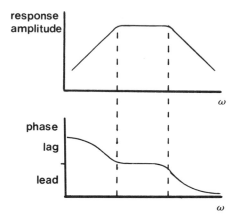

Figure 15.9
Schematic representation of the semicircular canal response to rotation. Response amplitude and phase shift of the semicircular canal response are plotted as a function of angular frequency. (Phase and amplitude are referenced to controlled velocity cycles.) For low-angular frequencies, the response lags and thus better approximates displacement, whereas for high-angular frequencies, the response leads and thus better approximates acceleration. In the midrange, which includes most physiological movements, the response best approximates velocity.

The vestibular receptors of the semicircular canals respond to movement of the head in a complex manner (figure 15.9). When the head is stationary, the receptors fire at a constant rate. If the head is rotated in a direction that includes a vector in the plane of that particular semicircular canal, the receptors may fire more rapidly. Rotation in the opposite direction reduces the firing rate below the level of its stationary response. The firing pattern depends on the magnitude and pattern of the movement. Because it has been most commonly tested with a quickly started, brief constant rotation followed by an abrupt stop, the receptor has become known (inappropriately) as a receptor of angular acceleration. Using this test, the perception is of rotation at about the time of the start and a reverse rotation following the stop. A broader range of stimuli shows the response of this receptor to be more complex. With very slow rotary movements, the closest single term from Newtonian physics to describe the response is *acceleration*. During moderate speed back and forth rotary movement, the response is more nearly described as a response to angular *velocity*. During very fast, cyclic rotary movement, these receptors respond very nearly to angular *position*. On the other hand, the vestibular receptor might be considered to be a position transducer with complete adaptation. Although this receptor has a mechanism of adaptation similar to that of the Pacinian corpuscle, adaptation terminology generally has not been applied to vestibular receptors. No simple, Newtonian term describes the stimulus that determines this receptor's output. Although the response characteristics may sound confusing, the nervous system effectively uses the information in motor control. Perhaps the problem is that the terminology that we are trying to use is not suitable for the biological system. We might do better to call the vestibular canal system simply a sensor of head movement and if more information is needed, then describe in detail what is observed instead of trying to find a simple term from physics.

15.16. Problem: An extensive study of vestibular receptor output dynamics has been made using sinusoidal back and forth rotation of the head in various planes and at various frequencies. As expected, the firing rate response from a particular semicircular canal nerve increased as the plane of the rotation approached the plane of the canal from which the nerve originated. As we have seen, the cyclic firing rate is dependent on the angular velocity of rotation, following successively acceleration, velocity, and then position as the angular velocity is increased. In these experiments, it is most convenient to define the input to the vestibular receptors as cyclic velocity. How would the phase of the position and acceleration cycles compare with the velocity cycle? Draw graphs of the cyclic amplitudes of position at different frequencies of constant amplitude sinusoidal velocity cycles.

Individual semicircular canals have been mathematically modeled as hollow circular tubes filled with fluid that exhibit inertia and viscosity. The tubes are blocked by an elastic plug, the displacement of which determines the output. Solving the resulting equations, with realistic values for the various parameters, produces a response pattern that is quantitatively very similar to the pattern measured from animal data. Sinusoidally oscillating movements with different frequencies but with a constant maximum velocity produce displacements that decrease with increasing frequency (figure 15.10). The acceleration cycle of the stimulus leads the velocity cycle by a quarter cycle (90°) and the displacement cycle lags 90° behind the velocity cycle.

The auditory receptors also have several adaptation-like processes. At very low frequencies of pressure change, the eustachian tube causes adaptation of the tympanic membrane by balancing atmosphere pressure across it. Within the auditory frequency range, very intense sound pressure is attenuated by an adap-

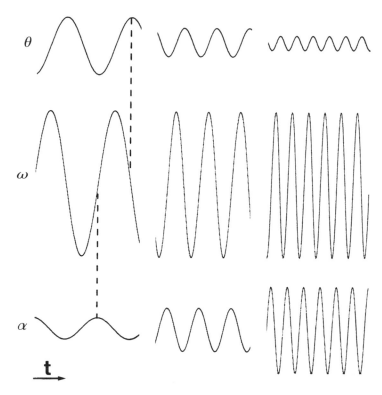

Figure 15.10
Sinusoidally oscillatory movements. Constant amplitude velocity cycles at increasing frequencies are related to increasing amplitude acceleration cycles and decreasing amplitude displacement cycles. Acceleration leads velocity by 90° and displacement lags velocity by 90°.

tive process of reflex contraction of muscles that alters the mechanical coupling between the outer ear and the inner ear. Further adaptation-like effects occur as sound-induced reflexes send neural signals back to the cochlea from the brain-stem. Although each of these functionally important actions has the characteristics of an adaptive process, they have not usually been so named.

The fine nerve endings that respond to noxious stimuli are usually considered nonadapting. The response may be terminated by actual destruction of the receptors although this would not usually be considered as adaptation. Tissue damage can cause the local release of chemical agents that cause an increased sensitivity of nociceptors to any stimulus. In some conditions, this *hyperalgesia* will obscure any counteracting effects of adaptation. Local tissue damage releases chemical agents, such as histamine, that diffuse and decrease the threshold of adjacent nociceptors. Thus, a normally innocuous stimulus may become painful. Here, the effect of a previous stimulus causes an increase of the response over time. Remember the sensation generated by contact of sunburned skin with normal clothing and compare it with the normal sensation of clothing contact. Variations in central processing can further alter the perception of nociceptive information.

With nociceptors, as with Pacinian corpuscles, the definition of the stimulus may affect the meaning of adaptation. It is not clear whether the stimulus should be considered the damaging process itself or the tissue alteration resulting from that process. After burning a finger, has the stimulus ended or does it continue? Perhaps biological receptors were not designed for convenience in classification of their adaptive processes!

Dynamic effects in structures that affect neural signals provide both predictive and cumulative information about stimuli.

In the first part of this chapter we saw that, especially with dynamically changing signals, delays occur due to fiber conduction and due to the lag produced by summation. Lag also modifies and smoothes signals after transmission as impulses on nerve fibers. In the latter part of the chapter we have discussed several mechanisms that introduce adaptation. These result in a type of signal prediction, an adjustment to the current operating range, an emphasis on change, and a loss of absolute measures of stimulus magnitudes. Together, the actions of adaptation and summation provide part of the filtering mechanism by which different nerve fibers carry information about the frequency range of a signal. The most interesting temporal function is not understood, that is how multidimensional stimuli are compared to experience so that when similar patterns are recognized, predictions of probable future situations can be made reliably.

Chapter 16

Neural Network Operations

When neurons interact in simple networks, functional properties can emerge from the network that do not exist in any of the individual neurons.

In several earlier chapters, we have examined functions that occur within individual neurons or parts of neurons. In other chapters, we have considered functions accomplished by the nervous system as a whole. These two types of operation only partly overlap. Complex systems such as the nervous system often include major aspects that, although originating in the combination of parts, are not properties of any individual part. It is generally assumed that many properties of the nervous system are such *emergent properties*. We will deal in this chapter with some general principles by which significant functions can emerge from combinations of neuron-like components. Although some investigators have examined neural network models containing a few thousand cells, we will limit our discussion here to networks of only a few cells. In fact, a simple loop of two neurons introduces many new functions that are not present in a single neuron and one is tempted to conclude that this minimal network is the basic element on which evolution of higher neuronal function is built. (Some current trends in this research are found the article by Getting in the *Annual Review of Neuroscience* 1989 and in sources such as *Computer Simulation in Brain Science*.)

As Sherrington (1941) implied in saying, "mind goes more ghostly than a ghost" (*Man on His Nature*), the human nervous system may be forever beyond full description, and even if one nervous system was fully described, there probably would never be another one exactly like it. We are in the position of accepting, without proof, the assumption that the operating principles of the nervous system can be extrapolated from representative simple subsystems. This chapter will take this assumption as its first premise.

In spite of a large volume of information about the structure of the nervous system, and an increasing rate of acquisition of new information because of recently developed tools, even the wiring diagram of the nervous system is far from known. Still, before examining any reduced models, it is important to have some idea of the nature of the information that is now known about real nervous networks.

1. Long pathways involving large numbers of fibers have been traced by both morphological and functional means. It is important to remember, though, that this is information about fiber pathways rather than about single fibers. Information about some of the best known trunks of nerve fibers is attractively summarized in the *Ciba Collection of Medical Illustrations* by Netter (1986).

2. The ramifications of a single cell's branching have been described using special staining techniques. Silver staining methods, related to silver-based photography, were developed by Camillo Golgi late in the nineteenth century. These methods, with subsequent modifications, made it possible to visualize individual whole neurons. Although it was not understood how these methods stained some cells and not others, silver stains supported most of the early understanding of the fine structure of the nervous system (see, DeFelipe and Jones [1988], *Translation of the Writings of Cajal on the Cerebral Cortex*).

3. Neuron-to-neuron connections through nearby cells have been traced in considerable detail. Early study of the exact connections making up nerve networks is illustrated by the work of Lorente de Nó. He studied closed pathways of individual neurons that could be traced within a very small series of histological sections. These neurons then had one dimension restricted to less than 0.1 mm. It has recently become possible to trace pathways that involve multiple successive histological sections by using confocal microscopy with computer reconstruction techniques. These computer reconstructions can then be rotated and viewed from any angle (figure 16.1). There is a wide range of cell configurations among neurons. Many of these shapes are so characteristic that the shape alone is sufficient to identify the locus in which a neuron is found. One is inclined to suspect that these configurations have functional significance.

Sometimes connectivity patterns, found in one small area of neural tissue, are repeated throughout a considerable volume of the nervous system. For instance, the monosynaptic reflex pathway is repeated hundreds of thousands of times throughout the length of the spinal cord and parts of the brainstem. A more complex network, including several different cell types, is typical over the whole of the cerebellar cortex. Still other characteristic networks are localized in many cerebral cortical areas and in central cell clusters of the brain (figure 16.2). One must make such spatial generalizations with caution, though, because subtle

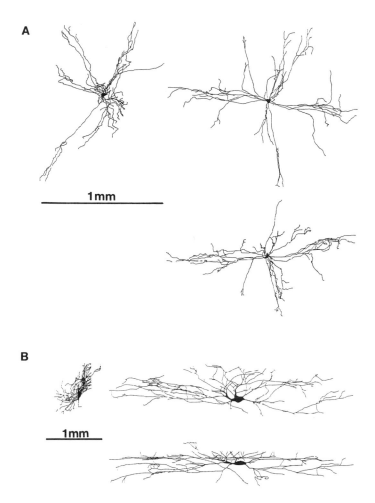

Figure 16.1
Three views of each of two neurons from a cat spinal cord, digitally reconstructed from multiple histological sections. (A) Data from 18 sections, each 60 μm thick (courtesy W.E. Camron and He-Fang). (B) Data from 12 sections, each 80 μm thick (courtesy M.J. Sedivec, L.M. Mendell, and J.J. Capowski). Right angled rotations were accomplished by J.J. Capowski using facilities of Eutectic Electronics, Inc.

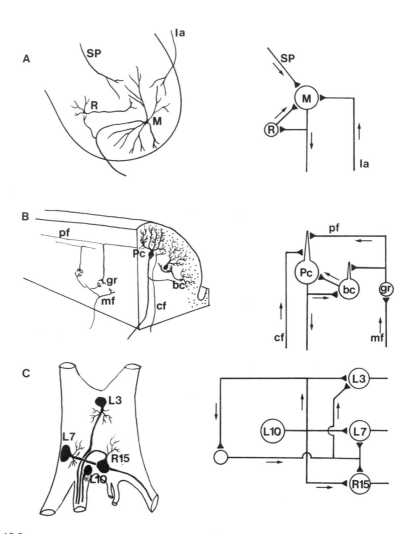

Figure 16.2
Examples of neural networks. The left hand figures show semipictorial representations of
neuronal morphology; the right-hand figures show circuit representations for the same networks.
(A) Spinal reflex arc: SP, descending spinal tracts, M, spinal motoneuron; R, Renshaw interneuron; Ia, primary afferent from muscle spindle. (B) Cerebellar cortex circuits: Pc, Purkinje
cell; bc basket cell, pf, parallel fibers of the granular cells; gr, granular cell; mf, afferent mossy
fiber; cf, afferent climbing fiber. (A and B are after similar figures in G. Shepherd, *Synaptic
Organization of the Brain.*) (C) Invertebrate (*Aplysia*) neuronal circuit. Identified *cells* in the
abdominal ganglion are numbered with an L and R prefix depending on the side of the ganglion
(after similar figures in E. Kandel, *Cellular Basis of Behavior*).

structural differences among generally similar networks may have major functional significance.

The opposite extreme, nonrepeated networks, is found in the nervous system of several invertebrates. The structure of many of these networks has been described in considerable detail and often their unit function has been equally well characterized. In marked contrast to the typical case in the mammalian brain, invertebrate nerve networks often consist of a few, individually identified afferent neurons, an equally small number of interneurons, and often only one efferent neuron. Even these very simple networks can, however, control complex responses.

4. Extensive functional studies have been carried out to probe the inputs to, and outputs from, single neurons in vertebrate nervous systems. When such a cell operates within the nervous system, it can receive a multitude of inputs so that its output can be significantly influenced by many other neurons. Microelectrodes inserted into individual neurons (see chapter 10) can be used to record the effects of individual inputs on the cell's electrical activity. Such information has provided us with information about interactions between small regions of the nervous system and specific cells. In addition, it is possible to place a microelectrode into a cell and, while recording its electrical activity, introduce dyes that spread throughout the cell. Such methods are valuable in relating structure to function in specific types of neurons that are part of known networks.

Qualitatively divergent activity patterns in a network may arise out of differences in input pattern or in changes of the effectiveness of connections.

In parallel with the growth in understanding of the structure of the brain from the work of Cajal, has been a similar growth in the understanding of the network function of the brain. A collection of 43 papers tracing one line of these studies from 1890 until 1987 has been assembled by J.A. Anderson and E. Rosenfeld (1989).

Although anatomical connections impose absolute limits on what a neural network can do, the network can accomplish very different results depending on the effectiveness and dynamic properties of each connection. As a result, similar connections may produce quite different effects and, conversely, similar effects may be generated in very different circuits. The possible functions of a network span a far greater range than the known variations of anatomical connections.

To keep the topic within manageable limits, we shall consider only a few general patterns of connections and of interactions found within nerve network components. Even simple networks have a complexity of function that has not yet been adequately explored and can provide the foundation for an understanding of many neural functions that cannot be explained in terms of isolated unit properties.

Several important properties combine to determine the response of neurons or receptors to driving signals. *Threshold* sets a lower limit below which no response occurs, whereas *saturation* sets an upper limit to the response (see figure 6.6). Nerve fibers, while transporting information from one site to another, introduce conduction *delay* without otherwise altering the temporal pattern within the impulse signal. Branching in axons causes the same signal to be often delivered to more than one site. The energy inputs from a variety of sources *converge* to produce changes in the electrical potential of a receptor. Likewise, signals carried by different axons can converge on the cell body or dendrites of an individual neuron and signals from the central nervous system can converge with external inputs in some receptors. Additional convergence occurs when the endings of one axon terminate on a second neuron's presynaptic termination on a third neuron (e.g., presynaptic inhibition as discussed in chapter 13). These converging signals eventually produce a new signal in which the incoming contributions are inseparably combined. Because of interactions, both the dynamic interpretation and the scaling of the effect of a particular input signal are commonly different from one instance to the next, even in the same neuron or receptor.

The functional implications of theories about simple networks of neurons are sufficiently complex that formal modeling studies are essential for understanding network behavior.

Intuitive interpretations that may seem reasonable can be totally wrong when applied to systems that operate on signals. A formal examination of the properties of a dynamic system is generally essential to avoid such errors. Various methods have been used to simplify the treatment of either the dynamic or the nonlinear properties of biological systems. Unfortunately, when both nonlinear and dynamic properties are combined, many of these methods fail. Simple computers can be of considerable use in exploring properties of moderately complex systems. It is important to keep in mind that the discontinuous representation of time that is used in all digital computer models can sometimes introduce serious errors into models of dynamic systems.

In one of the most direct approaches, simple components are first described with algebraic and first-order difference equations to determine the rate of change of the output as a function of inputs and internal signals within that component. Larger systems can then be represented simply by linking the outputs (after necessary integrations over time) of the appropriate components to the inputs of other components. The whole set of equations is evaluated at one time and then these values are used iteratively to evaluate the system at successive time intervals. In spite of the apparent simplicity of this method, there are many technical problems that await the unwary modeler. One problem is that in nonlinear operations, the exact order of successive operations is critical. The sequence of linear and nonlinear operations becomes especially important. The length of the time intervals in the iteration is also critical. Intervals that are too coarse miss important fast changes whereas intervals that are too fine not only add excessive time to the calculations but lose sometimes critical small differences. When these two time restrictions overlap, special "stiff system" methods are required.

Many very instructive computer representations of models can be constructed with elementary programming ability. The student with some programming ability is encouraged to try modeling but is advised to start with what may appear to be absurdly simple partial models. Even these are usually found to have some unexpected characteristics. Only after the partial models have been tested thoroughly should an attempt be made to assemble several partial models into a more extensive system. A stepwise development is advisable because those effects that commonly appear as surprises in extremely simple models may be totally unaccountable when first encountered in a complex model. Although the purpose of modeling is to build up an understanding or to verify theories of complex systems, extensive models can function just as obscurely as the real system, unless approached in small steps.

Models of neural networks generally make use of the following four signal-modifying actions.

1. *Convergence,* in which signals from different sources are combined;

2. *Serial sequence,* in which the output of one operation becomes the input of the next operation;

3. *Parallel operation,* in which the same or a related signal is delivered simultaneously through multiple pathways; and

4. *Feedback* in elementary networks, in which a closed pathway brings the output of an operation back to determine at least part of the input to that same operation.

Block diagrams, a formal algebra that defines acceptable manipulations, are a convenient tool for representing functional relationships in a neural network.

To treat systems in a general way, formal *block diagrams* are used to represent the connections of the systems under consideration. Although block diagrams are frequently used casually, their effectiveness depends on the specific and consistent use of each symbol. The simple, but sufficient, version that we will use is defined in appendix J. A few restrictions, manipulations, and implications of certain diagrams are also discussed in appendix K.

16.1.* Problem: Draw a block diagram equivalent to the schematic diagram of one Purkinje circuit as shown in figure 16.2B. Draw a second diagram of the cerebellar circuit representing multiple individual circuits as a single block but show that many parallel outputs exist and that many granular and climbing fiber inputs are involved. You will probable need a stack of scrap paper or a blackboard to organize these block diagrams.

Many neural functions are not generated exclusively through neural components but require mechanical, chemical, or endocrine processes to complete the function. Thus, in passing through the system, a signal may be carried in one part by endocrine agents, in another part by mechanical action, and in another part by local depolarizations or nerve impulse trains. Block diagrams represent information processing and do not deal with exchanges of materials or with any specific energy exchange.

By itself a block diagram represents only the connections involved in signal processing. Parts of the operation on these signals often can be combined without modifying the overall function by using specific rules of block diagram algebra. One example of this process is shown in appendix K.

A given stimulus can act on many receptors and afferent nerve fibers. Thus one stimulus can provide different inputs with different eventual uses.

The representation of many types of information within the nervous system is not defined by the activity of individual cells but exists only in a spatiotemporal

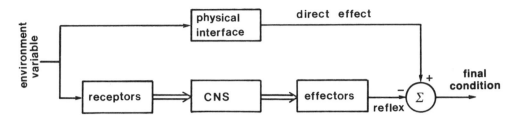

Figure 16.3
Block diagram representation of prototypical feedforward circuit. Environmental variable is shown as acting on both a sensory receptor and on a physical parameter within the body. The sensory receptor activates a reflex response that compensates for the effect of conditions sensed in the environment. Resulting internal conditions are determined by a combination of direct influence and the compensatory reflex.

distribution of parallel signals over an array of cells. Neural signals that originate in similar, adjacent receptors and then travel on adjacent nerve fibers to similar second-order neurons are examples of nearly parallel systems. Usually the signals on such pathways have close functional relationships. A similar type of parallelism occurs when a single nerve fiber bifurcates and the branching fibers carry identical signals to different but related destinations. Often pathways that are not geometrically parallel are functionally parallel in that they carry similar signals and accomplish similar results. When different pathways, carrying signals originating from the same stimulus, finally converge on the same output, the pathways are topologically parallel, although they may not be geometrically parallel or even functionally equivalent. Some pathways extract different types of information from the same multidimensional stimulus and then transmit those signals to the same or adjacent units. Feedforward control is one special case in which information, which is carried by different means from a common input, reaches a common output (figure 16.3). In the most general sense, all neurons have a certain parallelism in that afferent neurons operate independently to process part of the total world information whereas efferent fibers operate in parallel on the total effector drive. The commonality of one or another form of parallelism across the whole nervous system leads one to suspect that the survival of parallel connections, in spite of added metabolic cost, represents an appreciable functional value.

16.2.* Problem: List several functionally important results of different types of parallelism in neural operation that could contribute to the survival of both the individual and the species.

We will illustrate the many parallel pathways of the nervous system with several examples.

Signals on the axons in a muscle nerve originate in a motoneuron pool of the spinal cord and travel over parallel fibers through the nerve branches that finally form the muscle nerve. These signals can eventually accomplish similar results on the individual motor units that they supply. Furthermore, most muscle nerves branch extensively near their terminals and these branches drive functionally similar muscle fibers in parallel.

16.3. Problem: Under what circumstances would a single nerve fiber supplying all the motor fibers of a single muscle be less satisfactory than the system of multiple parallel fibers?

Adjacent retinal photoreceptors act on visual signals producing information that is carried on several parallel pathways. Even within the traditionally color-specific cone system, there is evidence for three parallel information processing systems. One system extracts wavelength information from the multireceptor signal. A second system extracts high-resolution spatial information that is necessary for static form perception. Finally, a third system extracts information about movement and stereoscopic depth. Individual receptors can contribute to all three of these sets of extracted information (Livingston, 1988).

In and just beneath the skin are found a variety of receptors that respond differently to natural cutaneous stimuli. These receptors supply separate nerve fibers, sometimes having both different conduction velocities and different central connections. Often branches of the fibers, carrying signals from different kinds of skin receptors, travel along somewhat parallel pathways and eventually converge onto cortical regions that are more characteristic of the location of the receptors than of the type of stimulus to which that receptor responds. Thus, signals representing different types of stimuli, occurring in adjacent regions of the skin, can act on a contiguous region of the cerebral cortex. The absolute size of these cortical areas is not fixed but can change with usage (Merzenich et al., 1984).

16.4.* Problem: Under what circumstances might it be important for different types of information from adjacent skin areas to be brought into proximity in the brain?

Those bundles of fibers, which are named as tracts of the central nervous system, provide parallel pathways from one group of neurons to specific clusters of somewhat similar target neurons. Even if the connections were exactly known, there would be an inadequate basis for identification of tract function without also knowing the quantitative and dynamic actions of individual fibers. It is unlikely that any two fibers in a given tract will always carry the same signal nor is it likely that two neurons in the target nucleus will produce exactly the same effect or be driven only by branches of the same tract fibers.

16.5.* Problem: Describe ways in which both the similarity and the differences in signals on individual fibers in a tract might be of value. Be as specific as you can about particular examples of information that might be involved.

A complex type of parallelism is apparent in the structure of the cerebellum. The cerebellar cortex is distinguished by a very uniform-appearing network of connections with only one type of output cell, the Purkinje cell. Purkinje cells receive inputs from a few cell types, two of which are the *parallel fibers* and the *basket cells* (see figure 16.2B). Of particular interest is that much of this regular organization is in the form of a strict array in the three Cartesian coordinates. The dendrites of Purkinje cells spread over parallel planes that are intersected perpendicularly by parallel fibers. Each parallel fiber makes one excitatory contact with one Purkinje cell as it passes through the plane of its dendrites and then goes on to synapse with 300 to 500 other Purkinje cells. A single Purkinje cell will receive parallel inputs from perhaps a quarter of a million different parallel fibers. Basket cells make a powerful inhibitory synaptic input onto the cell body of a Purkinje cell. Each Purkinje cell receives input from but one basket cell but a single basket cell has parallel outputs to about 20 different Purkinje cells. For an introduction to this highly parallel structure see the *Handbook of Physiology,* section 1, chapters 16, 17, and 18. Those familiar with matrix algebra might surmise, correctly, that cerebellar function could be investigated as a matrix operation. One tensor transformation theory that has been recently examined is described in *Cerebellar Functions* by A. Pellionisz (1985).

 The parallelism of a feedforward system (figure 16.3) differs in an interesting way from that of the systems that we have been describing. For example, in the regulation of body temperature, an external thermal environment is interpreted by thermoreceptors in the skin in terms of neural signals. This set of neural signals, after combination with other signals and processing within the nervous system, regulates biological processes that modify both heat production and heat dissipation by the body. The energy gradients that produced the stimulus also appear as information in the entirely different form of gradients for heat transfer between the body and the environment. This common source information passes by different pathways to converge finally in the resultant body temperature. The neural signal and its effect produce feedforward regulation of body temperature.

16.6. Problem: Modify figure 16.3 to include the effects of internal body temperature. Is this feedforward control?

Neurons are often treated as a simple convergence point at which synaptic inputs are added. In some cases the dynamic differences associated with different dendritic locations of synapses are trivial, but in other cases they may not be (see figure 13.8). Threshold and impulse encoding action can add significant nonlinearities. The nature of the postsynaptic ion channel will have marked effects on the postsynaptic potential change. Synaptic inputs can alter the postsynaptic effectiveness of other synaptic inputs. Presynaptic inhibition or facilitation can presynaptically alter the effectiveness of a synaptic input. The interactions of these nonlinear combinations of signals give more functional capabilities to a network than would exist in neurons with only the simple additive convergence of signals.

16.7.* Problem: Draw a block diagram of signal processing in a single neuron that provides specific representation of these aspects of convergence. How can this diagram be reduced without misrepresentation?

There are many examples in which threshold nonlinearity following a convergence of signals contributes to function. Some regions of the CNS are called *activating systems*. Activity of these systems converges on reflex pathways to increase the level of excitation of the reflex. Many modulatory effects of neurons that we have considered are examples of nonlinear convergent combinations. This is analogous to the combination of signals that is represented in figure K.7 in appendix K.

All signals, while being processed by the nervous system, are subject sequentially to a variety of operations, each of which changes the way in which the initial information is represented.

Frequently, some of the information content of the signal is lost in the process by which information from multiple sources is combined at a central nervous system junction. Serial operations occur even within individual receptors and neurons as well as within neurons connected in a serial network. The minimal neural sequence of a receptor, a central neuron, and an effector introduces serial operators into all neural pathways. In any such series combination, the output of one element is the input of the next element, so that effects accumulate as the signal passes through the sequence of elements. Although most junctional regions both operate on an incoming signal and serve as a point of convergence, it is convenient to look first at what would happen to a single input because of series-connected operators if no other converging signals were involved.

Several effects of serial operators, applied to continuous signals, are illustrated in appendix K. Corresponding effects can occur in neural pathways, but are sometimes less obvious because of the pulse coded form of some of these signals. The simplest series action in a neural pathway is a conduction delay. Serial delays change the time of arrival of the signal without altering the pattern of successive impulses in the signal. On the other hand, lead and lag operations alter the form of the signal and its timing and as in the serial combinations of figure 16.4, can be cumulative or compensatory. Serial combinations that include nonlinear components interact in a way that makes the dynamic and amplitude operations cross-dependent (see figure K.5). Unless a linear approximation is used, it is essential to recognize the appropriate sequential position of any nonlinear operator. This can present a difficult problem even for the set of operators that represents a single neuron.

Feedback pathways are ubiquitous to neural structures ranging from pathways involving only local connections to those that involve the longest fibers.

Within the nervous system, and in its interactions with the world, the output of individual components frequently contributes to the input of those same components. This is then a *feedback system*. Some properties of feedback systems may not be intuitive and, in fact, may come as a surprise. The complete properties

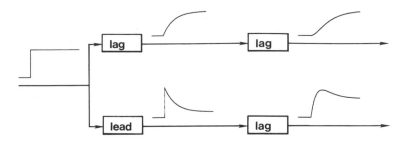

Figure 16.4
Comparison of serial combination of two different operators acting on the same input signal. The effect of a single lag or a single lead operator appears as the output of the first block of parallel pathways. These outputs are in turn the inputs to a second block in each pathway. The second block in each case is the same lag operator. The combination of two lags in series operating on the step input results in a lag that is greater than either operator alone and results in a slow initial rise of the signal. The lag following the lead operation results in an overall response in which neither the lag nor the lead effect is as great as when acting alone. One dynamic operator in this case partially compensates the effect of the other.

of a feedback system usually exhibit dynamic characteristics and patterns of response that differ from those of any of the component parts or even from any simple sum of the component properties. Feedback systems may generate periodic or complexly varying behaviors that emerge from the system. Many properties of feedback systems can be illustrated in simple examples, but most real neural examples involve details of sufficient complexity that it may be hard to recognize the underlying general principles. The present discussion will deal with properties of greatly simplified models.

The simplest cases of feedback by way of nerve fibers in the central nervous system are in a variety of neurons in which collateral branches return and synapse directly on the same neuron. Presumably, conduction delay in these connections is very short. Such feedback circuits have been identified in both cerebral and cerebellar cortical areas and in many deeper nuclei of the brain. Functional, rather than anatomical, evidence was used to first identify one simple pathway, the *Renshaw pathway,* driven by a motoneuron and acting back onto that same motoneuron. Although Cajal's microscopic studies showed what appeared to be closed circuits of individual cells and between nearby cells, there was very little interest in the functional significance of these observations. In 1939, Lorente de Nó (one of Cajal's students) went to considerable effort to show the existence of closed neuron pathways that he called *reverberatory circuits.* He attempted to explain sustained responses to a brief stimulus as resulting from pulses circulating in a closed pathway. At that time it was not yet recognized that the effect of an impulse is extended by the dynamic effects of the lags at junctions (see figure 9.3). We will see later that lag can be greatly accentuated by some feedback pathways.

Neural feedback circuits in sensory and effector systems have been identified both by functional tests and by anatomical tracing. Although many local feedback pathways can be identified anatomically, long feedback pathways are considerably more difficult to identify because of the difficulties in tracing individual fibers over long distances and specific connections through multiple junctions. Feedback pathways that pass outside the central nervous system have generally been traced only functionally. As a minimum, such a neural feedback pathway that involves an effector action must include a nonneural element and a sensory component to return information to the neural parts of the loop.

The stretch reflex involves a closed loop in which the stretch of muscle spindle receptors within the muscle generates a signal that causes excitation of motoneurons, which, in turn, drive contraction of the muscle containing the spindles. In this instance, the mechanical response closes the loop from the efferent to the afferent signal. A similar feedback pathway is found with tendon organs that respond to tendon tension and reflexly inhibit the muscle fibers that drive the muscle acting on that tendon. Two other feedback loops involving muscle and mechanical movement are seen in the eye where the visual image provides neural information that feeds back onto the muscles that rotate the eye, thereby changing the image location on the retina. These same visual inputs also are employed through other pathways to control the muscles that adjust the pupil diameter in response to total light flux. Other feedback systems with portions of the loop outside the nervous system depend on blood-borne agents. For example, the kidney responds to endocrine agents to regulate Na^+ excretion in response to changes in blood osmolarity sensed by osmoreceptors in the brain. Similarly, both O_2 and CO_2 levels in the blood are sensed to produce reflex signals that drive respiration changes that alter those blood gas levels.

Feedback systems are generally classified into *negative* and *positive* feedback depending on whether a static input change at one point in the loop returns a signal to that point with an effect that *increases* the original change (positive) or that *decreases* the original change (negative). In passing through a reflex pathway, there may be more than one inhibitory action, but it is the sign of the action taken around the whole loop that determines the sign of the feedback. A sequence of an even number of inhibitory steps around the loop will produce a positive feedback and an odd number results in negative feedback. It is necessary to define feedback in terms of a static signal because, when a cyclic signal is delayed as it passes around the loop, phase shift causes an instantaneous change of sign that depends on signal frequency. Oscillations can result when the feedback signal from one cycle lags enough to drive the next cycle of oscillation.

16.8.* Problem: Explain why the stretch reflex is a negative feedback system when stretch of the muscle spindle, in parallel with muscle fibers, excites motoneurons that then excite the muscle fibers to contract.

Positive feedback occurs when a small static change in a signal acts around a closed loop so that it tends to increase the original change in the loop.

With positive feedback, the response to a small input can be much larger than it would have been in the same system without the feedback (figure 16.5A). In a positive feedback system, a small change of input produces a response that is fed back as a further change of the input in the same direction. The output will be determined by the sum of the original input and the further input that is added by the feedback. If this added input is smaller than the initial input, the feedback loop has a gain of less than one and the final output will settle to a value that, although larger than the output without feedback, is determined by both the input and the system responsiveness. On the other hand, if the positive feedback is greater in size than the input that generated it (loop gain > 1), then the output will run away to the limit of what the system can produce (e.g., as in the Hodgkin cycle in the generation of an action potential.)

One approach to analyzing feedback systems is to use a simple algebraic calculation for steady-state relationships after all the transient effects of a previous change have died out. The input amplitude of each component is related to its output amplitude by a response ratio. The input signal, multiplied by the response ratio, determines the output amplitude of that component. For a linear system, a set of simple algebraic equations can be written to express this relationship. Solving these equations simultaneously defines the values that would exist in a steady-state equilibrium. In the feedback system diagrammed in figure 16.5B, the steady-state response ratio (gain) of the forward element is G and the response ratio of the feedback component is H. Thus the output of the feedback

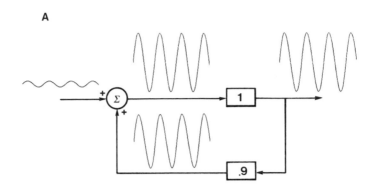

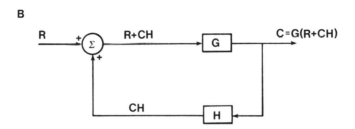

Figure 16.5
(A) Positive feedback system response to a small input signal. Feedback adds a response that changes in the same direction as the input signal. (B) Positive feedback system with forward operator, *G,* (gain) and feedback operator, *H.* The system responds to steady-state input, *R,* (reference) to produce an output, *C* (controlled variable).

operator, H, is simply the product $C \times H$. After summation with the input signal, R, the input to the forward operator, G, is $R + (C \times H)$. The output of the forward element, C, is again the product of its inputs and its response ratio:

$$[R + (C \times H)] \times G = C \tag{16.1}$$

This can be rearranged to give:

$$R \times G = C - C(H \times G) \tag{16.2a}$$

$$= C[1 - (H \times G)] \tag{16.2b}$$

and

$$C = R \times \frac{G}{1 - (H \times G)} \tag{16.3}$$

As is seen in equation 16.3, when $H \times G$ is greater than 0 but less than 1, the output, C, is proportional to R and is greater than $R \times G$. Thus, the output is not only sensitive to changes in the input, R, but also is sensitive to small changes in the system parameters, $H \times G$. This is especially true for values of $H \times G$ only slightly less than 1. Substitute different values for G and H into equation 16.3 to satisfy yourself that you understand how responsiveness in the forward and the feedback elements affect the overall responsiveness, C/R, of a positive feedback system.

We will discuss the case of $H \times G < 0$ (negative feedback) later, but mention needs to be made of the case of $H \times G = 1$. When $H \times G = 1$, the equation for the output involves division by zero. No real feedback system can have an open loop gain, $H \times G$, equal to 1 because this would require that the system produce infinite outputs when the loop is closed. Real systems have output limitations that produce nonlinearity such that, at large amplitudes, the effective gain is reduced to some value slightly less than one. Under these conditions, the system can go to a limiting output that is maximal or minimal depending on the sign of the reference input.

One frequently sees diagrams of neuronal circuits (e.g., figure 16.6A) that are, in fact, positive feedback circuits although this feedback aspect is usually ignored or not even recognized. Such circuits may include reciprocal activation of antagonistic outputs, mutual inhibition between inputs, and central organization of reciprocal activities. In each case, two neurons, or two pools of neurons (*half centers*), are each subject to varying excitation and in turn provide an output that has a branch that inhibits the other neuron or pool. When these are redrawn in the topologically equivalent block diagrams (e.g., figure 16.6B), it becomes apparent that for either input there exists a positive feedback pathway (two inverses). Whenever the positive feedback circuit causes an increase in the output from one neuron pool, the resulting inhibitory action will decrease the output of the other neuron pool. If one neuron pool is driven slightly more than the other, there will be a greater relative difference between the outputs of the two pools. A simple reciprocal inhibitory network can act as a discriminator that responds strongly to small differences in the relative effectiveness of two simultaneous inputs. When one input arrives before the other, it will have precedence.

A

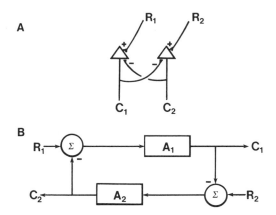

B

Figure 16.6
Pictorial (A) and equivalent block (B) diagrams of two reciprocally related neurons. Input signals, R, minus the signal from the opposite unit provide the input to the operators (A). Each output, (C) depends on the circuit characteristics and on both inputs. The operators can be simple multipliers or they can include threshold effects. A more complete representation of the neuron includes the effects of different input signal sizes and timings.

16.9.* Problem: The neuronal circuit in figure 16.6 could represent two motoneurons whose outputs drive antagonist muscles that determine the angle of a joint. (Do not be surprised if this is more difficult than appears on first inspection.) Using the same type of fixed-gain calculation that was used in describing the responsiveness of a simple positive feedback system, write an equation relating the output joint angle of the system shown in this figure as a function of the two inputs and the system parameters. Consider the effect of thresholds. Assume that the product of the two gains is less than one. Determine how either of the motoneuron outputs is related to changes in the corresponding input. Decide how one motoneuron's output is related to changes in the opposite input. When one motoneuron is driven to exactly zero, is the other output zero, positive, or negative? What would happen if the gain were to be exactly one?

16.10.* Problem: Speculate on the possible significance of reciprocal circuitry in the problem of spatial localization of sound. This function involves a trade-off between intensity information and the phase differences between sound arrival at the two ears. Would your speculation fit with the known frequency dependence of the trade-off?

Whereas positive feedback usually accentuates the effect of inputs and of changes in the elements in a loop, negative feedback can compensate for changes in elements and reduce the relative effectiveness of some input signals.

In 1927 Heymans and Heymans described the chemoreceptor reflex that regulates respiration in a way we would now call a negative feedback system. In 1924, Liddel and Sherrington clearly described what we would now call a negative feedback system in the stretch reflex. They recognized both its corrective and its oscillatory possibilities. They applied the term *myotatic reflex* to this loop and *clonus* to the oscillation well before feedback was an established term. The engineering term "feedback" was not ordinarily attached to such biological systems until 1948 when Wiener pointed out the similarities among technological and biological control problems and proposed that similar mechanisms might be employed. He recommended the common study of these systems as a means to advance both subjects and called such study *cybernetics*. Independently Merton (1953) pointed out that the stretch reflex had characteristics of a servo system with negative feedback properties.

In a negative feedback loop, any small change in the signal at some point in the loop results in an effect that will be returned to that point and then subtracted from the initial signal. This simple change in sign of the feedback results in qualitatively different properties from those of a positive feedback loop. A negative feedback system is less responsive to input changes than is the isolated forward component of the system. The output is less sensitive to changes in the responsiveness of the forward component and less sensitive to interfering actions that enter certain parts of the pathway.

Frequently, the inverse effects in a signal-handling pathway are shown by using a negative sign in the input to a summing point. On the other hand, it is often more appropriate to place the inverse operator within a block. For example, activity on the vagus nerve inhibits the heart so we might draw the cardiac pacemaker in a block with the vagus nerve as an input. The relationship between the input (vagus nerve firing) and the output (heart rate) has a negative slope. Over some ranges, this might be approximated by a constant multiplier with a negative value. In practice there is a nonlinear limiting relationship so that, even in the presence of a strong inhibitory input, the heart rate never takes on a negative value nor can nerve firing rate be negative. An inverse operator, as much as a negative combination at a summing point, results in a single sign change when determining whether a feedback pathway is negative or positive.

16.11.* Problem: Review equations 16.1–16.3 and make the necessary changes to represent a negative feedback system in the steady state. Is there now any problem with the equation 16.3 when $G \times H$ has a magnitude of one? When the reference signal, R, changes by ΔR, does the controlled variable, C, change by $\Delta R \times G$, or more, or less? Again, examine the effect on the output of separate changes in the magnitude of G and H. Does the output change in the same direction as the change in G? Is the output affected in the same way by changes in H? Are there any discontinuities in the effect of changes in values of G and H as long as $G \times H < 0$?

The effects of feedback are the same in technology and in biology but may differ in the relative magnitude and importance of different parts of those effects on function.

Since the introduction of cybernetics by Wiener, there has been a tendency to describe reflex systems with ideas and terms from engineering feedback systems. It has been assumed that the function of reflex feedback is to linearize the effect of nonlinear components, suppress disturbing interference, compensate for changes in load, and reduce response sensitivity to variations of component characteristics. Although there is no reason that negative feedback should not operate in biological systems as it does in technological systems, it does not follow that the relative benefits of these different effects would be the same. Biological systems often have quantitative differences from their engineering counterparts and similar effects are not necessarily of equal value in the two instances. Since it is much easier to analyze linear than nonlinear systems, it is generally desirable to make engineering components behave linearly. Negative feedback can be used to give a poorly controlled but powerful motor a more linear and consistent performance by using precise sensing and controlling elements that, unlike biological sensors, do not introduce significant errors of their own. Biological feedback systems differ from their engineering counterparts in that suppression of noise is less effective and ease of analysis offers no functional advantage. Although it is convenient to take advantage of the extensive information about engineering feedback systems in the study of biological parallels, one must always be cautious of the validity of the analogies.

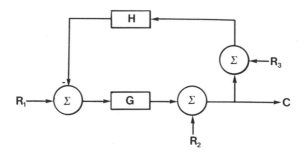

Figure 16.7
Closed-loop negative feedback system with three inputs, R_1, R_2, R_3. A nonlinear transformation following a summation can produce a situation in which one input signal is acted on differently as another varies.

Figure 16.7 illustrates a simple feedback system with inputs at three functionally different points. The static balance for these different inputs exemplifies that of neural feedback loops where each neuron in the feedback pathway serves also as an additional input point. It requires only algebra to show that the effect of an input on a particular output may be reduced or even reversed in direction depending on where it enters the feedback system. The response to an input at some points in the loop may be somewhat insensitive to changes in some parameters while being sensitive to changes in other parameters. Likewise, increasing a parameter can increase the sensitivity of the output to one input while decreasing its sensitivity to another input. Since it is common for a closed loop pathway in the nervous system to have both multiple inputs and multiple outputs, it is probable that multiple effects are being accomplished simultaneously. For example, a simple loop, such as that in figure 16.6, might coordinate reciprocal activity in a flexor-extensor pair of muscles.

16.12. Problem: The static equilibrium point in a linear feedback version of figure 16.7 has different sensitivities to the different inputs. The partial derivatives of the output to each input are

$$\frac{\partial C}{\partial R_1} = \frac{1}{1 + (G \times H)} \tag{16.4}$$

$$\frac{\partial C}{\partial R_2} = \frac{-G}{1 + (G \times H)} \tag{16.5}$$

$$\frac{\partial C}{\partial R_3} = \frac{-(G \times H)}{1 + (G \times H)} \tag{16.6}$$

For each of these derivatives, determine the partial sensitivity of the output to changes in G and in H. In each case, is adjustment of G or H more effective in determining the magnitude of output response to signals entering at each of the inputs? If you cannot answer one of these questions, what additional information do you need?

Not only does negative feedback tend to reduce nonlinear effects in the forward component of a loop but, when nonlinearities appear in the feedback pathway, the total response takes on a characteristic that is the inverse of the feedback component's behavior. This can give a neural pathway a response pattern that does not exist in any individual neuron—an *emergent property*. The convergence of signals within feedback loops, along with nonlinear behavior, greatly increases the variety of possible combinations of signals.

Nonlinearities and feedback together complicate even the static characteristics of very simple networks. Real neural feedback loops are more complex than the models that we have considered, yet the effects discussed in these simple models can be expected to be part of the rules of the more complex biological systems (figure 16.8).

Feedback produces quantitative alterations of both static signal amplitudes and the temporal scale of dynamic responses of the whole loop as compared to those of the individual components.

Since much of the nervous system's function involves time-varying signals, the dynamic characteristics of neural networks become critical to functional analysis. In closed pathways, dynamic details determine the temporal relationships between changing input signals and the returning feedback signals. Even small quantitative differences in dynamic properties can lead to qualitatively different patterns of activity in feedback pathways. As they do in static balances, positive and negative feedback systems give different results in dynamic relationships. Lag in summation at neurons, temporal discontinuities in pulse coding, adaptation in receptors, and delay in nerve fiber conduction are the principal dynamic factors that determine the behavioral patterns seen in neuronal feedback loops. A simple

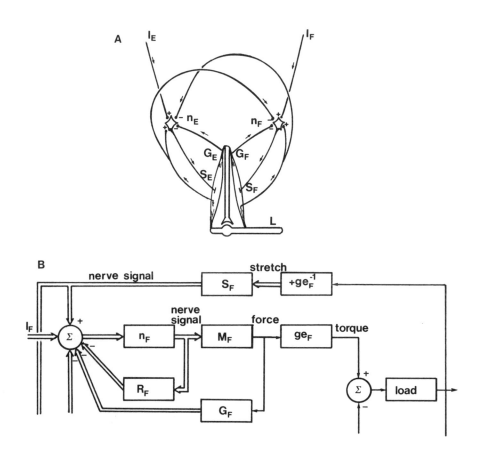

Figure 16.8

Diagrams of spinal reflexes operating at a single joint in pictorial form (A) and the flexor half in block diagram form (B). These diagrams show the response to Golgi tendon organs (G) and muscle spindles (S) in a flexor (F) and an extensor (E) reflex operating on muscles. These both act through the geometry (ge) of the attachments of the muscles on the load (L) on that joint. Inputs (I) from higher centers act with signals from receptors, summing on the neurons (n) of the motoneuron pools of the two muscles. The summed signals are acted on by the operators of the neurons in the two pools producing multineuronal outputs that drive the motor units of the associated muscles (M). The outputs of motor units of each pool act back through Renshaw paths (R) to inhibit motor units of the same pool (the interaction of position on the muscle is not included). From the pictorial diagram in (A) you should be able to complete the extensor half of the block diagram. Examine this figure closely and identify the different signals and the different types of sub pathways that are involved.

knowledge of the connections within a network tells little of how it would operate without the addition of quantitative information about dynamic details.

Lag and delay in a positive feedback circuit result in a time shift of the signal that is fed back around the loop. A change in the input leads to an additional change, in the same direction, in the output that follows the delayed return of the positive feedback signal. At the point where the input and feedback signals are combined, the total drive is determined partly by the input and partly by the result of the signal that was fed back through the lagging pathways. This combined signal is, in turn, subjected to further lag as it again traverses the loop. The cumulative effect is that the total lag of a neural network with positive feedback can be much longer than the lag of any of its component neurons. For example, whereas the lag in a single vertebrate synapse has a time constant of only tens of milliseconds, the lag in a positive feedback circuit containing such synapses might theoretically exhibit time constants up to seconds. A short, and relatively simple, neuronal pathway with only small lags in its parts can account for large temporal effects because of feedback actions. As we mentioned earlier (see figure 9.2), prolonged actions of a stimulus were once thought to be the result of a series of isolated impulses circulating in a "reverberatory circuit." One serious problem with this idea was that because it explained the decay of a response after stimulus termination as fatigue, it did not explain the subsequent increase in the response of the system to a new stimulus. Lag in positive feedback dynamics much more accurately accounts for these characteristics.

Negative feedback affects not only the static properties introduced by elements in the loop but also the manifestation of dynamic properties. Negative feedback through a neuron can result in a complete system that does not lag as much as does the isolated effector element. If lag occurs in elements in the feedback pathway, the effect on the whole loop will be the introduction of an adaptation-like property between the input and the output (figure 16.9). An easily observed example can be seen in the pupillary light reflex. Light striking the retina produces signals in both the neural network that accomplishes image analysis and the network that reflexly adjusts the pupil diameter. That this pupillary reflex is subject to lag can be easily shown by watching the contraction of the pupil following an abrupt increase in light level. This lag lies in both the neural pathways and in the muscles that directly determine the diameter of the pupil.

16.13.* Problem: How might the pupillary reflex response to an abrupt change of light intensity on a subject's eye be expected to modify the temporal pattern of light intensity in the observer's eye?

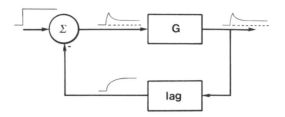

Figure 16.9
Lag in the feedback pathway of a negative feedback system results in a delayed reduction of the driving signal. The effect of lagging feedback is shown for a step input with a simple forward gain, resulting in a system response that corresponds to that of a partial adaptation operator.

Oscillatory activity often emerges from negative feedback loops that have no oscillation in their inputs or in their internal components.

The nervous system generates a variety of signals that control periodic actions such as walking, breathing, and playing vibrato on a stringed instrument. There is a variety of pathologic conditions in which the functional problem involves abnormalities of oscillatory neural signals. Such phenomena include hippus, an oscillation of the pupillary reflex, clonus, an oscillation of the stretch reflex, and Cheyne-Stokes respiration, an oscillation of respiratory control. In these and many other examples, the neural basis for generation of both useful and detrimental oscillatory outputs is thought to result from a feedback process.

Mutual inhibition between opposing neural pools with a common drive (as in figure 16.6) will produce a selective response of one of the two opposing outputs. Such activity is seen in the interaction between inspiratory motoneurons and expiratory motoneurons. The stronger or earlier input influences the way in which the output is driven. Once a choice is initiated, the crossed inhibitory action generally drives the output more strongly in that direction (*precedence of stimulation*). Under some conditions the same kind of interconnections will cause an oscillatory alternation between the two extremes. Graham-Brown proposed in 1911 that the alteration between flexion and extension of walking involved a fluctuation of the drive to opposing motoneuron pools that he named *half centers*. Gesell (1939), again using the half center terminology, found evidence that alternating respiratory movements were the result of excitability of one half center maintaining its activity until taken over by the other half center with a subsequent repetition in alternating half cycles. Recently, several variations of the concept of mutually inhibitory half centers have been revived in attempting to explain different types of alternating neural activities (see, for example, Shepherd, 1988; Shik et al., 1968; Smith, 1978; Grillner, 1975).

The operation of neuronal half centers is similar to that of a class of electronic circuits called *flip-flops*. These circuits have topological similarities to neural systems; in addition, their three functional varieties have certain neuronal parallels. *Astable flip-flops* use adaptation-like transient interactions to produce a continuous alteration between two output conditions. The oscillatory frequency in such systems can be influenced by the level of a nonoscillating input and can be entrained by the frequency of an oscillating input to one or both sides of the circuit. *Bistable flip-flops,* when driven, produce either of their two possible outputs depending on the relative intensity and arrival time of signals at the two inputs. Once the decision-making circuit produces one output, it requires a considerably greater input to the opposite side to switch it to the other output state. *Monostable flip-flops* respond to an above-threshold input by transiently changing from their resting output state to their active output state and then automatically returning to their resting state (like a neuron's action potential). These important electronic circuits can provide a valid model for some elements of neuronal information processing.

With the development of cybernetics came a particular emphasis on negative feedback as a basis of oscillation in neuronal systems. In technological systems involving negative feedback, transient or continuous oscillation is common, either as a problem or as a useful function. Closed loop pathways are found widely in the nervous system or in the combination of neural and effector components. It is not possible, however, from information only about connections to determine whether a particular closed loop will behave as a positive or negative feedback system or whether it might be subject to transient or sustained oscillation. Although the theoretical requirements for oscillation in negative feedback systems have been well established by those who design technical systems, it is difficult to obtain the necessary information to apply these criteria to neuronal systems and further complications arise because of nonlinearities and changing parameters in neural feedback components.

In a negative feedback system that generates an internal oscillation, an oscillatory signal is necessarily returned to the input by way of the feedback pathway. In any cycle, the size of the returned signal determines the size and timing of the subsequent output oscillation. Oscillation of the output depends on two factors: (1) the inversion of the feedback signal inherent in negative feedback circuits, and (2) a one half cycle lag in the feedback signal provided by lags and delays around the loop. If, in one passage around the loop, the size of the returned signal is exactly that needed to drive another identical cycle (and if the phase is appropriate), the loop has an (open loop) gain of one and will sustain oscillation at a constant amplitude. Otherwise the amplitude of successive cycles will grow or decrease, depending on whether the gain is more or less than one. If the oscillation has a nonsinusoidal time course, the corresponding set of timing and amplitude requirements may differ in detail although not in principle.

16.14.* Demonstration: Locate two points in front of you that are separated horizontally by an angle of 30° to 120°. Point first at one and then, moving your whole forearm, point at the other. Observe the movement pattern when the change is made slowly and again when it is made as rapidly as possible. Sketch a graph of angle vs. time to represent the patterns of movement that you saw. These movements involve interaction between a driving signal, motoneurons, muscle contraction, muscle dynamic properties, inertial load, and reflex modification of the activity of the muscle.

Even in feedback systems that do not exhibit sustained oscillation, a transient disturbance will often initiate a damped oscillatory activity.

Biological oscillations are frequently damped. That is, oscillation begins following a transient input, and then the oscillation decreases in amplitude with successive cycles (figure 16.10A). A freely swinging pendulum shows a damped oscillation with each cycle becoming smaller than the previous cycle. The relationship between acceleration, velocity, and position produces the necessary half cycle lag. One biological example that obeys similar rules is the elastic-inertial oscillation that is found in loaded muscle systems. Here the decrease of amplitude per cycle is considerable—more like a pendulum swinging in water than in air—because of the large amount of energy that is absorbed by the muscle in each cycle. Reflex oscillations originate in appreciably more complex systems but often respond in a pattern that is almost indistinguishable from that of simpler mechanical systems. Purely neural feedback pathways also can produce oscillatory activity that involves negative feedback and shows dynamic characteristics similar to a pendulum.

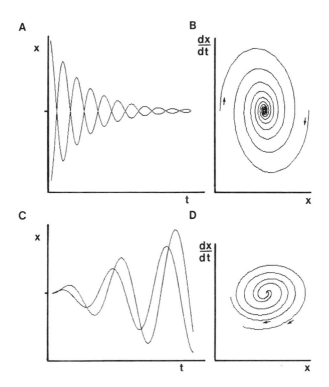

Figure 16.10
Oscillations in a simple feedback system following initial transient inputs. (A) Time graph of the magnitude of two different damped oscillatory responses following different initial displacements. (B) Graphs of the same two damped oscillations superimposed on the phase plane. (C) Time graphs of two expanding oscillations starting at two slightly different initial conditions. (D) Trajectories on the phase plane of the same two oscillations shown as time graphs in (C). The system parameters apply to both trajectories on each graph, only the starting conditions differ.

The position and velocity of a swinging pendulum correspond to signals in the feedback system, and, since the direction of the force is opposite to the displacement, force represents the negative action in the feedback pathway. Each cycle of the pendulum decreases because some of the energy that would sustain equal and opposite swings has been lost through various forms of resistance. In a feedback system, the loss of signal amplitude in successive cycles results simply because the ratio between the inputs to and the outputs from the pathway is less than one so the signal returned is not equal to the starting signal. In either a reflex or a pendulum, an external disturbance can alter the smooth progression of normal oscillation. In neural parts of a reflex, converging neural signals from outside the loop can alter any neural oscillation. In the absence of external interferences, the future trajectory of the pendulum's or reflex's feedback oscillation is entirely determined by the current conditions and the rules by which the system operates. In the pendulum system, the current conditions of importance are position and velocity, whereas in the reflex, the current excitations and their rates of change are critical. The pendulum differs from the neural loop in that the signal that governs the pendulum's oscillation is identical to the energy involved in movement, whereas in the neural loop the energy originates outside the signal-handling system and is governed only by the signals. For motor reflexes, the signals can control the flow of large amounts of energy while themselves operating with low-energy consumption.

16.15.* Experiment: Galileo is credited with the first quantitative description of a pendulum's properties in 1583, although Leonardo da Vinci had hinted at these properties a century earlier, and it took another century after Galileo before Christian Huygens actually provided definitive proof of Galileo's description. To investigate some of these properties yourself, hang a simple pendulum from a stable, *but movable,* support and use it to answer the following questions. Can you manually override the pendulum's oscillatory properties? Can you start similar oscillations from different initial positions and velocities? How does the response to a slow, smooth horizontal change in the support position differ from that to an equal but rapid displacement? Is a quick displacement of the support and its immediate return to the starting position equivalent to no movement? How does the direction of the initial swing of the pendulum relate to the initial change of support position? With a constant support position and manually started pendulum swings, do different starting conditions (position and velocity) produce either different final positions or different oscillatory frequencies? If two moves of the support are accomplished in succession, how critical are the direction, velocity, and timing of the second move with respect to the first in determining the resulting combination of responses?

16.16. Problem: Although the characteristics of a simple pendulum probably present no surprises, can you transfer these intuitively familiar effects to applications in neural feedback systems? Compare the input to a neural loop to a movement of the point of support of a pendulum. What possible feedback effects might account for the problems encountered when a person terminates a period of strenuous exercise by sitting down with an iced drink, when blood pressure-reducing medication is abruptly discontinued, or when a rapidly flashing light triggers an epileptic seizure in a sensitive subject. Why is a second stimulus sometimes followed by a response that is different from the response seen after the first stimulus? Identify other analogies between biological feedback systems and a pendulum. What limitations are there in extrapolating from a pendulum to applications in biological feedback systems?

Under conditions in which there are no external disturbances, the immediate future of many systems is entirely dependent on the magnitude and rate of change of one variable. Many such systems, including the simple pendulum, are *second-order systems. Pseudo-second-order systems,* including many biological feedback systems, are those in which the external behavior looks like that of a second-order system, although more complex internal processes are actually involved. Although time graphs of responses of these systems are probably familiar (figure 16.10A), their dynamic behavior is perhaps better characterized in a *phase plane graph* (see appendix L and figure 16.10B).

Damped oscillation loses information about the starting conditions as time progresses. Under some circumstances, oscillation in feedback systems can generate new information while behaving in a completely determined manner.

Damped oscillatory feedback systems, like a swinging pendulum, will eventually run down to a stationary final condition that is represented by a point on the phase plane graph. If the same system is restarted to produce repeated damped oscillations, the resulting trajectories will all converge on the same point, known as a *point attractor.* The velocity and position information at any point during the oscillation carries information that is related to the starting conditions but, as the trajectories converge, the distinction between trajectories decreases and information is lost until, at the final point, no information remains about the initial trajectory. In feedback systems, however, it is equally possible for the returned signal to grow instead of decrease in successive cycles (figure 16.10C, D). This is shown on the phase plane as trajectories that follow increasing spirals as time progresses. Such expanding trajectories, although initially indistinguishable, will diverge over time and thereby gain information about differences among trajectories. This type of generation of new information by a system that obeys exact rules has interesting implications to neural systems.

Negative feedback systems can produce either damped or expanding oscillation depending on the effectiveness of the feedback pathway. Between these two there should theoretically be conditions that would sustain a constant amplitude oscillation. Since this would require an exact balance of the return signal, the common existence of feedback oscillators that maintain a constant amplitude most certainly results from something other than perfect adjustment. When the loop contains nonlinear elements, it is possible for small-amplitude oscillations to occur in a phase plane region where oscillations expand and for large-amplitude oscillations to occur in a region where oscillations are damped. The result of this combination is a system in which the oscillations adjust themselves to an intermediate magnitude where the returned signal is just sufficient to sustain a constant oscillation. The oscillation produced in this way changes until it traces a closed loop trajectory, in the phase space, that is called a *limit cycle* (figure 16.11A).

The response properties of neurons are even more nonlinear than is necessary to produce a limit cycle oscillation. Very small signals are typically limited by threshold whereas large signals are limited by saturation. Between these extremes is the region of greatest responsiveness (see figure 6.6). When such elements are found in a feedback system, very small or very large oscillations will be damped and intermediate sized oscillations can expand (see figure 16.11B). The trajectory of small oscillations will approach a point attractor. All larger trajectories will expand or contract toward a *limit cycle attractor*. In simple cases, one or the other of these end conditions would be the ultimate result of any starting conditions that fell within a region near that particular attractor—the *basin of the attractor*. The input starting conditions need not be exactly on an attractor for the response ultimately to reach that attractor; they need only fall somewhere within the attractor's basin. When a system is operating within one basin, a subsequent input can drive its activity from that basin into another basin (see

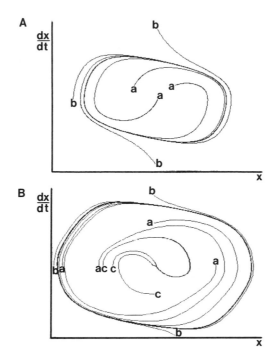

Figure 16.11
Phase plane graphs of trajectories of nonlinear systems. (A) System with one basin leading to
a single limit cycle attractor. Responses starting at points marked *a* expand to the limit cycle
while those starting at points marked *b* contract to the same limit cycle. (B) Nonlinear system
with two basins, one (including points marked *c*) leading to a point attractor and a second
(including all points marked *a* or *b*) in which trajectories either expand or are damped to a limit
cycle attractor.

figure 8.9). Such a change of basins places less strict requirements on an input than does the precise movement from one attractor to another.

There has been recent fascination with the mathematical theory describing dynamic behavior in strictly deterministic but nonlinear systems. The complex, nonstationary, and unpredictable behavior that these systems can produce is sometimes called *chaos*. Applications of chaotic theory have been found in meteorology, physics, engineering, ecology, epidemiology, neurophysiology, and sociology, but proof that a specific real system is truly chaotic is difficult or impossible to obtain. All systems that behave chaotically must be at least slightly more complex than those described by simple second-order dynamics. This complexity can be in the form of functional discontinuities in time or in the presence of higher order terms in the controlling functions. Chaotic behavior is held within bounds, and is constrained to a nonrepeating *strange attractor*. Such behavior continues to generate new information. Chaotic systems can enter one or more basins within each of which all trajectories converge on a specific strange attractor. Chaos is best defined in very simple systems, but its applicability to complex systems is based on observations of behavioral similarities and extrapolations rather than on rigorous theory. (A popular account of the history of the idea of chaos can be found in *Chaos* [Gleick, 1988]. For a more applied account, see the special issue on chaos of the *IEEE Transactions* [Chua, 1987]. A technical examination of some issues is found in *New Directions in Dynamic Systems* [Smith, 1987] and *An Introduction to Chaotic Dynamical Systems* [Devaney, 1989]. A review of graphic representations of nonlinear dynamics is found in *Self Organizing Systems* [Abraham and Shaw, 1987].)

The complex variability seen in repetitive neural activity may originate deterministically rather than as a random process.

Although real neural systems often behave approximately as if their response depended on only the current magnitude and the rate of change of one variable, their future behavior generally depends on additional information about past conditions and about other current variables. When the system behaves like a simple system it is either because some factors are of only minor importance under the conditions of the observation or because effects are hidden by compensation. Even those neural systems that produce simple trajectories over the phase plane may, under other circumstances, show a more complex nature in

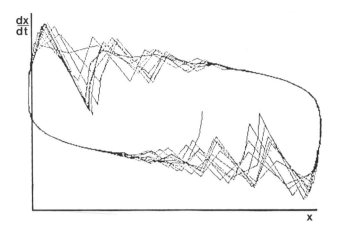

Figure 16.12
Phase plane trajectory of response of a nonlinear and second-order system in which trajectories are determined only at sampled points. This trajectory repeatedly crosses the limit cycle that the same system would have followed if the trajectory had been determined continuously. Sampling rate is approximately 25 samples per orbit.

which successive orbits of their trajectories cross each other and in which oscillations occur with regions of damping and other regions of expansion. The nonrepetitive, complex nature of successive periods in walking or breathing may be solely generated by the rules of a simple neural network without any interference by a random process. These activities also may involve a chaotic component and in any case they are not strictly periodic.

A simple, nonlinear system that uses feedback to generate regular and constant limit cycles is converted to very complex behavior if the feedback information is not delivered continuously but rather is sampled periodically. The effects of the sampling rate and the delays that are involved in the generation of a pulse code in neurons are more than sufficient to produce this type of complexity. As previously described, small oscillations increase in amplitude and large oscillations decrease in amplitude, but with pulsatile signals, information about a current oscillation acts to determine the trajectory until the next impulse is generated. Depending on the shape of the limit cycle and the nature of the adjustment, it is possible for delayed information to produce a trajectory that wanders back and forth across the ideal limit cycle (figure 16.12). Because of relationships between the sampling interval and the period of one orbit of the trajectory, the start of a new orbit may not occur under the same conditions as those under which previous cycles started. Sometimes successive orbits may never return exactly to the starting point of any previous orbit so that the pattern becomes only quasiperiodic. An analog computer model of feedback in two neuron-like elements can develop an oscillation that sustains a complex pattern. These oscillations can exhibit the whole range of patterns seen in EEG recordings. Although the EEG in an intact individual involves activity in at least 10^5 neurons, this simple model demonstrates that it is not necessarily the number of elements that is responsible for the complexity of the output.

Three important principles arise from the analysis of the dynamics of nonlinear systems.

1. Complex behavior does not require the presence of an underlying complex structure.

2. It is important to establish that a variation is random and not chaotic before applying statistical methods to measurements that seem to vary unpredictably.

3. Although the bounds of a measure of behavior of a chaotic system may be precisely defined, the specific trajectory that the activity will follow can be so sensitive to the initial conditions that its course within those bounds is completely unpredictable. Like expanding trajectories in simple feedback, the unpredictability leads to a generation of new information as the actual trajectory is revealed over time.

Transient responses are more important in nervous system function than are the undisturbed chaotic activities that have been of central interest in nonlinear dynamic investigations. The nonlinear dynamics that lead to chaotic behavior can, however, complicate transient and input-driven responses. The study of nonlinear dynamics probably will provide major insights into neuron function of which chaotic behavior may be only a small part.

Real neural networks include branching and converging pathways, multiple interlaced feedback pathways, parallel and sequential neurons each with its own nonlinearities, and the complications of impulse generation. To extrapolate from the simple systems that we have been discussing to neural networks ranges from a trivial task to a completely unexplored area of investigation. One point of extrapolation is that neuronal pathways normally have multiple independent inputs. A loop with inputs to more than one neuron will exhibit interactions that depend on temporal differences in the inputs arriving at the entry points. The concepts of temporal sensitivity that we have considered in the pendulum model are directly transferable to neural networks and to loops with many neurons. Although feedback loops involving many neurons still exhibit many elementary feedback properties that are found in the simplest loops, the higher order equations needed to describe these loops accurately have been described extensively in the mathematics of dynamic systems. We have already considered, for reciprocal innervation patterns, the extrapolation of these principles to multiple outputs. Nonlinearities generated by different thresholds and saturation values of parallel neurons in a pool will behave like the nonlinearities of a single unit. Multiple feedback pathways behave in different ways depending on how strongly they are interlocked and on the details of their interrelationships. The number of potential interactions grows exponentially with the complexity of the system and the resulting possibilities of new emergent properties have hardly been explored. There is little theoretical basis to predict how a potentially chaotic system would interact with the continuously changing inputs that are seen typically by neural systems in normal activity.

The new functional properties that emerged from the introduction of closed loop pathways in neural systems may have been a critical increment in the evolution of higher neural function.

The limited processing capabilities of individual neurons form the basis for all neural functions as we understand them. However, several additional and useful reflex responses can be accomplished by simple combinations of as few as two neurons. These can be extended by the addition of parallel pathways of the same type. On the other hand, most of the processes accomplished by human nervous systems are completely impossible without a complex network. It is hard to imagine the evolution of higher brain functions without the development of some precursor modules that, in themselves, proved to be useful. In simple reciprocal pathways we see a combination of individual neurons that, with quantitative variations, leads to a diversity of complex functional capabilities. Perhaps the feedback loop is one primitive module that, after proving useful, was then incorporated into more complex, refined, and specialized processors of neural information. It is, at least, a module for building an understanding of neural processing at a level appreciably more complex than that of the individual neuron.

Feedback can prolong the effect of an input either as an oscillation or through a long-duration lag. Only quantitative differences in the same circuit are needed to generate such actions as the comparison of inputs that is necessary to make decisions between responses, or the alternation of responses to successive inputs. Emerging from simple feedback circuits are oscillatory signals that are capable of producing new information. Feedback loops can convert one spatiotemporal pattern of inputs into a different spatiotemporal pattern of outputs. These closed loop systems can generate specific output patterns in response to a variety of spatiotemporal inputs. Although simple operations are far from the basis for intelligence, they do offer a richer repertoire of functions than do single neurons. If each addition of a layer of interactions in successively more complex systems expands the capabilities as much as does the combination of neurons into simple loops, recognizable intelligent behavior should emerge without many more layers of subsystems.

Chapter 17

Combined Neural Operation

In the introduction we suggested that the nervous system exists because of the survival value to individuals and species that results from an ability to adjust to a changing environment. Subsequent chapters have dealt with the specific details of neural function. We will turn now to review some aspects of the interaction of these details in supporting survival. Although there is a temptation to limit the important consequences of nervous system function to consciousness, art appreciation, eloquent speech, scientific innovation, or textbook writing, these products are necessarily of secondary importance to survival. Although realizing that some "higher functions" have emerged from systems that evolved for survival, higher functions, per se, are not the subject of this chapter. Survival functions encompass a broad spectrum of responses and we will limit the discussion of this chapter to energy balance and its control. Our selections of examples are intended to illustrate the types of relationships that are of general importance in neural operations.

The routine activities that support survival use a wide range of neural functions and have presumably been important in their evolution.

Ordinary physical systems are subject to a relentless process of degradation (increasing entropy) by which structural organization decays along with a decline in the energy available to do work. Living systems have periods of increasing organization and increasing available energy to which the term *negentropy* has been applied. This does not imply a deviation from the laws of physical chemistry but merely represents the fact that life exists as an open part of a larger system from which the living entity draws both energy and structured materials. These external supplies are degraded as they pass through the living system leaving behind local reverses of degradation, structural growth, the increased organization. Although some biological systems can survive nearly static periods (e.g., dehydrated fairy shrimp or frozen gametes), life depends on significant periods of increased organization and of available internal energy.

17.1. Question: How do the statements in this last paragraph relate to the what happens to a protozoan that reproduces by cell division? Relate your answer to the biomass of the earth.

The nervous systems of higher animals contribute to and depend on the control of the internal conditions that make coordinated life processes possible.

The chemical processes that are the basis for life are possible only in the presence of specific substrates and can operate only under restricted conditions of temperature, pH, dilution, light energy, enzymes, and so on. Most terrestrial environments do not support these complex reaction systems. A controlled environment, such as is maintained within the bounds of a cell membrane, is usually required. Metazoan cells can exist in a more diverse external environment than can single-celled organisms because the intracellular environment has a two-stage isolation. The individual cells in a multicellular organism must cope only with the more stable internal environment of the organism. To maintain this inner uniformity in the presence of necessary exchanges of energy and material with the external environment, these exchanges must be carefully controlled. Both feedback and feedforward control require a sensor, a variable effector, and a communication link between the two and the nervous system performs these three functions. Stable internal conditions and effective neural control are interdependent since neural controllers are most effective when they operate under stable conditions.

Philosophers have recognized, with varying degrees of clarity, that the living body can modify the conditions of its own existence. Hippocrates, for instance, believed that the body could cure its own diseases. With the rise of the experimental method and the development of the measurement tools of the nineteenth century came a growing recognition of the constancy of conditions that are associated with life (Pflüger, 1877; Frédéricq, 1884). It was the clear statement and later development of the idea of constancy of the internal environment by Claude Bernard (1878) to whom we owe our modern acceptance of this idea. In the years following Bernard, many investigators described reflex mechanisms that contribute to the maintenance of the constant internal environment (e.g., carotid sinus reflex for blood pressure, Herring [1927], and the carotid body reflex for blood gasses, Heymans and Heymans [1927]. Barcroft (1928) promoted the importance of Bernard's idea and Cannon (1929) gave it the name *homeostasis*.

The widespread acceptance of the principle of homeostasis has led to a tendency to think, without justification, that biological variables are fixed at an ideal value (e.g., body temperature = 98.6°F) and that deviations, although sometimes tolerable, are undesirable. It is both theoretically and observationally apparent that internal conditions are adjusted within bounds rather than being held absolutely constant. For many functions, there is no ideal condition. For example, the body temperature that is most favorable for conserving energy is different from that for providing the fastest response. The energy-conserving low temperatures in resting muscles would cause a slow response in those muscles that are necessary for the movements involved in capturing food. Biological control systems do adjust internal variables to levels that change with the needs of the moment.

17.2.* Question: Name some examples in which biological control is maladaptive.

Adjustment of energy and materials exchange with the external world must be based on the accumulated quantity present internally.

The free quantities of substances are regulated through control of intake, output, internal storage, release, and synthesis. It is the cumulative effect of the combination of these effects, rather than their individual rates of change, that determines the available amount of the substance. Regulation or control of specific substances is accomplished by adjustment of a combination of the different rates in a pattern that is characteristic of the particular quantity in question. For example, CO_2 and urea accumulation are controlled largely by adjustment of removal rates, O_2 deficiency is compensated by intake adjustment, and temperature regulation can be dominated by either changes in heat removal or production.

Following a change in the rate of utilization or loss of a substance, the supply rate must be adjusted inversely or the accumulated quantity will change continuously. The adjustment of material acquisition that contributes to the regulation of critical substances in the body involves several neural processes. The cumulative nature of internal quantities dictates that for the intake control of a substance to be effective in maintaining a constant internal value, the related intake rate must be modified based on information about the quantity already present that must be sensed and then fed back.

Deviations of different internal values are sensed by various interoceptors whose outputs provide both the basis for unconscious (autonomic) control and for conscious perception. Both low blood glucose and contraction of an empty stomach are stimuli that lead to the perception of hunger. An increase of blood osmolarity is one of several stimuli that initiate the perception of thirst. In other cases, a recognizable sensation is initiated by the reflexly driven correcting response as for hyperventilation driven by elevated blood CO_2. Hyperventilation also provides compensation for low blood O_2, although much of the sensing is based on blood CO_2 level. This is an effective reflex response because low O_2 usually accompanies high CO_2. Energy supply can be sensed through internal temperature and through blood glucose levels, although there is no evidence that these two types of information are used in any combined form.

The control of internal conditions involves interactions among the sensing requirements, acquisition means, and removal that are related to different variables, some of which are independent of direct control.

Control of a particular quantity requires first that a deviation is sensed and then that there is a specific adjustment of a variable that regulates that quantity. For neural control, deviation of a variable must be represented by a distinctive pattern of activity in central neurons, and this information must be carried through to the effectors. Signals from equivalent receptors must converge on neurons, the output of which represents the particular deviation. One well-studied controlled variable is the body temperature of homeothermic animals. Some differentiation must be maintained between signals from skin temperature receptors and those from sensors of central body temperature since the responses to these two inputs are not identical.

Biological regulatory systems generally deal with only part of a particular homeostatic control problem. A regulating system, designed by evolutionary chance, need only provide an important contribution over part of its range to be acceptable for its survival value. There is no reason that it might not, by chance, also duplicate part of a regulatory action already provided by another system. Theoretical study of feedback control systems has shown that multiple parallel controllers may provide closer control of a variable without oscillation than can a single controller. This property is a further benefit that is supported by the development of controls with overlapping functions.

To be effective, the controlled compensatory actions must be specific for the particular deviation that requires correction. Correction is accomplished by an alteration of one or more of the rates of addition or removal of the particular variable involved. For a koala, the selection of a target for nutritional intake correction is rather simple since a koala responds to all such deficiencies by consuming eucalyptus leaves. There is one appropriate corrective action in response to sensing a deficiency. On the other hand, a variety of foods is consumed by humans to meet metabolic demands. For a human, a sensed blood glucose deficiency can suggest a wide range of foods that can be used for an appropriate corrective response.

Presumably, humans do not inherit a genetic basis for identification of all possible sources for dietary input. Indiscriminate consumption is not acceptable; it is necessary to learn distinguishing information. "Intentionally taught" and "accidentally observed" food identification are possible sources of learning criteria. It is unlikely that many individuals would discover the nutritional value hidden in a clam or a nut shell, but these are important food sources for whole communities. Individual experimental discovery must form a basis for identification of food sources in a changing environment. A milk-fed mammalian infant can explore orally a variety of substances without the risk inherent in consuming a whole meal of an unproven substance. There seems to be an inherited bias for sweet and against bitter and this can be used to help identify samples that could provide nutritional value while rejecting potentially toxic substances. The strong aversion to materials, the odor or taste of which has been associated with nausea, is a further foundation for experimental learning of safe selections. Regardless of how the stored information about intake selection originated, it must be activated by sensed need and other information about local conditions to be useful in the adjustment of intake as a control of an internal variable.

For any system to make a value-based decision, that system must have been provided with some form of initial criteria. These criteria may be final criteria for the evaluation or only a basis from which the final criteria are developed. The initial criteria for a computer are entered as a program that reflects some value judgment made by the programmer. Without initial limiting criteria, a system cannot learn specific criteria by trial and error if an error means destruction of the system. In the absence of an external programmer, a set of traits conferring differing survival probability can act within a species to provide initial criteria. Loss of individuals due to high risk traits generates an inverse image of those traits in the surviving individuals and perhaps eventually within the inheritance of the species. These initial criteria can, in later generations, either directly specify the final criteria (e.g., eat eucalyptus leaves) or provide the basis criteria (e.g., accept sweet and reject nausea) for developing the final criteria (e.g., eat grapes but do not eat rotten meat). Initial criteria capable of identifying specific actions are immediately available for use in decisions identical with those on which they were based but provide no means of dealing with new problems. Basis criteria, on the other hand, provide a foundation for developing a multitude of specific judgments that are related to experiences but are not usable until adapted to their environment by "learning experience."

Inherited identification and control mechanisms can deal with situations that are consistent across a species. Learning is, however, necessary for those situations that require adaptation to existing environmental or individual characteristics.

Once the need for a class of food has been identified, response to that need requires the selection and acquisition of one or more known examples of that class. Available examples of a class of foods may depend on location, season, or ease of acquisition. To take advantage of the flexibility provided by an omnivorous diet, it is necessary to choose specific target foods from a set of alternatives. This choice is affected by need, sensed availability, and the idiosyncrasies of the individual. The specific selected target is first symbolized as a pattern of neural activity. To be effective, the target food must be associated with a plan for finding and acquiring that food. This too is symbolized by a neural activity pattern that precedes any motor command. If the food source is remote, conversion of an acquisition plan to motor drive involves recall of route information (long-term memory), locomotor signals (motor pattern generation), changing proprioception (sensory transduction), motor correction (via feedback), and perceptual identification of the target vicinity (pattern recognition). Within the target vicinity, further sensory information must be processed to isolate and identify (basin entry) the sought food signal from all the sensory background. Actual identification uses information from the original target selection (short-term memory). Only at this point can sensory information about localization be used to generate the goal-directed motor signals for acquisition. If the food is in the form of a living animal, an initial prediction of some response requirement may be quickly outdated. With a rapid and irregularly moving target, successful capture depends on a continual update of sensory information and reorganization of the motor control plan.

Let us examine parts of a common activity. One of a variety of possible combinations of physiological and sociological factors activates the mental basin that calls for food acquisition. When activated, this basin initiates a selection process through which the student "decides" on a hamburger. The selection is an idealized hamburger since the one that will be eaten does not yet exist. Currently sensed information processed with neural activity based on past experience leads to neural activity related to the fact that the probability of getting any hamburger in the library is low. Quickly this distributed neural activity enters the basin that initiates a general route plan. So far the simple acquisition of food exists only as abstract thought. Next a centrally generated, quasiperiodic sequence of muscle actions underlies a stepping sequence that is continually modified by addition of local feedback and feedforward signals along with signals from higher brain centers. As the vague route is converted to specific movement, details are resolved and deviations are generated that are based on local traffic details. On arrival, new information about a specific advertisement leads to modification of the original intention and a milk shake is consumed with the hamburger. The abstract has been actualized and the ideals approximated while an elementary survival function was served.

Higher functions of the nervous system often override simple reflex actions to produce adjustments that depend on complex factors that are related to predictable costs and benefits.

An identified need, coupled with the recognition of a source, is not sufficient information to justify pursuit of a particular food object. Giving priority to the acquisition of food has both costs and benefits. The most successful individuals will include a value judgment before initiating pursuit. Energy expenditure will certainly be required and risks of exposure to a hostile environment, accident, or contact with hostile individuals are all possible costs that should be balanced against the product of the value of success and the probability of success.

17.3. Problem: Compare the neural processing that is necessary for optimization of energy replacement with the neural processing used to optimize the chance of forcing a checkmate in a game of chess.

The metabolic cost of acquiring energy replacement not only reduces the general yield of the activity, but affects the regulation of various other internal variables. The energy that is consumed is in the form of chemical energy released in reactions within the active nerve, gland, and muscle cells. These reactions use precursors (e.g., glucose and O_2) and produce wastes (e.g., CO_2 and heat) with a resultant alteration of their quantities in the internal environment. Thus, the acquisition of energy cannot be accomplished in isolation but must be coordinated with other exchanges so that internal conditions stay within acceptable bounds.

The complexity of the interactions of components in a nonlinear system often increases faster than does the number of components. Changes in a particular variable depend both on changes in the other variables (multifactor effects) and on the relationships among those variables (cross-term effects). Often the complexity of the system increases exponentially with the number of variables involved and centrally organized control of a system grows in complexity similarly. (If each variable was independently controlled, the complexity would increase only as fast as the number of independent controls.) When calculated from information about the actions of all the variables on the system, control can require prohibitively complex computation even with relatively few variables. Feedforward control, although inherently stable, allows an increasing error in any cumulative quantity being controlled. A simple feedback control corrects cumulative error and avoids the need for dealing separately with each driving variable because adjustments are based on the combined effects on the controlled variable. Multiple, independent feedback controls of all the variables in a system allow a system to be partitioned into independent controllers with a consequent reduction in the general complexity. The partitioned feedback controller is subject to a trade-off between instability and residual error in each variable (chapter 14). Most advantageous is a combination of feedbacks on all cumulative variables, supplemented by feedforward anticipatory compensations for the most important driving variables. Combined control minimizes cumulative error by using feedback and reduces the residual effect of load-dependent factors by using feedforward control.

Direct actions within a biological controller usually produce side effects that activate compensatory reflexes outside the primary controller.

Increased activity of a muscle that is associated with food acquisition leads to local depletion of the energy supply and an accumulation of waste. Modification of these conditions is minimized by circulatory transport of materials between the local site and the rest of the body. Since the blood flow that provides this transport requires further energy expenditure, it is inefficient to maintain the local flow necessary for maximal activity at all times. Resting blood flow is far below the maximum flow. Local chemical changes in active muscle lead to local vasodilation and increased blood flow to the muscle. This is a nonneural local feedback control that minimizes change in local chemical conditions.

Local vasodilation not only leads to a shunting of blood from other tissues, but decreases the total peripheral resistance, which, in turn, has the effect of reducing the blood pressure drive. If there is no correction, there will be a decrease in blood supply to other tissues including the brain. A decrease in blood pressure is sensed by baroceptors (Herring, 1927) in the major arteries and provides the afferent drive for the reflex increase of heart rate and vasoconstriction (except in the brain). Baroreceptor reflexes, combined with local vasomotor responses, minimize local chemical changes in the active tissue at the expense of a decreased supply to inactive tissues while maintaining a stable metabolite supply to the brain. This transport control is not directly dependent on the control of muscle activity but it results from the consequences of activity of the muscle.

17.4.* Experiment: Measure heart rate and blood pressure and other physiological responses that are associated with different aspects of exercise. How do these variables change between rest and either considering exercise or actually performing exercise? Is there evidence for feedforward adjustment of circulation in anticipation of exercise? How do your measurements relate to an auxiliary support for exercise? Is there any evidence for error in this description? What additional measurements or improved experimental design would help you to define the details of what happened? What extraneous factors might have influenced the values that you measured?

Effector activities consume energy and materials and produce heat and waste; this requires appropriate adjustment of both acquisition and disposal.

Circulatory exchange with the rest of the body can only buffer the changes that result from local activity. Ultimately the materials used and the wastes produced must be exchanged with the exterior. The extra O_2 extracted from the blood and the extra CO_2 added to the blood must be compensated through exchange between blood gases and gases in the lungs. The same "final common pathway" is used for both O_2 and CO_2, although these two gases generate independent sensory information. It is the CO_2 level that dominates the control of exchange of both O_2 and CO_2 between the lungs and environment. Exchange of one variable (O_2) based on another variable (CO_2) is not typical of engineering design but is effective in the biological system where O_2 deficiency is generally associated with a CO_2 excess. The control of muscle activity results in blood gas changes that are sensed and compensated by reflex feedback, so this motor control is ultimately subservient to a controller of energy supply.

Metabolic heat production in endothermic animals is necessary to maintain body temperature within narrow limits. If the balance of production and removal is not maintained, body temperature will change. The motor and chemical processes associated with replacing expended energy consume chemical energy and produce additional heat. Passive heat dissipation minimizes temperature change but is not sufficient to maintain a tolerable internal temperature in the face of changing heat production and changing environmental thermal conditions. Even the process of energy replacement contributes to the need for a feedback from internal temperature to the regulation of heat dissipation and production. Besides feedback information, the regulation of heat exchange is subject to feedforward sensing of the load imposed by skin temperature.

17.5.* Problem: Is it reasonable to design an insulated space suit based on constant heat dissipation? What additional variables might need to be considered? Use the following calculations to help answer these questions. Determine the rate of heat production (calories per hour) under basal (resting) conditions and during heavy work. Draw graphs of the rate of temperature change vs. the rate of heat dissipation for the two levels of work. Use the same coordinates for both lines and thus define a range of expected values. If this calculation leads to a constant rate, what assumptions might you have made that could have caused an error? Why is it more important to check the validity of a constant rate design than of a variable rate design? What type of controller might you use in a variable dissipation design? How does this problem relate to temperature regulation in normal activities?

The control of internal temperature is accomplished by the modification of energy exchanges and heat transfers, all of which originate in signals from one or more of three types of receptors. Several neural modifications of energy exchange and three neural modifications of heat transfer are involved in short-term adjustment whereas neuroendocrine modifications of metabolism play a role over longer periods of time. This control is complicated because the relative effectiveness, in temperature control, of the different operations varies widely depending on several environmental conditions. Under different environmental conditions the same circulatory change can favor either heat gain or heat loss.

Behavioral relocation, with respect to radiant exchange, and wind exposure are used by humans and other animals to modify heat exchange. Postural change that alters contact and the amount of exposed surface affect the exchange rate with the local environment. Thermal receptors in the brain, as well as warm and cold receptors in the skin, provide the thermal information on which these adjustments are based. Both muscle activity and nonshivering thermogenesis are neurally controlled heat production pathways. Vasomotor changes in and near the skin modify the rate of transfer of heat between deep tissues and the surface. Neurally controlled sweating affects heat removal through evaporative heat loss. In nonhuman mammals piloerection provides a variable control of local air movement near the body surface and thus influences heat exchange. Transfer of heat by conduction and by evaporative heat loss within the respiratory passages allows further adjustment of exchange rate in some animals. In the control of this single variable, we find separate sensory information and multiple effector pathways producing a compound control.

Conflicts may occur when multiple sensor or effector systems deal with the control of a single variable.

Ventilation of the lungs is one example in which separate operations are dependent on having unique control of the same effector. The exchange of O_2 and CO_2 is adjusted by the same respiratory action that supports vocalization and, in many animals, is a major effector in the control of heat dissipation. In addition, the pharynx is shared between respiration and food passage. In humans, ingestion and vocalization controls are time-shared with the other functions, but can compete for control during periods of high demand for ventilation. Heat and gas exchange actions are partially separable since the depth and frequency of respiration act on gas exchange in a different way than they do on heat exchange. Because of the operating range on the hemoglobin saturation curve, short-term conflicts between O_2 and CO_2 exchange are small as long as CO_2 removal requires the movement of more air than does O_2 acquisition. An additional separation of CO_2 and O_2 exchange exists because CO_2 is influenced by renal removal of HCO_3^- in response to pH regulation.

17.6. Problem: Describe temperature regulation in conditions when the skin temperature is below and the central temperature is above normal. Describe the processing of thermal information from the skin when both hot and cold receptors in the skin are excited by trauma. Consider your subjective and objective reactions to exposure of one side of your body to a hot shower while the other side is still dry.

Homeostasis provides a relatively stable environment in which general biological function can operate effectively, whatever the combination of activities at the moment. The environment is made up of many variables; we have just considered temperature, blood oxygen, blood carbon dioxide, and circulatory transport, each of which is subject to control by relatively independent feedback systems. With variables held within certain bounds, complex operations such as organizing the acquisition of needed nutrients can be effectively undertaken. Homeostasis would be possible if each of these variables was controlled by an entirely independent controller, with all controllers operating simultaneously. However, since the controllers operate within the same body, they interact whenever one contributes to the load of another. There are also weak central coordinations in the form of feedforward signals that make some adjustments in anticipation of future loads and some that offset the controlled level in ways that are often favorable to the effectiveness of other simultaneously active controls. In general, though, these supporting controllers operate essentially independently and in parallel with each other.

The nervous system generally does not operate as a unified and monolithic controlling system.

The neural basis for the acquisition of energy, which we have been describing, involves a sequence of sensing, combining, selecting, and pattern generating operations in which each operation provides a part of the information that initiates subsequent operations and determines their details. These sequential operations may be accomplished in different neurons, but they are functionally a common system in which each neuron is effective only with signals from the others. The existence in the nervous system of independent parallel controllers has not been definitely established. It is, however, most likely that the organization of a visual search is accomplished in relative independence of the comparison of visual patterns with those patterns that show the presence of the desired food. Likewise, the generation of a walking pattern with its compensatory adjustments is most likely independent of the organization of a route plan. The locomotor task and the visual task need not be controlled in common, yet some critical information from one must be delivered to the other. The simplification accomplished by partitioning large problems would be of such value to the nervous system that it is expected that many nearly independent operations occur simultaneously and share only that minimal information necessary to prevent conflict. The complex operation of energy acquisition can be built around the coordination of a sequence of rather simple operations. The refinement of the result can be developed in a commonwealth of nearly independent systems that receive only general instructions from the core operation.

Ethologists have shown that the complexly organized activity of flocks of birds, schools of fish, hives of bees, and hills of ants emerges from the interaction of individuals each with simple rules for interaction. These systems operate with neither a leader nor a global rule for operation. (See, for example, *The Honey Bee* by Gould and Gould [1988].) A similar emergence of complexity from interacting simple parts is demonstrable in computer programs. Even the unabridged dictionary is built of simple interactions among a few letters. It is not necessary to assume that all complexity of neural activity grows out of intrinsically complex rules in a single unified system.

17.7. Problem: Draw a set of separate block diagrams for signals for each of the following simplified controlled variables as they have been described in this chapter: blood O_2, blood CO_2, blood flow to a muscle, and body temperature. Draw a minimal diagram of the food acquisition system showing the relationships among energy need, food location, O_2 consumption in muscle, heat production, and vasodilation in muscle. Add other variables and controllers as needed. For each variable that is modified by the food acquisition system and is regulated by a separate control system, use specific marks to show the points where the systems are joined. As a first approximation, can you justify omitting the action of the outputs of the separate controllers on the food acquisition system?

The ingestion of acquired food marks the beginning of the oral phase of the digestive process. This involves several related neural processes including the motor control of mastication, control of salivary secretion, and several types of mechanical and chemical sensing processes related to ingestion and the possible rejection of already ingested substances. Salivation is initially stimulated by reflexes that originate in exteroceptors, and then by mechanical, gustatory, and olfactory stimuli. Because of the separate effector nerves, the ratio of water, enzyme, and mucus in the secreted saliva is variable and depends on the stimulus pattern. Mastication involves biting and chewing and is coordinated with food manipulation by the tongue and facial muscles. This coordination must be accurately adjusted both temporally and spatially with variations based on the changing mechanical properties of the material involved. Texture, compliance, and chemical composition are monitored by receptors on the tongue and adjacent surfaces as chewing mechanically disrupts the food and mixes it with solvent, digestive, and lubricating saliva. Besides rapid distribution of food between the teeth, the tongue is simultaneously involved in sorting materials and forming a bolus to be swallowed. (This does not include its often almost simultaneous involvement in speech!) Three-dimensional shaping of the tongue in these overlapping operations is accomplished by longitudinal and vertical movement by activation of selected muscle fascicles from a large set, oriented in three general directions (see figure 7.1). The tongue participates in injecting the formed bolus into the pharynx. At this point further reflex interactions suspend respiration during bolus passage through the intersection of the digestive and respiratory passages. The complex activity, associated with the oral phase of digestion, makes this one of the most complex of neural controls.

17.8. Problem: It is not known in detail how independent the various parts of the oral phase of digestion are. Describe experiments that could help to identify differences between unified and partitioned control of the oral phase of digestion.

The neural signals that control digestive functions, such as in the complex nervous system of the gut, are largely, but not entirely, independent of the CNS.

The act of swallowing provides a clear example of a reflex sequence. The reflexes that start the bolus down the esophagus involve somatic nerves and can be voluntarily influenced. As food enters the lower part of the esophagus, it comes into the territory of autonomic and local plexus innervation. Arrival of the bolus, driven by somatic reflexes, stretches the lower esophagus, thereby initiating a reflex pattern that generates a peristaltic wave of cyclic relaxation and contraction that moves the bolus along the esophagus to the stomach. Thus a continuous effect is accomplished by locally organized actions, made up of an alteration of mechanical and neural components each driving the next. Such sequences also occur in many somatic activities but dominate control of mechanical actions throughout the rest of the gastrointestinal tract.

As the bolus of food passes from the mouth to the gastrointestinal tract, the nature of the actions and the role of neural control change quantitatively. The function becomes largely chemical with mechanical action taking on a supportive role. Exteroceptive information becomes almost irrelevant and the location of a stimulus becomes less important. The speed of response and the combination of multiple types of information are less necessary. Neural processing often gives only simple stimulus-response relationships with many control functions taken over by local nerve networks and the endocrine system.

The gastrointestinal tract contains a network (the *enteric plexus*) of nerve fibers and cell bodies that is arranged in two layers along most of its length. The fibers of this network lie in proximity to the longitudinal and circular smooth muscle fibers—their mechanical effectors. Sensory signals in the gut act in a reflex-like manner through this plexus without the signals passing through the central nervous system so that this network is similar to the most primitive nervous systems. Besides these local networks, the gastrointestinal tract receives fibers from both the sympathetic and the parasympathetic divisions of the autonomic nervous system. These autonomic fibers act both directly on the glands and the muscles of the tract and indirectly to modulate activity in the local neural networks. Sensory fibers with direct connections to the central nervous system are also found within the gut.

Neural control of gastrointestinal function deals with the internal operations of the gut as distinct from control of homeostasis.

The gastrointestinal system accomplishes three general functions. It provides the storage that allows fast and discontinuous ingestion of food to supply a slower and more continuously acting digestive process. The digestive process converts many ingested materials into forms that are less diverse and more nearly ready for use by individual cells. Finally, the digestive process separates dissolved and colloidal materials that can enter the bloodstream from a residue that is further processed or simply eliminated. Optimal conditions for the various reactions are rather different and are attained by a spatial separation. This separation is supported by mechanical movement of the gut contents, local addition of reacting enzymes, and local pH adjustment. Endocrine and neural control of the timing and intensity of the various contributing actions accomplishes control of the environment in the gut rather than controlling homeostasis. The conditions controlled in the gut are generally unfavorable for cell life so local control is critical. Failure of this control can lead to either failure of digestion or to digestion of the cells of the digestive tract.

The control sequence in the gastrointestinal tract begins with secretions in the mouth and stomach that are initiated by afferent signals associated with visual, olfactory, and gustatory identification of food. This initial feedforward reflex is supplemented by reflexes from mechanoreceptors stimulated by the arrival of material in the stomach. The pH optimum for gastric digestion is provided by neurally driven HCl secretion accompanying the secretion of gastric enzymes. When the acidified chyme enters the upper end of the intestine it is mixed with enzymes that function in a neutral or alkaline environment. The required pH change is effected by the addition of HCO_3^-. Throughout the intestine information about osmolarity, acidity, distention, and chemical composition is sensed, and this provides the basis for neural control of secretion, mixing, and movement. As mixing and digestion progress, the mixture is slowly moved forward. However, while the duodenum is filled, a combination of endocrine and neural responses to the stretch and to the acid in the chyme slows further delivery of chyme from the stomach. An exception to the general rather local action of gastrointestinal reflexes is the gastrocolic reflex (well demonstrated in some infants) that initiates movement of feces in the colon in response to gastric filling.

Although these processes within the digestive tract generally are not consciously perceived, there are circumstances in which they are. Filling of the stomach leads to termination of the contraction waves that are perceived as hunger pangs, whereas further stretch gives the sense of fullness. Abrupt and strong stretch of parts of the gastrointestinal tract, local hypoxia, inflammatory products, or damaging chemical conditions lead to conscious perception of visceral pain. Such stimulation can alter both circulatory function and somatic motor activity and can interfere with the food acquisition process. When, as is common, the conscious localization of the source of these noxious stimuli in the gastrointestinal tract is inappropriate it is called *referred pain*.

Nerves associated with the vascular system do not only modify the circulatory transport of nutrients from the gut but are also associated with sensing the level of some of those nutrients in the blood.

Materials introduced through the digestive system enter the circulatory or lymphatic systems rather than passing directly to the environment of the cells of the body. Transfer through the vascular system gives most cells three stages of isolation from the external environment. The regulation of the contents of this middle compartment is, in part, under neural control and its sensors even contribute to perception. We will consider four examples of materials in this space that are processed in different manners: (1) materials that are used in large quantities by metabolism and are subject to feedback regulation (e.g., glucose), (2) substances that have a detrimental effect but pass from the gastrointestinal system into the circulation (e.g., *Salmonella* toxin), (3) substances that are not used in metabolism but are of importance to cellular function (e.g., Na^+), and (4) substances from the diet that are important but are not regulated by any direct controller (e.g., vitamin C).

Glucose, directly absorbed from the digestive tract, replenishes the supply in the blood and thereby provides a direct energy source for many cells of the body. As blood glucose rises, its action on brain glucose receptors leads to a sensation of satiety that usually terminates eating behavior. Glucose is converted to a ready reserve of glycogen in the liver and in muscle. Less directly, glucose can be converted to triglycerols and stored in adipose tissue from which it can be retrieved later to maintain blood glucose levels. The regulation of blood glucose levels by feedback regulation of insulin with further modulation by substances such as cholecystokinin and glucagon is well described in general physiology texts and will not be further considered here.

A variety of toxic materials may appear in ingested food or may, like *Salmonella* toxin, be produced by bacterial action within the digestive system. If these agents are absorbed from the digestive tract and excite cells in the brain that drive the emesis reaction, a reflex elimination of the source of the toxin remaining in the stomach will occur. The learned aversion to foods associated with the period immediately before emesis allows adaptation of the individual to local conditions but can lead to avoidance of innocent foods by association. All toxic agents do not produce emesis and among mammals there are differences in response to different agents. Thus, some poisons that do not produce emesis in rats but do in other small animals have been used to selectively eliminate rats.

Sensed deficiency of a nutrient is likely to drive ingestion of a mixture of materials including other nutrients in a variable ratio that is usually not proportional to the relative needs.

When food is ingested in response to a glucose deficiency, it is likely that it will, besides glucose, include in variable quantity other substances of importance. Most natural foods contain Na^+, K^+, Ca^{2+}, and Cl^- ions, and may contain various vitamins, amino acids, and lipids. In spite of variable intake and continuing depletion, it is generally important for these materials to be maintained in the internal environment.

Since Na^+ ions are not consumed or exchanged with inactive storage within the body, the intake must, over a period, be balanced by elimination. Different foods contain different amounts of this ion so a constant output rate would lead to changing accumulation with variations in the source. The passive disposals into urine, through the lower digestive tract, and in sweat fluctuate somewhat with the internal concentration, but these are an insufficient control to maintain a constant internal concentration. Since Na^+ ions effect osmolarity, body fluid distribution, pH, and cell excitability, the Na^+ ion concentration must be held within a narrow range. Severe depletion leads to a specific "salt hunger" and will initiate an active attempt to increase input as is seen in animals that travel great distances to a salt lick. When supply is sufficient, removal becomes the point of control. Na^+ ion concentration in the blood is sensed directly by brain neurons and indirectly through effects on osmoreceptors and baroreceptors in the vascular system. This information is used, through hormonal responses, to act on renal function to modify Na^+ ion retention. Again, detailed accounts of renal mechanisms can be found in standard general physiology texts.

Vitamin C, like many other essential dietary substances, is not selectively acquired, stored, or conserved. The quantity in consumed foods varies from none to many times the needed quantity. The only accommodation to this variability seems to be that an intake variability over at least a 100:1 range is tolerated. In the absence of modern vitamin substitutes, vitamin C's sufficient presence in the body is dependent on the probability that it will be adequately supplied in the available food. Cases in which an adequate supply was not available are well documented in scurvy deaths.

Simple physical or neural inputs lead to complex interacting processes in the body, whether the initiating action is a normal or a pathologic event or even if it is introduced as a therapeutic intervention.

In accomplishing one neural function it is possible that variables are altered that modify activity in other regulating or control systems. These controls involve both nonlinearities and feedback, characteristics that can be the source of unpleasant surprises when an attempt is made to intervene directly in a targeted function. As a result (1) intervention in one system can cause changes in other systems that may have very different functions; (2) a transient change in the intervention may initiate oscillatory behavior in either the intended target or in an associated function; and (3) although feedback may make it difficult to alter the targeted variable, the intervention may have a profound effect on an associated function or even on the targeted variable once the feedback saturates.

This chapter has been concerned with one cycle of a relaxation oscillation. An internal, continuous process depletes blood glucose, eventually initiating an external, transient process that restores blood glucose. The cycle is completed with the system returned to its nonrestorative state. Changing signals from internal sensors of glucose modify certain ongoing activity in the central nervous system until that activity switches into the basin of the restoration operation. In the glucose restoration basin, signals from certain exteroceptors (vision, olfaction, etc.) and central processing elements are used in a way that is characteristic of that basin.

17.9.* Problem: Reduce the controls described in this chapter to a matrix and a descriptive table. Make the matrix a grid with a labeled column for each variable that contributes to determining the future value of other variables (and that same variable). These variables may be signals in either neural or endocrine form, information stored in memory, or quantities of materials. Each affected variable should be assigned a separate row. Except for inputs, many variables will appear in both a row and a column. Mark each intersection where an action occurs. After identifying each interacting intersection, make a table in which each interaction is defined as well as possible. Continue to use this matrix and table to organize your future knowledge about neural interactions.

An essential foundation for the relative independence of humans from conditions in their environment is the ability to acquire energy in a more varied form than is acceptable to individual cells. This diversity depends directly on functions of a nervous system that are most reliable under relatively stable (neurally controlled) local conditions. The internal state is sensed to produce signals that are carried to central nervous networks where they initiate characteristic activity. Signals from this activity are combined with signals from receptors that respond to external conditions and with signals fed back from internal activity of the nervous system. These combined signals, acting in a network whose detailed properties depend on results of past activity, lead to external motor activity, an altered basis for interacting with current input signals, and long-term alterations of the functional rules of the system. Neural activity, both directly and through motor response, alters other internal conditions that directly and indirectly modify neural and endocrine controls that act in parallel with the energy acquisition system. Energy acquisition is not accomplished in isolation, but is cross-linked and coordinated with most of the homeostatic systems through effects of non-neural variables. The process of energy acquisition uses sensory, communication, feedback, and motor functions of the nervous system and accomplishes pattern recognition, object classification and generalization, symbolic representation, value judgment, adaptive adjustment, and memory storage and retrieval. The feedback in multiple and somewhat independent loops introduces self-driven activities that need not be dependent on sensory input although they may be modified by it.

The evolution of the neural tools necessary for sophisticated energy acquisition has left us with a commonwealth of loosely coordinated mechanisms capable of both homeostasis and intellectual activity.

Appendixes

A. Electrical terms

The use of the word *current* often leads to confusion. In metallic conductors, current results from the movement of electrons in one direction whereas in electrolyte solutions, current results from the movement of charged ions. In the presence of a voltage gradient, current flows from the anode toward the cathode by the action of cations moving in the designated current direction and anions moving in the opposite direction. A confusion in nomenclature sometimes arises from the close relationship between current and voltage. Voltage gradients cause current flow and the flow of current produces voltage drops. Terms such as endplate potential and endplate current have been used interchangeably without recognition of the parameter being measured. Important distinctions do exist and the proper terminology should be used so that the parameter named is the one that was actually measured. The different terms do not, however, imply differences in the underlying biological phenomenon.

B. Animal models

Much of the original study of mechanisms underlying the action potential used the giant axon of the squid. This unusually large nerve fiber can have a diameter of almost a millimeter. Frequently, as with the squid axon, the species used has been a critical factor in the success of the investigation because of some peculiarity of that species. After ideas and methods have been refined in animal experiments it is sometimes possible to confirm the results in human tissues. In other cases, only indirect evidence is possible to support the extension of ideas derived from animal study into human application. The basis for many neurological procedures used today has never been fully confirmed by studies of the appropriate human tissue but relies merely on an acceptance of the conservative nature of evolution. It is encouraging to note, however, that the theories developed from the study of squid nerves have been successfully applied to mammalian nerve, muscle, and heart cells with only quantitative modifications.

Early experiments on the nervous system used animal (and human) procedures that today would be considered cruel. It is important to realize that at that time surgical amputations were undertaken using only strong restraint of the patient. Some useful, but crude, observations were made with these preparations, but nowadays such methods would be both ethically and scientifically inexcusable. Today important research depends on experimentation with animals. These animals are often strays that have been held in animal pounds for a period beyond which they would normally have been euthanized. Strict local and federal regulations require that experimental animals receive proper veterinary care and that they are anesthetized during any surgical procedures. For the more refined information presently sought especially in neuroscience, not only pain but minor disturbances such as unaccustomed handling can introduce effects that will totally mask crucial information. Further, the argument of "similarity within limits" that is used to justify the application of results of animal experiments to humans applies to comparable humane considerations. Scientists involved in animal experimentation must justify the benefits of animal research and they do not make these planning decisions lightly. If you should work in a laboratory engaged in animal research, you should realize that inconsiderate treatment of research animals, although acceptable to some pet owners, can be cause for dismissal from employment.

C. Graphics

Although the functional relationships between various physiological parameters can be represented in many ways, physiologists have historically preferred graphic representation. A large part of our knowledge of neural function has been acquired as graphs such as figure 2.3 that relate a *dependent variable* (e.g., current, voltage, or muscle force) to an *independent variable* (e.g., time). Very often both clinical and experimental data are displayed directly as time graphs on a cathode ray oscilloscope, a pen recorder (e.g., a polygraph), or a computer screen. When properly read, a graph can be an efficient way of acquiring and communicating information. With time graphs, as with any other graph, a critical detail for understanding is the recognition of the scale used on each axis.

Some graphs, including that in figure 2.4, have time on the abscissa but are not the result of a record obtained during a single time sequence. These graphs are built up from data obtained in repeated independent sequences. This type of graph is used in the study of a process that occurs after a repeatable initiating event but when sampling of that process alters its subsequent course. In the example in figure 2.4, it was necessary to use an adjustable second stimulus to test the threshold at various times after a fixed intensity initial stimulus. The second stimulus alters the time course of further changes in threshold so that no further tests can be made in that particular trial. The data in this graph are the results of testing at a series of different intervals after each of a series of initial stimuli. It is important that the initial stimulus for each trial is separated sufficiently in time so that any residual effect of the previous stimulus has disappeared. Since the refractory period is nearly constant from one test to another, the superimposed records show how the threshold varies in time after an initial stimulus. The final graph defines a continuous underlying process, although this process was not directly measured on any of the individual tests.

It is frequently important to determine thresholds although, by definition, threshold cannot be directly measured. Threshold is the demarcation between those stimulus intensities that generate a response and those that do not. Since threshold itself includes neither group of stimuli, individual test stimuli will be either suprathreshold or subthreshold. Threshold is also subject to small changes in an unpredictable and apparently random way from one test to another. As a practical matter, multitrial experiments to find threshold are improved when the effect of the test sequence is reduced by choosing the sequence of stimulus intensities and intervals in a random order.

Figure 2.7A introduces a common variation of the time graph. Here different, but related, processes are shown as parallel graphs. Each graph has its own scale on the ordinate but they share the time axis. Since each graph shares the independent (time) axis it is important to compare temporal relationships among the lines at critical points. Sometimes, the function plotted on one y axis (in ths graph *input*) can be an independent variable that drives the other responses. Figure 2.7B shows the information of input and $1/t$ redrawn from figure 2.7A. This redrawing shows better the complex relationship between the two functions but it loses the easy recognition of the total time pattern.

D. Temperature coefficient

The temperature coefficient, Q_{10} is

$$Q_{10} = \frac{R_{T+10}}{R_T}$$

where R_T is the rate at $T°C$ and R_{T+10} is the rate at 10°C higher temperature. For temperature differences $(T_2 - T_1)$ of other than 10°C, an exponential relationship is used:

$$Q_{10} = \left(\frac{R_{T_2}}{R_{T_1}}\right)^{10/(T_2 - T_1)}$$

E. Pulse codes

In digital computer communication, pulses can be sent at regular intervals along a single pathway between two devices. Each interval may or may not contain a pulse and thereby carries one bit of information. The bits are arranged into groups in which the relationships in a string of intervals carry information. Although there exists here a tempting analogy with the nervous system, there is no evidence of binary encoding of information in the pulsatile signals of nerve fibers. Also the amplitude and duration of nerve impulses can vary under some circumstances. For example, in some nerve cells the duration of the action potential increases at high firing rates. Since this change depends on the changes in pulse recurrence, it may be a redundant source of information about the encoded signal.

Using a pulse code to transmit information about analog physiological signals produces characteristics that are similar to a sampled data system. These include high-frequency attenuation and limited aliasing. In addition, the pulse rate code introduces an amplitude-dependent rate of sampling.

The Nyquist criterion states that *to define a signal it must be sampled at over twice the highest frequency present in that signal*. This criterion has restrictions that are not appropriate in a biological system. Namely, the Nyquist rate is based on an instantaneous and uniform sampling of a function that contains no higher frequencies and the information retrieval requires a more involved signal analysis. When considering neuronal function, it is more appropriate to apply the older, and more conservative, rule that 10 samples are necessary to represent a simple wave. Even this ratio may introduce complex effects in some systems (e.g., figure 16.12). The modulated pulse rate used in nerve signaling further complicates the Nyquist analysis that refers to a fixed sampling rate.

F. Graphics

Information about neurophysiological threshold is presented in two inversely related graphic forms: threshold vs. test dimension and sensitivity vs. test dimension. It is important to note which is being used in a particular case. Figure 4.3 is an example of a sensitivity graph. Here the sensitivities have been normalized so that each curve is drawn with respect to its maximum point to compare the relative responses of different receptors at specific wavelengths. This graph does not show that the minimum threshold for rods is much lower (higher sensitivity) than that for cones.

G. Terminology of sensation and stimulation

Some parts of this table have been left blank due to lack of information.

Sensation	Major physical dimension	Receptor
Mechanical Relations: Location, Direction, Magnitude, Distribution of Force, Position, Angles, Velocity, Acceleration		
Touch	Location of small forces	[a]
Contact	Location of force	[a]
Vibration	5–200 Hz oscillation	Pacinian corpuscle
Movement	Angular and linear velocity	Vestibular and retinal
Acceleration	Angular and linear acceleration	Vestibular
Posture	Joint angles, gravity direction	[b]
Smooth/rough	Smooth or rough surface	
Slippery	Low coefficient of friction	
Hard/soft	Mechanical compliance	
Tickle	—	
Perceived shape	Geometry of object	
Tactile object	Mechanical and other information	

Sensation	Major physical dimension	Receptor
—	Visceral pressures and distension	
Sound	Pressure oscillation	Hair cells
Loudness	Amplitude of oscillation 0–120 dB SPL	
Pitch	Frequency of oscillation 16–16K Hz	
Timber	Distribution of superimposed oscillations	
Localization	Phase, comparative amplitude (intensity)	
Phoneme	Brief period of changing pattern of oscillation	
Sound object	Sound and other inputs	
Chemical Composition: Concentration of Ions, Molecules, and Mixtures		
Taste	Dissolved chemicals in mouth	Taste buds
Flavor	Chemicals and temperature in mouth and nose	
Smell	Dissolved airborne chemicals	Olfactory hairs, facial
Chemoreceptors		
—	O_2, CO_2, Na^+, pH, glucose	Carotid, aortic bodies, central neurons
—	Osmolarity	Brainstem neurons
—	Endocrine agents	Central neurons
Pain	Noxious stimuli	Fine nerve endings
Localization	Specific endings	Nociceptors
Itch	—	
Burn	—	
Ache	—	
Stabbing pain	—	
Throbbing pain	—	
Light	Electromagnetic radiation	Rods and cones
Brightness	Light intensity	
Color	Wavelength 400–700 nm and mixtures	
Saturation	Energy distribution over wavelength	
Image	Spatial distribution of light	
Localization	Image, eye position, focus, parallax, experience	
Visual object	Light pattern class	
Heat	Temperature, heat conductivity	Fine nerve terminals
	Humidity, air flow	

Sensation	Major physical dimension	Receptor
Cold		Fine nerve endings
Warm		
Hot		Fine nerve endings
—	Internal body temperature	Central neurons

[a]Several receptors in skin and deeper soft tissues.
[b]Eyes, vestibular system, skin and soft tissue, joint receptors, and motoneurons.

H. Use of a seven-node collective computation circuit

This example will be developed as a stimulus to the student's thinking about associative memory. Although it is presented as simply an illustrative model, it does have some striking similarities to certain biological memory processes.

1. It is distributed, that is, multiple memories can be discretely represented in an overlapping manner over the same set of general purpose nodes (neurons).

2. The retrieval process is associative, since part of the stored information pattern (memory) can be used to identify the rest of the pattern.

3. The decision-making process can be an analog process with a threshold. As we will see in chapter 12, neurons integrate continuous inputs to a threshold, at which point an output is produced.

4. Information storage (learning) results from modification of the strength of connections (synapses) between nodes (neurons).

Establishing the collective memory

1. Encode the memory information into the appropriate binary code. In the example of a seven-segment number, specific segments are either activated ($+1$) or not activated (-1).

2. For each memory, connect those nodes with the same value with a $+$ (solid) line and nodes with opposite signs with a $-$ (dotted) line. Overlay all the memories on the same seven nodes.

3. Reduce the connections by canceling any parallel $+$ and $-$ connections. This is now the collective computation circuit.

Retrieving a memory

1. Fill in the known nodes ($+1$ or -1).
2. Fill in the unknown nodes with 0s.
3. Calculate values for the unknown nodes using the following scheme:

a. For every solid line to a node, add the value at the node at the other end of the line.

b. For every dotted line to a node, subtract the value at the node at the other end of the line.

c. Divide the summed value at each node by the total number of lines entering that node. This gives the probability, for each unknown node, that the node is $+$ or $-$. Zero can now be used as a threshold to find which of the unknown nodes are $+1$ and which are -1.

Try filling in three of the values for a memory (one of the three seven-segment numbers represented in figure H.1) and calculating the other three. Do you get the correct seven-segment number representation? If not, draw the seven-segment figure that you get. Can you still make a good guess from that description?

In the example with "1," "2," and "3" stored in seven nodes, and with only three known segments, the four remaining correct segments are predicted 74% of the time for "3," 83% of the time for "2," and 29% of the time for "1." With four known segments, the retrieval of the remaining three segments is improved to 80% for "3," 85% for "2," and 45% for "1." A distributed, associative memory such as this works reasonably well for storing up to about 15% of the maximum different memories. Given that the human brain has about 10^{13} neurons, each of which makes perhaps 10^3 connections with other neurons, there is potential for storing an exceedingly large number of memories with such a distributed, associative memory scheme. Probably only some synapses that are interposed between a sensory receptor and the effector neuron are modified in a particular instance of learning. Little is known about the process of selection of which synapses are to be modified in order to learn a particular input pattern.

I. The Nernst-Planck equation

The Nernst-Planck equation is a way to combine the diffusional effect on an ion, which is a stochastic, thermal process, and the electrical force on the ion, which

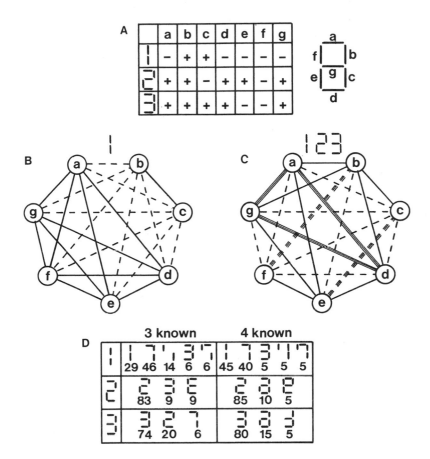

Figure H.1
Seven node collective computational circuit. (A) Truth table for seven-segment numerals 1, 2, and 3. A + or − indicates whether a specific segment is lighted or not to form a specific numeral. These represent +1 or −1 in the computational circuits below. (B) Computational circuit containing information for the numeral 1. (C) Computational circuit containing the information for numerals 1, 2, and 3. (D) A "retrieval table" that shows the percentage of times that each indicated figure is retrieved when all possible combinations of either three or four known segments are specified. See the text for further information concerning this figure.

is the result of its residence in an electrical field. We start with a definition of ionic *current*, I_s, for ion S equating it to the valence of the ion times Faraday's constant times the flux of the ion:

$$I_s = z_2 \, FM_s$$

Now consider two separate conditions of the flux, M_s. First, when there is a concentration gradient but no electrical field, we have for the flux

$$M_{s(c)} = -D_s \frac{\partial C_s}{\partial x}$$

where C_s is the local concentration of S and D_s the diffusion coefficient of S. (This is *Fick's equation*, which is used in a variety of diffusion situations.) Second, when there is an electrical field and no concentration gradient, we have for the flux

$$M_{s(E)} = -z_s u_s C_s \frac{\partial E}{\partial x}$$

where z_s is the valence of S and u_s the mobility of S. (This is the *electrophoretic equation*, which is applied in cases where a charged ion is moved under the influence of an electric field.) The *total flux* is simply the sum of these two fluxes:

$$M_s = M_{s(c)} + M_{s(E)} = -\left(D_s \frac{\partial C_s}{\partial x} + z_s u_s C_s \frac{\partial E}{\partial x}\right)$$

We can eliminate the u_s term using the Nernst–Einstein equation:

$$u_s = \frac{D_s F}{RT}$$

and solve for *ionic current*:

$$I_s = -z_s F D_s \left(\frac{\partial C_s}{\partial x} + \frac{F z_s C_s}{RT} \frac{\partial E}{\partial x}\right)$$

At equilibrium the net $I_s = 0$, so

$$0 = \frac{\partial C_s}{\partial x} + \frac{F z_s C_s}{RT} \frac{\partial E}{\partial x}$$

Rearranging this equation yields

$$\partial E \partial x = \frac{-RT}{F z_s} \frac{\partial C_s}{C_s} \partial x$$

and integrating between $x = 1$ and $x = 2$ gives the *Nernst equation*:

$$E_1 - E_2 = \frac{RT}{F z_s} \ln \frac{C_{s_2}}{C_{s_1}}$$

J. Block diagramming

To make effective use of a set of symbols to represent the organization of an information processing system, it is necessary that the symbols are used in a consistent and well-defined manner. In the study of nervous systems, many pictorial diagrams have been used without the acceptance of a single formal pattern. These pictorial representations often tie function to specific anatomical examples. A means for representing topologically and functionally equivalent classes of local circuitry is needed for our discussion of networks. We have chosen to use a small, but adequate, set of block diagrams for this purpose. This format allows representation of the pathways and the operations on signals while the underlying energy supply system and the synthetic and dissipative pathways for materials involved are concealed. We suggest that you use these forms for your organization of knowledge about signal processing.

Four different symbols are needed to represent formally the different operations that occur within a variety of information-processing systems. It is important to recognize that block diagram symbols deal with functional divisions of the system that do not necessarily have the same boundaries as the related anatomical structures. Adherence to the strict rules for manipulation of block diagrams not only simplifies explanations, but forces the user of the diagram to think consistently about the system being diagrammed. Even with the application of rigid rules, the same system can be represented by different block diagrams for different purposes. Thus, a single neuron may be represented by several symbols in one case, whereas in another case thousands of neurons may be represented by only a single symbol.

Figures J.1 to J.6 provide a set of block diagram symbols and their significance.

x(t) →   x(t) x(t) →
                               ↓ x(t)

Figure J.1
Transmission of a scalar signal from one source to one or two destinations with no modification or delay.

In figure J.1, the single line represents transfer of an unidimensional signal (scalar function of time) from a single source to an element on which that signal acts. Arrowheads show the direction of transfer. Branched lines always represent divergence in the signal pathway with the same signal delivered by each branch. No signal modification, not even conduction delay, is represented by a line. However, the physical nature of the signal can be any form that is relevant, including nerve impulse trains, neurotransmitter concentration, or mechanical action.

In figure J.2, the broad (double) line represents transfer of more than one separable signal dimension (i.e., a vector signal) between the joined points.

In figure J.3, the circle represents additive convergence of signals with the converging signals and the resultant single output signal distinguished by arrowhead directions. Two or more single (scalar) signals can be summed to yield an output in which the separate inputs are no longer separable. Alternatively, the two inputs can produce a vector output, the components of which remain iden-

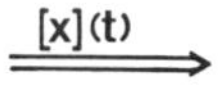

[x](t) ⇒

Figure J.2
Transmission of a vector signal with no change.

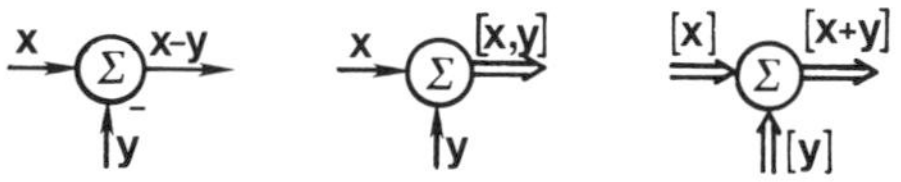

Figure J.3
Additive combination of two signals producing a single output signal. Examples are shown of (1) two scalar signals combined after inversion of one (shown by negative sign) producing a scalar output, (2) combination of signals of different dimensions into a vector signal made up of those dimensions, (3) combination of separate vector signals producing a vector output with appropriate dimensions.

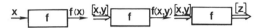

Figure J.4
Operators that act on their input producing a modified output signal. Included are (1) unidimensional operator that modifies the signal magnitude, temporal aspects, or both of its unidimensional input, (2) an operator that combines terms in a vector input into a scalar output, and (3) an operator that modifies its input vector producing a vector output with components organized in a different coordinate space.

tifiable and can still be treated independently at any point that receives that vector signal. At the junction of arrows and circles, the use of $-$ and $+$ signs can be used to show subtractive as well as additive combinations. The additive combination of vector signals also can be represented by the circle figure. It is important to require dimensional compatibility at these summation points. Analysis of the dimensions can reveal internal inconsistency of the theory being represented.

In figure J.4, the block shows that there is a modification of the input signal. This is called an *operator* in that it operates on its input signal to produce its output signal. There is but one input and one output signal for a block, but either or both may be multidimensional vectors. The output may not be definable in the same dimensions as the input nor need the input and output be carried in the same physical form. Block operation on a scalar signal $x(t)$ can include conduction delay, transduction, temporal summation, adaptation, threshold, saturation, or scale modification. When the input to a block is a vector (more than one variable), the block can represent multiple operations on the individual scalar component signals and can produce a new vector as an output. The block with a vector input also can represent operators in which individual signals within the input vector interact to produce an output that is a scalar time function.

There is no limit to the complexity of the operation that is represented by a block signal as long as that block is provided with the necessary input and output. Thus, a single block with a vector input and vector output might even represent the whole nervous system with all of its sensory input pathways and effector output pathways. Generally block diagrams represent only part of the system modeled and its usage is restricted by what is included in that part. Relationships among operators can be represented by a diagram without definition of the properties of the individual blocks, although without that definition, the understanding of function remains very limited.

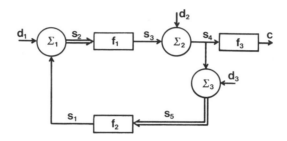

Figure J.5
A closed loop feedback system with two operators, f_1 and f_2, within the loop and another, f_3, on its output pathway. This system has input signals, d, that are added to the local signal in three functionally different locations of the system. Classes of signals and operations are designated by standard symbols. Qualitative details are not restricted by the diagram.

J.1. Questions: To review of the use of this set of symbols, examine figure J.5 and answer these questions.

1. How are the operations of Σ_1 and Σ_3 similar to each other but different from Σ_2?

2. How are the operators f_1 and f_2 similar to each other but different from f_3?

3. How do the f operators differ from the Σ actions?

4. What happens only with signal s_4 but no other signal?

5. What dimensional relationship must be found between s_3 and d_2 and s_4 that may not be found between d_1 and s_1, or between s_4 and d_3?

It is often convenient either to reduce or to expand a block diagram while dealing with a particular system. In the process, if separate operators are combined in a single block, that block will have an operator that combines the action of the parts included. Thus the block diagram shown in figure J.5 can be drawn as shown in figure J.6.

J.2. Problem: Draw an alternate diagram using a different operator to represent some part of the same system.

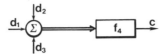

Figure J.6
Alternative representation of the circuit of figure J.5 that defines the operation of f_4 so that it incorporates the effects of the components and network of the more detailed functional diagram.

K. Block algebra

For systems with only linear operators, there is a formal algebra available to reduce the many operators of the network to a single operator that is exactly equivalent. For nonlinear systems, linear approximations may have only limited usefulness. In this book, nonlinear systems are treated sometimes by approximating them as linear systems and in other cases by intuitive examination of their nonlinear aspects without recourse to formal analysis. Extensive study of nonlinear systems requires a background in engineering control analysis or advanced mathematics (see, for instance, *New Directions in Dynamical Systems*, *An Introduction to Chaotic Dynamical Systems*, or *Analysis of Nonlinear Control Systems*).

When dealing with linear operators or linear approximations, f, of real systems, it is permissible to shift blocks across summing points and this may help clarify the nature of some connectivity patterns. The two block diagrams in figure K.1 are equivalent.

Nonlinear blocks, Φ, also can be shifted across branch points as is shown in figure K.2.

When blocks are connected in series, with no branching, the presence of several simple, but separate, time delays, τ, can be reduced to a single equivalent delay as is shown in figure K.3.

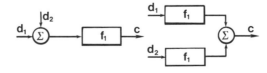

Figure K.1
Functionally equivalent block diagrams, applicable only for linear operators.

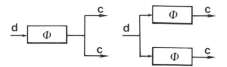

Figure K.2
Exchange of the order of operators and a branch point for either linear or nonlinear operators, indicated by the symbol φ. Note that this is possible because the same signal is found on both branches after the path separation.

When A and B are simple scalar multipliers or when used only to calculate the steady-state response ratio of an operation that may have linear dynamic properties, the blocks in figure K.4 are all functionally equivalent.

For dynamic, linear operators, it is necessary to combine the differential equations that represent the separate operators by appropriate methods such as convolution, frequency response methods, or the use of Laplace transformations.

Systems involving nonlinear elements are not easily manipulated, especially if they also involve dynamic operations. As in algebra, the sequence of operations is not interchangeable when any operation is nonlinear. The signals associated with the block diagram in figure K.5 illustrate one example of the differences resulting from sequence reversal.

For relatively simple systems, including nonlinear operators, it is often impossible to reduce the diagram beyond the so-called *sandwich model* (figure K.6). A nonlinear block is used both before and after a block that represents all the linear dynamic parts of the system.

A threshold type of nonlinearity following a point of convergence (figure K.7) can act like a switch in which the steady magnitude of one input sets the bias of the system so that another signal may act in either the low or the high responsiveness range of the operator.

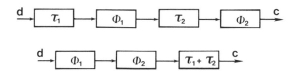

Figure K.3
In a strictly series-connected system in which no internal signals are of interest, representation of time delays can be combined or moved along the series, between input and output.

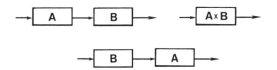

Figure K.4
The operation of linear elements in a strictly series connection can be combined into a single block with an appropriate combined effect or the sequence of operations can be reversed while preserving the same input-output relationships.

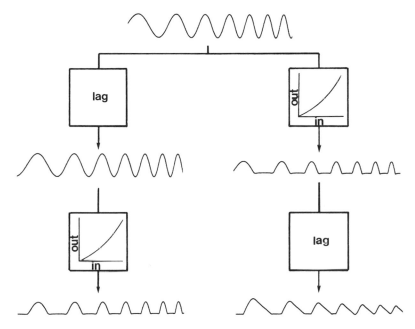

Figure K.5
The relationship between input and output of a series of elements, consisting of a dynamic and a nonlinear operator is dependent on the order of their connection.

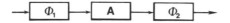

Figure K.6
The "sandwich model," in which two appropriate nonlinear operators are presumed to be located one before and the other after a linear operator. This often provides the minimally useful model for describing an unknown nonlinear system.

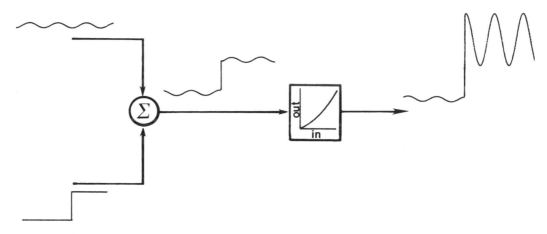

Figure K.7
When two signals are combined before passing through a nonlinear operator, the part of the output of that operator that represents one of the input signals can be modified by details of the signal with which it is combined.

Methods of describing and analyzing the behavior of systems that have both nonlinear and dynamic properties have had considerable attention under the mathematical discipline of nonlinear dynamics. One reference to applications in nervous systems was published by Marmarales and Marmarales (1978).

L. Phase plane

A graph in which the horizontal axis represents the magnitude of some function and the vertical axis represents the rate of change of that function, is called the *phase plane*. Every point on that plane represents a unique combination of rate and magnitude and each combination is represented by only one point on the plane. Further, a change in magnitude or of the rate of change of magnitude is shown as a point moving over the phase plane. A trace of sequential phase plane locations of that point over time is spoken of as its *trajectory*. Because of the relationship between magnitude and rate of change of magnitude, all trajectories on the phase plane will progress with time in a clockwise direction. (Convince yourself of the truth of this statement.) The phase plane graph is especially useful to show the dynamic behavior of second order systems, including very nonlinear ones. For this class of systems, if the rules of the system do not change between trials and if the system is not driven by external inputs, the trajectories on successive tests will be related. At any point on the phase plane, the rules are always the same so from that point the direction of the trajectory also will be always the same. Consequently, in successive trials, starting from different initial conditions, the second trajectory may travel over the same pathway as its predecessor or, if it does not, the two pathways will not cross. In a damped oscillatory response of a system, trajectories that are not superimposed will follow converging spiral pathways (figure 16.10B).

Concepts

Chapter 1. Introduction

The nervous system has a special controlling or modifying action over most body functions although its cells depend on the same metabolic processes as do other cells.

Any course of neurophysiology should be considered no more than a foundation on which to build further study of the ever-changing details of our understanding of neuroscience.

The nervous system generally has little value in dealing with stationary conditions but provides an animal with the ability to adjust to changing conditions.

The nervous system contains certain elements that are specialized to move information from a site of origin to more remote points of utilization.

Information is distinct from the form in which it is represented. Transduction is the process of translating information from one physical form to another.

Effectors transduce neural signals into physical responses and contribute significantly to the combination and processing of these signals.

Neural control requires that there be a prediction of future needs and conditions.

Normal neural function requires the combination of information entering over a period of time and by way of multiple pathways.

Nervous systems and computers both deal with information in a pulsatile form, but the organization and processing details are markedly different.

Chapter 2. Transmission Phenomena

Coordination of activities in different locations implies communication, whether by neural or other means.

Mechanical, chemical, and electrical phenomena, by which conditions in one location influence conditions in another location, are capable of communicating information.

Specialized properties of the membranes of excitable fibers provide for the renewal of spatially decrementing signals. This allows nondecremental communication at a distance with relative independence from intervening local conditions.

Once initiated, an impulse will travel the length of a fiber but generally it does not affect activity in other fibers.

The conduction velocity of nerve impulses can be fast, although slow enough to be measurable in a length of nerve of only a few centimeters.

The pattern of successive impulses on a nerve fiber and the relationship of the activity on different fibers, rather than single nerve impulses, define the information communicated.

Nerve impulses are relatively immune to varying conditions but their discontinuous nature limits a nerve's ability to communicate information about continuous processes.

Multiple fibers carrying related information provide a safety factor in case of fiber loss but cannot eliminate some effects introduced by the discontinuous nature of pulses.

Although both digital computers and the nervous system use pulses to communicate, the way that these pulses are used is rather different in these two cases.

Chapter 3. Information Inputs

The nervous system controls processes that adjust both internal operations of the individual and relations between the individual and the external environment.

Humans experience continually a vast array of stimuli from the environment. An extensive, but arbitrary, set of classifications and quantitative measures has been developed for use in describing the status of, and changes in, these conditions of the environment.

Besides an external environment that is shared with unicellular animals, most multicellular animals have an internal environment the status of which is of major importance.

Objects and conditions that make direct contact with the surface of an animal have an immediate effect on the future of that animal.

Important quantitative information must be obtained regarding objects that contact the body surface. Besides object identification, this information is necessary to predict how the contact will change on its interaction with the surface.

The relationship between geometry of an external object and its pattern of contact with the surface is dependent, in part, on the configuration of the part of the animal making the contact.

Information about changes at a remote location (e.g., sound, light, and air-borne chemical substances) provides a basis for prediction of possible future direct interactions.

Characteristics of the light source are usually of less importance in light-transmitted information than are those modifications that result from intervening reflecting and transmitting media.

Characteristics imparted by the sound source are usually of more importance in sound-transmitted information than are those modifications that result from intervening reflecting and transmitting media.

Biologically important sound distinctions commonly involve time-variant patterns of changing intensities over multiple frequencies.

Information from specific, remote sources can be modified in transmission through intervening media and mixed with information from extraneous sources (noise).

All of the sensory receptors together provide a characteristic response to only a small fraction of the information from internal and external sources.

The information reaching the body from many sources is both redundant and too extensive to be processed and stored by any finite system. The amount of information required to represent changing conditions increases as the required temporal resolution of detail increases.

Chapter 4. Receptor Selectivity

Common to all information-handling systems is the requirement that information enter the system. This usually entails a change of the form in which that information is found.

Sensory receptor systems differentiate between different sources of energy.

Encoding with pattern codes and transmission over labeled lines are two means by which distinct types of sensory information are differentiated.

The various modalities of sensation represent the dimensions of sensory space.

Mechanoreceptors provide sensitive responses to a wealth of different mechanical stimuli.

Chemoreceptors respond when specific chemical agents come in contact with the receptor cell.

Although all neurons are affected by temperature, certain neurons respond principally as temperature receptors.

Mammalian photoreceptors respond to light signals relative to the dimensions of intensity, wavelength, and spatial coordinates.

Sensitivity to electric currents and fields, although common in many neurons, is not a well-developed sensory system in humans.

Extreme conditions are likely to damage any cell and as a result will affect the behavior of any neuron. Certain neurons, however, are especially responsive to conditions that are likely to lead to damage.

The exchange of more than a certain minimum amount of energy must occur before a sensory receptor will respond.

Our perceptions of the world are limited by the sensitivities of those sensory receptors with which we have been endowed by evolution.

Information arriving at the body, especially that from remote sources, often has considerable redundancy.

Sensory receptors limit the response range of the input information.

Sensation occurs within specific sensory coordinate systems.

When receptors respond to more than two dimensions of physical input, the response of a single receptor is necessarily ambiguous in those dimensions.

Sensory encoding recurs at multiple steps as sensory information is conveyed centrally. Specific sensory information is selected in this encoding process.

Stimulus amplitude is typically encoded in a nonlinear manner.

Spatial and temporal boundaries are emphasized in sensory encoding.

Our familiar sensations result from information in many physical dimensions that originates from a multitude of sensory receptors.

Chapter 5. Accessory Structures to Sensory Receptors

Receptor properties determine the response to the energy that reaches a receptor, whereas other structures selectively affect what part of the energy from the environment reaches each receptor.

Differential selectivity, as a result of accessory structures, can impart unique response patterns to a set of nearly identical receptors.

Accessory structures protect the individual mechanically sensitive hair cells of the auditory system from stimuli other than a specific range of air-borne vibration.

Enhanced responsiveness to a particular stimulus energy can be produced by structures that either increase the energy converging on the receptor or increase the effectiveness of coupling of a particular type of energy to the receptor.

The specific location of action and source of energy that causes a particular sensory neuron to respond is the receptive field for that cell.

The information reported by a single receptor is reduced, because of the transduction process, to a single dimension. This reduction occurs regardless of how many dimensions are required to define all of the variations of the energy that are delivered to, and absorbed by, that receptor.

Efferent neural signals often effect alterations in the relationship between an individual receptor's response and the conditions in the environment to which the receptor responds.

Although prolonged changes in accessory structures can alter the response of sensory receptors, sometimes the central processing of signals from those receptors is altered in a compensatory manner.

Different species, having evolved in different environments, have sensory systems that respond to stimuli that are important in those environments. Often one species will respond to conditions that are not sensed by another species.

Chapter 6. Convergence

Information is almost always carried in the nervous system by multiple nerve impulses that can be distributed over time on individual fibers and over multiple fibers in the same time period.

Junctional regions between different nerve cells are usually the site of computation and signal modification.

Multiple, separate nerve pathways generally converge on each neuron in the central nervous system.

Successive nerve impulses, when delivered to a neuron in the central nervous system over a short period, usually lead to a nonlinear cumulative result.

The receptive field of a neuron in the central nervous system includes all types and locations of stimulation that directly or indirectly produce an identifiable alteration of the response of that neuron.

Both the facilitory effectiveness and the time course of the action of an impulse delivered to a neuron are subject to variation depending on where the impulse arrives on the neuron.

Inhibition is at least as important as excitation in the action of nerve signals arriving at a neuron in the central nervous system.

Both the facilitory and the inhibitory actions of nerve impulses act over a period of time that is appreciably longer than the initiating action potential.

A reflex is usually a somewhat stereotypic motor response to one of a restricted range of stimulus variations.

A pair of motoneuron pools that innervate muscles with antagonistic actions are frequently reciprocally innervated.

While the overall reflex response may be stereotypic, the response detail may vary depending on the "local sign" of the stimulus.

The nonlinear properties of reflex pathways often lead to interactions among different inputs such that the responsiveness to one input varies with the magnitude of the other inputs.

Feedback pathways are common in the nervous system in which the response of a neuron acts directly or indirectly as part of its own input.

Very different types of stimuli often produce responses that interact to generate specific neural responses.

Interactions in the relationships between sensory input and motor responses can also lead to activity patterns that emerge from the system rather than from any individual part.

The output of neural systems depends on the previous conditions (state) of the system as much as it does on the current input.

Chapter 7. Effector Actions

The transduction, processing, and transmission of signals in the nervous system impart a survival value to the organism only after these signals have been further modified and transduced by effector organs.

The coordination of chemical processes probably has been a major drive toward the general development of neural communication and organization.

Neural signals are responsible for modifying the rate of production, the composition, the secretion, and the transport of the products of a variety of glands.

When neural signals modify the output of endocrine glands, the endocrine product forms another signal with the final result occurring in the target tissue of that endocrine agent.

Neural control of motor activity of skeletal muscle is accomplished entirely by the modification of muscle excitation. The response of skeletal muscle to neural excitation involves changes in velocity, length, stiffness, and heat production.

Muscle contributes a major portion of the total basal production of heat in the body and is the principal source of neurally controlled heat.

The force produced by muscle is the usual, but not only, variable controlled by efferent nerve signals.

Although the nerve impulses that drive a muscle are discrete events, the much longer duration of muscle twitches allows their responses to overlap and produce a relatively smoothly changing output.

The relationship between the pulse rate of excitation and the intensity of muscle contraction is a nonlinear, sigmoid function. The results of muscle excitation are determined by the mechanical properties of the load along with the forces coupled to that load.

When the force generated by a muscle acts on a load there is a requisite exchange of energy between the muscle and the load.

The relationships among force, movement, and stimulation rate in a muscle depend only on those conditions that act directly on the muscle.

For muscle to generate the same movement with different loads, it is necessary that the force generated by the muscle change with the load. This requires a change in neural excitation.

Activity of a prime mover muscle, to be effective, usually requires coordinated activity of a number of other muscles.

Human movement starts and ends with muscle-controlled posture.

The control of movement with one degree of freedom often still requires action of a pair of antagonistically acting muscles.

Only under very special circumstances does a muscle act against a constant force and on a constant load impedance.

Reactive forces, resulting from activity in one muscle, generally require stabilizing contractions in other muscles.

Muscles are three-dimensional, complexly organized structures whose structural details are important to their varied functions.

Muscle tension is not converted simply to torque on a hinge because of complications of articulation patterns and muscle connection geometry.

Normal motor control depends on periods of dynamic equilibrium in positions that would not be statically stable.

Although it complicates motor control theory, a body geometry that allows alternative ways of accomplishing the same manipulation provides adaptability to variable motor problems.

Chapter 8. From Reception to Perception

Both the motor response to and the perception of the environment involve central processing of information about the world that has been transduced into signals on sensory nerve fibers.

The identification of an object in sensory space results not from discretely localized information but rather from a spatiotemporally distributed pattern of incoming nerve impulses.

The information content of a pulse rate code is theoretically infinite but practically it depends on how well the receiver is able to distinguish differences in the continuously variable interval between individual pulses.

Events that involve changing relationships among objects depend on spatial and temporal information about object identification and interobject relationships.

The utilization of current information to predict future conditions is critical to the function of the nervous system.

Ordinary cognitive processes are developed through experience and are based on stored information as well as on recent sensory input.

Object recognition may result from first recognition of individual features and then the combination of these features.

Percepts in the nervous system can exist only as patterns of activity distributed over many neurons.

The limitations imposed by computer models have biased current interpretation of the nervous system.

The relationship between sensory input and internal signals is shaped by connections that are determined by genetics and then modified by experience.

Many of the effects of signal combination that are essential for perception are comparable to combinations known in reflex function.

As with spatial convergence, the temporal sequence of successive impulses onto a neuron influences the response of a simple reflex or perception.

Neural function makes exchanges between the temporal and spatial patterns of neural activity.

Because perceptions are usually relative rather than absolute, current details are associated with a transient frame of reference.

The reflex or perceptive outcomes of particular stimuli depend on the state of the nervous system at the time of arrival of the stimulus.

Perceptual processes can be conveniently described using the concept of perceptual basins.

On different occasions the same percept may be extracted from the total sensory inputs that contain not only different critical information but different background information.

Sometimes similar sensory inputs are sharply partitioned and excite different perceptual basins depending on small but critical temporal or spatial details.

Diverse inputs activate individual basins the uniformity of which is shown by the constancy of the perceived objects.

The rules by which a sensory input is converted to a response are plastic. On different occasions the same input can activate different basins or one basin can be activated by different inputs.

The naive brain, exposed to neural inputs from sensory stimulation, must organize its own activity in a way that discovers the existence of consistency in the source of these stimuli.

Chapter 9. Information Storage

We will presume that memory resides in the effectiveness of the interactions between neurons.

Memory is the maintenance over a period of time of an alteration of function as a consequence of previous experience.

Human learning represents a specialization into certain specific areas of a general ability of all animals.

Learning that involves the association of two stimulus patterns is distinguished from learning of the specific properties of a single stimulus pattern.

Short-term memory lasts for only a period of conscious awareness whereas long-term memory can last a lifetime.

Short-term memory relies on functional modifications of the synapses between neurons.

Synaptic efficacy can be modified transiently by a number of different biochemical processes.

One important mechanism by which short-term memory can occur is through the alteration of existing protein molecules.

Memory consolidation depends on arousal and stimulus repetition and probably requires protein synthesis.

Long-term memory persists through alterations of consciousness and depends on protein synthesis.

Human memory retrieval is associative and distributed.

A network of elements can be constructed with functionally simple nodes that allow associative retrieval of information that has been stored in a distributed manner.

The genetic code provides an effective memory of ancestral experiences.

Chapter 10. Neuroelectric Phenomena

In tissue, electrical current is carried by the movement of charged ions in opposite directions with the arbitrary designation of current direction being that of movement of positively charged ions.

Current flowing outward across the membrane of an excitable cell tends to stimulate that cell.

Electrical stimulation of excitable tissue in the clinical setting is usually accomplished by the delivery of current between an external anode and cathode so arranged that part of the current passes across the excitable membrane.

The variation of current density in different parts of a volume conductor can be used to localize the tissues that will be most effectively stimulated.

Although electrical stimuli can be used to excite either sensory or motor nerves, it has been extremely difficult to generate and deliver appropriate spatial and temporal patterns of activity to substitute for defective physiological excitation.

Appropriate input signals are a necessary prerequisite to the generation of motor control stimuli.

The activity of excitable tissue results in local currents and potential changes.

Temporally overlapping activity in multiple nerve or muscle fibers generates local voltages that result from the addition of the separately generated currents in the shared volume conductor.

The time course of the recorded action potential from a single nerve fiber depends on changes in differences in potential between the two electrode sites as the nerve impulse moves along the fiber.

The spatial and temporal distributions of the electrical event of an action potential are related by the conduction velocity of the nerve impulse.

The most precise measurements of the electrical properties of excitable cells come from single cell recordings.

Muscles are a second category of excitable cells whose electrical activity is commonly measured.

Local activity in the brain produces a low voltage that changes relatively slowly. Recordings of these potentials can be valuable in evaluating certain aspects of neural activity.

Synchronous peripheral stimuli produce characteristic and local electrical changes (evoked responses) in the cortex that can be extracted from the underlying EEG activity.

Chapter 11. Generation of the Membrane Potential

Excitable cells have a potential difference between their inside and the solution bathing their outside.

The Nernst equation describes the relationship between a concentration gradient and a voltage gradient at which a particular ion will diffuse without a directional bias.

Ion channels provide the means for selected species of ions to cross the hydrophobic cell membrane.

Energy-requiring pumps are necessary to maintain concentration gradients across membranes.

Membranes with permeabilities to several ions maintain a potential difference that is determined by the concentration gradients of and the permeabilities to the various ions for which ion channels exist.

Calcium ions enter the intracellular compartment of cells through selective channels as a result of their electrochemical gradient. Once in the cytoplasm, these ions regulate numerous important cellular processes.

Chapter 12. Alterations of Membrane Potential

There are three basic characteristics of electrical current flow: (1) current tends to flow whenever unlike charges have been separated; (2) current always flows in a closed circuit; and (3) current flow can be either resistive or capacitive.

Except under certain experimental conditions, potential changes across the membranes of excitable cells are localized to one region of the membrane and decrease to insignificance at more distant regions of the cell.

Passive electrical properties of the cell, including the membrane resistance, capacitance, and cytoplasmic resistance, determine its space and time constants.

The space constants that depend on geometric characteristics of various cell types are important in determining the effect of local potential changes in those cells.

The ability to generate all-or-nothing action potentials sets excitable cells apart from all other types of cells.

Ion channels, protein molecules in the lipid cell membrane, are responsible for both resting and action potentials.

The function of ion channels depends on certain highly specialized properties of these protein molecules.

The action potential shares with various electronically generated time-marking pulses two important and related properties: it has a threshold, and once that threshold is exceeded the resultant potential change is *all-or-nothing*.

During an action potential, sodium channels open by the process of activation and subsequently close through the process of inactivation. With a somewhat slower time course, potassium channels also open as a result of their own activation process.

Local current flow permits action potentials to propagate along long fibers.

Saltatory conduction provides rapid, efficient conduction of action potentials over relatively small diameter fibers.

Chapter 13. Chemical Effectors

Most cell-to-cell communication results when a presynaptic cell releases a neurotransmitter that acts on a postsynaptic cell.

The neuromuscular junction is a highly specialized region of contact between a motor nerve and a muscle fiber.

Even when it is not conducting action potentials, the presynaptic nerve releases quanta of neurotransmitter that produce small depolarizations of the postsynaptic cell.

In the presence of Ca^{2+}, presynaptic action potentials initiate the release of a large number of quanta of neurotransmitter.

The coupling between depolarization of the membrane of the presynaptic terminal and the release of synaptic vesicles is accomplished by a rise in intracellular Ca^{2+} concentration.

Acetylcholine initiates electrical events in skeletal muscle cells by binding to ligand-gated channels in the postsynaptic membrane.

Nicotinic acetylcholine-gated channels open following the binding of two acetylcholine molecules to binding sites that are part of the channel molecule.

Nicotinic acetylcholine-gated channels are nonselective among many small cations.

The enzyme acetylcholinesterase is responsible for the rapid degradation of acetylcholine.

Neuron-to-neuron synaptic transmission utilizes a multitude of different neurotransmitters whose postsynaptic effects can be excitatory, inhibitory, or modulatory.

There are three general categories of neurotransmitters that fall into a natural hierarchy. The first category includes amino acids, the secondary category includes biogenic amines (e.g., acetylcholine), and the third category includes peptides.

Chemical synapses are sites of amplification, susceptibility to drugs and toxins, unidirectionality of transmission, and integration of information.

Not all synaptic effects are the result of a direct action of a neurotransmitter on a postsynaptic receptor–channel molecule. A very important aspect of the operation of synapses in the function of the nervous system stems from the modulation of synaptic and electrical properties by neurotransmitters.

Presynaptic inhibition occurs because of a reduction of the amount of excitatory neurotransmitter released by the presynaptic neuron.

Second messengers act intracellularly in postsynaptic cells.

In addition to the effects of postsynaptic potentials, neurotransmitters can have a variety of other effects in postsynaptic cells.

Chapter 14. Mechanical Effectors

A major aspect of nervous system function is its physical expression through muscle activity.

The motor unit is the effector unit of neural control in skeletal muscle.

The nerve signals that drive skeletal muscles regulate the intensity of response in two ways: by changes in the firing rate of individual motor units and by variation in the number of motor units that are active simultaneously.

The neural control of cardiac and smooth muscle is generally modulatory and a particular nerve fiber can be either excitatory or inhibitory.

Electrical excitation of a muscle fiber occurs when an action potential propagates over the sarcolemma.

Excitation of cardiac and smooth muscle fibers can originate in the muscle cells themselves.

The coupling of electrical excitation with mechanical contraction is accomplished through the action of Ca^{2+} ions.

Movement is a common feature to many living cells including those of animals, plants, and microorganisms.

The primary contractile proteins of muscle are actin and myosin. In skeletal muscle, contraction is regulated by troponin and tropomyosin.

Muscle shortening results from the sliding of interdigitating thin and thick filaments.

A single adequate stimulus to a muscle nerve or directly to a muscle will produce a single, rapid contraction of the muscle followed by a relaxation back to its resting condition.

The efficacy of muscle for a given change in enthalpy depends on how the output of that muscle is measured.

The contractile proteins are contained within a bag that has complex viscous and elastic properties.

The force that a muscle fiber can deliver at any one time depends on a very nonlinear interaction of the muscle length and velocity, its temperature, the level of excitation, and the recent history of the muscle's actions.

The relationship of length and force is generally investigated under isometric conditions.

The relationship between force and velocity can be investigated under several conditions of movement.

In normal activity, length, velocity, and force all change. This is a condition called *auxotonic contraction*.

Chapter 15. Temporal Modifications

Since the value of the nervous system lies in its contribution to the individual's response to changes, an understanding of dynamic processes is critical to an understanding of neural function.

The time consumed in conduction of nerve impulses along fibers is functionally significant, particularly in dealing with rapidly changing signals.

Correlations exist between function and fiber types so that functions involving rapid changes are generally signaled along the most rapidly conducting fibers.

Memory yields the longest delays between events and the neural consequences of those events.

An important result of summation is the smoothing (low pass filtering) of discontinuous signals.

Lags are produced by the temporal effects of summation on periodic inputs.

Adaptation has the remarkable and important effect of causing the output of the adapting system to lead in time any smoothly changing signals on which it operates.

Most sensory receptors show some form of adaptation to their adequate stimulus.

Receptors that adapt completely can produce signals to represent a changing stimulus but not a steady stimulus.

For receptors that operate over a large range of stimulus intensities, adaptation adjusts function into the current range of intensities.

Although adaptation has qualitatively similar effects in many receptors, the mechanisms of its production vary widely from one case to another.

Dynamic effects in structures that affect neural signals provide both predictive and cumulative information about stimuli.

Chapter 16. Neural Network Operations

When neurons interact in simple networks, functional properties can emerge from the network that do not exist in any of the individual neurons.

Qualitatively divergent activity patterns in a network may arise out of differences in input pattern or in changes of the effectiveness of connections.

The functional implications of theories about simple networks of neurons are sufficiently complex that formal modeling studies are essential for understanding network behavior.

Block diagrams, a formal algebra that defines acceptable manipulations, are a convenient tool for representing functional relationships in a neural network.

A given stimulus can act on many receptors and afferent nerve fibers. Thus one stimulus can provide different information with different eventual uses.

All signals, while being processed by the nervous system, are subject sequentially to a variety of operations, each of which changes the way in which the initial information is represented.

Feedback pathways are ubiquitous to neural structures ranging from pathways involving only local connections to those that involve the longest fibers.

Positive feedback occurs when a small static change in a signal acts around a closed loop in such a way that it tends to increase the original change in the loop.

Whereas positive feedback accentuates the effect of inputs and of changes in the elements in a loop, negative feedback can compensate for changes in elements and reduce the relative effectiveness of some input signals.

The effects of feedback are the same in technology and in biology but may differ in the relative magnitude and importance of different parts of those effects on function.

Feedback produces quantitative alterations of both static signal amplitudes and the temporal scale of dynamic responses of the whole loop as compared to those of the individual components.

Oscillatory activity often emerges from negative feedback loops that have no oscillation in their inputs or in their internal components.

Even in feedback systems that do not exhibit sustained oscillation, a transient disturbance will often initiate a damped oscillatory activity.

Damped oscillation loses information about the starting conditions as time progresses. Under some circumstances, oscillation in feedback systems can generate new information while behaving in a completely determined manner.

The complex variability seen in repetitive neural activity may originate deterministicly rather than as a random process.

The new functional properties that emerged from the introduction of closed loop pathways in neural systems may have been a critical increment in the evolution of higher neural function.

Chapter 17. Combined neural operation

The routine activities that support survival utilize a wide range of neural functions and have presumably been important in their evolution.

The nervous systems of higher animals contribute to and depend on the control of the internal conditions that make coordinated life processes possible.

Adjustment of energy and materials exchange with the external world must be based on the accumulated quantity present internally.

The control of internal conditions involves interactions among the sensing requirements, acquisition means, and removal that are related to different variables, some of which are independent of direct control.

Inherited identification and control mechanisms can deal with situations that are consistent across a species. Learning is, however, necessary for those situations that require adaptation to existing environmental or individual characteristics.

Higher functions of the nervous system often override simple reflex actions to produce adjustments that depend on complex factors that are related to predictable costs and benefits.

Direct actions within a biological controller usually produce side effects that activate compensatory reflexes outside of the primary controller.

Effector activities consume energy and materials and also produce heat and waste; this requires appropriate adjustment of both acquisition and disposal.

Conflicts may occur when multiple sensor or effector systems deal with the control of a single variable.

The nervous system generally does not operate as a unified and monolithic controlling system.

The neural signals that control digestive functions, through the complex nervous system of the gut, are largely, but not entirely, independent of the CNS.

Neural control of gastrointestinal function deals with the internal operations of the gut as distinct from control of homeostasis.

Nerves associated with the vascular system do not only modify the circulatory transport of nutrients from the gut but are also associated with sensing the level of some of those nutrients in the blood.

Sensed deficiency of a nutrient is likely to drive ingestion of a mixture of materials including other nutrients in a variable ratio that is usually not proportional to the relative needs.

Simple physical or neural inputs lead to complex interacting processes in the body, whether the initiating action is a normal or a pathologic event or even if it is introduced as a therapeutic intervention.

The evolution of the neural tools necessary for sophisticated energy acquisition has left us with a commonwealth of loosely coordinated mechanisms capable of both homeostasis and intellectual activity.

Notes

Chapter 1

1.1. *Library search methods: Backward search* starts with a known publication and looks at the references cited in that publication. The cited publications can then be used to track additional related sources. *Index search* is accomplished by using one or more indexes to find papers about particular topics, by authors known to work in the area, and in journals that deal with the subject of interest. Besides indexes such as *Index Medicus,* there are several abstract journals that provide short abstracts of many of the papers in a broad area. Some of these use a permuted index in which individual words in the titles of papers are arranged in order. Other indexes permit searching for word combinations taken from titles and from key word lists. A more recent development is the use of computerized search tools (e.g., Medline) that allows various indexed sources to be searched for words by using a Boolean definition of the desired topic. Access to these tools can be purchased or acquired from different libraries. *Forward search* can be accomplished by starting with one or more early papers in a field of interest. On looking up these papers in *Science Citation Index* it is possible to find papers in a more recent period that refer to the source paper. Presumably these newer papers deal with a subject that is related to the index paper. By scanning this source over many years, it is often possible to find support for and contradictions to the source paper.

1.3. An alternate method to using a stop watch takes advantage of computer programs that time intervals between a computer-generated signal and a manual response. The signal can be initiated by a random timer or by an operator action and the subject then responds by another action. The time interval should be displayed or stored for later statistical or graphic evaluation. Computational delay times involved in this measurement should be evaluated and corrected.

1.4. You might want to refer to a neuroanatomy textbook for information on sensory and motor pathways. (*The Ciba Collection of Medical Illustrations* provides clear simplified illustrations of major neural pathways.) Visual information leaves the eye on the optic nerve and with one intervening relay is transmitted to the visual cortex in the back of the brain. Motor information can originate in many locations, but one possibility is the motor cortex on the surface approximately half way between the front and back of the brain. This information is transmitted down the spinal cord to the appropriate level and then through a peripheral nerve to the necessary muscles.

1.6. We would not want to discourage a little rereading of physics textbooks, but in case your college mechanics text is lost in a box in the attic, the period of a pendulum is given by the equation:

$$T = \frac{1}{f} = 2\pi\sqrt{\frac{l}{g}}$$

where T is the period, f is the frequency, l is the length of the pendulum, and g is the acceleration of gravity (9.8 m/sec). In any problem it is worth doing a dimensional analysis, that is, insert the dimensions in the terms on the right-hand side of the equation to check that the correct units are obtained for the left-hand side of the equation.

Chapter 2

2.1. A reference to a human anatomy book would be very appropriate here. Muscles are attached to and move bones through tendons. These tendons can be rather long, even crossing joints. The human hand is a marvelous maze of tendons, muscles, and bones, the learning of whose names keeps anatomy students up late at night. At this point, though, you need to discover where the muscles are located that move the fingers.

2.2. Models generated on a digital computer are discontinuous in both time and magnitude. Thus digital models are only an approximation of essentially continuous processes. If you can solve the original equation for the quantity remaining as a function of time, substitution of a different time interval in that equation will give accurate theoretical values at each point calculated and this is the preferred approach. For equations that you cannot solve, a numerical approximation can be obtained for the change over a brief period. From this calculation, the approximate quantity at the end of the interval is derived and then used as the starting value for the next interval. Iteration of these steps gives a sequence of approximations over the desired period.

The simplest approximation assumes that the rate of change, as calculated at the beginning of an interval, remains a constant predictor of change throughout the whole period. More sophisticated calculations have been developed that use corrections based on higher time derivatives of the variable. These can be found in a variety of books on numerical methods. If you are comfortable with these refinements, they can be used for improved accuracy at the cost of more computation complexity and time.

In any case, numerical approximations require that the sampled intervals be short with respect to the time required to make an appreciable change in the variables. This is best evaluated if your program allows easy change of the sampling interval until one is found that is sufficiently accurate and yet does not take too much computation time. A particular time interval can be evaluated by comparing the results of that interval with results from shorter intervals. In more complex models, problems called *stiff systems* develop, but these will not be considered here.

It is usually worthwhile to develop computer models in stages, solving problems with one part before proceeding to more complex versions. If you have not done digital modeling before, we suggest that you might want to study the removal process (diffusion, renal excretion, respiratory removal, metabolic removal) first using a removal rate that is proportional to the amount still present. For this model, start with an initial quantity and follow its removal. This corresponds to the situation in which the initial quantity was added instantaneously at the time where the calculation started.

After this model is finished, proceed by adding the assumption that the agent is delivered at a constant rate over several time frames, while decay is also occurring. A more complex delivery pattern can be chosen to represent a continuous signal. You may want to consider more than one input pattern to represent different physiologically relevant situations. Extending the model by addition of noninstantaneous mixing leads to an appreciably more complex model.

2.3. Before deciding whether overlapping values represented true variations in threshold or were experimental artifacts, what are some sources of artifact that you should eliminate? As you study excitation further, refine and interpret the implications of your answers to these questions. Various methods of eliminating the effect of the time sequence can be used. Repetition of measurements of one point can be used to demonstrate that at that point the response is reproducible. If the repeated values show a change over time, it is not clear how measurement of other points should be corrected. One possibility is as a ratio to the reference point. A simple combination of a forward and a reverse sequence of values is sometimes used so that the average time to each pair of points is the same. This is satisfactory when change progresses at a constant rate.

   A random sequence of tests will remove the effect of a time trend and make individual values more variable. It is usual to use a pseudo-random sequence that can be easily generated by some well-defined method using a calculator or computer. Since these procedures begin with the insertion of a "seed" value, exactly the same sequence will be generated if the same seed value is used again. These sequences are usually decimal values between 0 and 1 with essentially uniform distribution within that range. An example of a simple pseudo-random number generator is called the *mid-square method*. The seed is added to π and the result is squared. Then a specified number of the middle digits is kept to be used for the seed in the next iteration. The number of digits that are kept determines how soon the series will repeat.

2.4. In fact, figure 2.7A does not have a single scale but represents a variety of scales as shown by the table in the legend. You might answer this question by calculating the width on the graph in units of 1 msec if the wavelength, λ, in the graph takes on each value listed in the third column of the table.

2.5. When electrical recordings are made from individual neurons, these neurons often exhibit electrical activity even when there is nothing obvious exciting the neuron. Whether this represents actual *spontaneous activity* is a difficult question to answer because (1) it is usually difficult to establish a condition in which there are absolutely no inputs to a neuron, and (2) it is probably impossible to be certain that the process of recording electrical activity from a neuron does not disturb the neuron and thereby excite it.

2.7. If you have been skipping some material presented in the appendixes, you should go back now and read the brief discussion of the Nyquist criterion (appendix E). One way of answering this question is to construct graphs of input magnitude against output pulse rate for encoding of different static inputs. With the appropriate graph, a brief explanation is all that is necessary. Intuitively you might expect the maximum and minimum averages to include the maximum and minimum of the encoded cycle. Starting with this it is possible to use numerical calculation to find the approximate value for those extremes. It is more elegant to set up approximate equations and to solve for the maximum and minimum values. How do you calculate maximum and minimum averages in a corresponding span of a sine wave that is offset by a bias of B? That is,

$$Y = \sin(\omega t) + B$$

when t is time and ω is π times frequency.

2.8. We do not want to offer any numbers as approximations for this calculation since we are inclined to think that the results are at best of questionable validity!

Chapter 3

3.2. Some useful definitions: *Temperature*, the condition of a body that determines how heat is transferred to or from that body. *Thermal capacity*, the quantity of heat necessary to produce a unit change in the temperature of a unit mass of some substance. *Thermal conductivity,* the rate of transfer of heat, for a given temperature gradient, across a given volume of some substance.

3.3. Some more useful definitions: *Compliance,* a measure of the resistance to a change of volume in response to a pressure change $C = \Delta V / \Delta P$. *Inertia,* a fundamental property of matter by which it resists any change in its current state of rest or motion.

3.4. A reliable and readable account of applications of light is available in *Light and Color in Nature and Art* by S.J. Williamson and H.Z. Cummings.

3.5. How might the usefulness of this information be improved if you, like a bat, had emitted the sound in the first place? What might be the basis of "sound sight" that blind people use?

3.7. Give special attention to an ordinary conversation and determine how far in advance of statements for which context is essential is the necessary context established. How dependable is the interpretation of individual words when they are out of context? Are there instances when the context is established only after the word has been uttered? How do such other sensory inputs as the identity of the speaker enter into establishing context?

3.8. While the oscilloscope settings will depend on the microphone used and some experimentation is certainly in order, you might start with an AC coupled input at 1 mV/cm at a sweep of 1 msec/cm. If you have an audio amplifier equipped for a microphone input, place it between the microphone and the oscilloscope to help reduce electrical interference. To stabilize the presentation of the oscillographic record, use an internal trigger to respond to a particular part of the waveform. Neither speakers nor microphones produce linear outputs with respect to input amplitude, but microphones tend to be more linear than speakers and probably should be used for approximate measurements. For a demonstration and discussion of some complications of sound perception, refer to the record provided with *The Science of Musical Sounds* by J.R. Pierce.

3.9. Our sensory systems are much better at comparisons than they are at absolute measurements. Why might evolution have selected for a specific temporal or spatial dimension for such comparisons?

3.10. The rate of sound absorption in its passage through air is available in tables relating absorption to pressure and to humidity (e.g., *Handbook of Chemistry and Physics*). Architectural handbooks provide interesting tables of sound reflection for use in designing acoustics of public rooms. An open window is set as the standard for no reflection and surfaces such as plate glass have high sound reflectance.

3.11. Should you be interested, the speed of sound in air is about 330 m/sec; the speed of sound as measured in the Seine River at 30°C is 1528 m/sec. Will these values help you in answering this question?

3.12. How good are you at localizing sound? Next time you go to a zoo make note of the various sizes and shapes of the external ears on the animals that you see. How might different size and shaped external ears vary in their effectiveness in extracting these two types of information? Since the ears of some animals have a major role in heat transfer, their structure may not be entirely explainable in terms of sound collection.

3.13. Both amplitude and phase relationships are important in this experiment. The peak-to-peak amplitude measurement on an oscilloscope is obvious, but phase measurement requires a reference. If a time-based display is used, the oscillatory output can be used to synchronize the sweep and immobilize the displayed location of successive cycles. If the oscilloscope allows simultaneous display of two signals, two microphones can be used and the timing of the test wave can be compared with that of the reference wave. If only one waveform can be displayed, measurements of successive samples can be compared as long as the sweep synchronization is stable. For the most accurate measurement of timing, you should measure the point of crossing of a magnitude where the waveform is changing most rapidly. Another useful method of display that shows both amplitude and phase is to use an X–Y plot and drive the abscissa with the signal from the reference oscillator and drive the ordinate with the signal from the test microphone. This display will have the form of an ellipse called a Lissajous figure. How do you use such a figure to measure phase and amplitude?

3.14. Some audio systems are provided with controls that allow amplification at specific narrow frequency bands. With such an amplifier you can model the frequency pattern found in various types of hearing loss. Use the equalizer controls to model various types of hearing aids. Pathological defects in hearing usually do not result in a modification of the pain threshold along with the depression of the auditory threshold. How can you use this fact in the design of your hearing aid?

3.15. It may be helpful to begin by considering an area that is so small that only one gas molecule can collide with it at a time. A larger area can be considered to be made up of many such small areas. At any moment, the total pressure over the large area would be the average of the pressures produced on all the small areas. This reduces the area problem to a question of statistical properties of the sums of multiple independent variables instead of being a molecular physics problem.

3.16. Information about mean free path, molecular density, and so on, can be obtained from handbooks. This problem, like problem 3.15, can be reduced to a question of statistics after assuming that collisions within an arbitrary small interval are not separately distinguishable. Would it be appropriate to assume that the pressure fluctuations over time would show a Gaussian distribution? The smoothing assumption is based on the fact that the membrane inertial and viscous properties damp the effect of individual collisions. Instead of assuming a series of time windows, it would be possible to set up a second-order equation for smoothing the effect of individual collisions. (Derivation of a predicted frequency distribution is not a trivial problem! You should identify your assumptions and then evaluate their probable validity.) For those who do not wish to attempt this derivation, an alternate problem would be to conduct a library search for a published treatment of the same problem.

3.17. You will find more information available about mechanical events such as respiration, heart rate, finger movement, walking, and fluctuations of sound and light than you will find about the dynamics of biological chemical or thermal, and visceral processes. Include entries in your table for those biologically important variables for which you have been unable to find adequate dynamic information. It may be of interest to keep this table and add to it in the future.

Chapter 3

4.1. You might want to draw some diagrams of a simple optical system to determine which parts of the visual world are projected onto each part of the retina. (This is similar to the consideration of how you put a slide into a slide projector for it to be projected the right way up and with the correct left-right orientation.) Stimulation of receptors in a specific retinal location is always *perceived* as a stimulus in a specific location of the visual field. Does your perception of the location of the spot relate to the corresponding location in the visual field with the eye rotated? To answer this question, you will need to test the relationship between visual field locations and the orientation of your eye using visual stimuli. When looking straight ahead, what are the limitations on the solid angles at which you can see objects?

4.2. Are the results of this experiment related to the results that you obtained in experiment 3.4 in chapter 3?

4.3. Just in case you have forgotten, Avogadro's number is 6.02×10^{23} molecules/mole.

4.4. Assume that the distance between the centers of receptive fields is inversely proportional to the distance between resolvable points. How would this relate to the density of receptors? The added requirement for receptors can be expressed as the relative increases of density times area rather than attempting to estimate the actual number of added receptors that would be required. Presumably, the increased density also would apply to the increase of fibers needed to carry the extra information to the brain. Would this increase be significant to the bulk of the nervous system?

4.5. $$\Delta R = k \log \frac{R_1}{R_0} - k \log \left(\frac{R_2}{R_0}\right) = k \log \left(\frac{R_1/R_0}{R_2/R_0}\right) = k \log\left(\frac{R_1}{R_2}\right)$$

$$\Delta R = k \log \left(\frac{0.1}{0.03}\right) = k \log \left(\frac{R}{10}\right)$$

$$R = 33.3$$

4.6. In scanning a stationary scene or in changing your gaze from one point to another when there is no moving target, your eyes make rapid, ballistic movements called *saccadic eye movements*. We do not perceive these movements because visual perception is depressed while the movements are made.

Chapter 5

5.1. *Archimedes' principle:* When a body is immersed in a fluid it is buoyed up by a force that is equal to the weight of the fluid displaced. *Pascal's law:* When a pressure is exerted at some point on a confined liquid it is transmitted undiminished in all directions.

5.4. Lens diagrams are useful in the various optics problems that arise in considering the visual system. Two general situations arise in such problems: (1) *Magnification* problems, in which an object, at a distance greater than the focal length of the lens, produces an inverted image on the opposite side of the lens from the object. A longer focal length lens used in this arrangement will produce a larger image and thus have more magnification. (2) *Power* problems, in which an object, at a distance less than the focal length of the lens, produces a virtual image that is not inverted and is on the same side of the lens as the object. A shorter focal length lens used in this arrangement will produce a larger image and thus has greater power. Use lens diagrams to convince yourself of the validity of these statements.

5.6. Children with *strabismus* (inability to align their eyes) can permanently lose the possibility of depth perception based on parallax even after the defect has been repaired. It would appear then that the necessary neural connections for this form of depth perception are based on experience. (In Chapter 8 we will discuss other visual information that can be used to determine depth.)

5.8. What must corrective lenses do to compensate for each of these visual defects?

Chapter 6

6.3. Remember that the area of a circle = $(\pi d^2)/4$. Light intensity, form a point source, falls with the square of the distance along any straight light path. Did you consider the effect of light reflected from the walls of the room? Did you observe adaptive changes in the pupil diameter to a constant light intensity? Did you correct for changes that, over time, affect the sequence of your measurements?

6.4. Hint: set up the algebraic equations in order and then combine them. "Effectiveness" is a multiplicative factor, e.g., $A \times E \to B$ means $B = E \times A$. Multiple inputs are added, e.g., $C \to E \leftarrow D$ means $E = C + D$. This problem assumes static values; it could be expanded to dynamic values of effectiveness and signal.

Chapter 7

7.1. Remember that the regulation of chemical processes must deal with the conservation of mass and energy.

7.2. Catching a ball requires that the processing is simple enough to be accomplished within the ball's flight time.

7.4. Pressure in a cylinder is directed outward in all radial directions. The effect on lateral force is the integral over one-half circumference of the vector components in one direction. *Hint:* This integral is equal to the force due to pressure on a plane with the length of the cylinder and a width equal to the diameter.

7.5. Examples could be horizontal and vertical movement of a joint. Approximate a limb as a cone of the same volume and length with a density only slightly greater than water.

7.7. When a crane is used to lift a load, a large counterweight is used for support. Where is your counterweight?

7.8. Have you attempted to correct for muscle length change for relatively constant tendon length contributions? It is known that some muscle fibers contract appreciably faster than others. Besides contraction speed, what information is needed to determine whether a particular muscle fiber is capable of participating in a fast movement?

7.9. Write separate equations relating muscle force in antagonist muscles to angular stiffness at the joint. Combine these equations. Since contraction increases both muscle stiffness and tension, how does cocontraction of antagonists affect joint stiffness and joint torque differently?

7.10. Refer to figure 7.1 for details of tongue muscle attachments.

7.12. Investigate different chair types and strategies of arising that could be advantageous for a weak or grossly overweight person.

7.13. A wide base often is used to increase standing stability, but this is exchanged for faster displacement during a single step in walking.

7.16. Note particularly the problems that you encountered in obtaining accurate data. Several computer programs are now available to calculate the changes in center of mass, moment of inertia, and velocity in these exercises. These programs are used by such groups as the U.S. Olympic Committee, trauma medicine, and sports medicine investigators.

Chapter 8

8.3. You were not expected to operationally define "triangle" so that your rules would recognize the intuitively obvious relationship between the geometric object and the social situation existing between two men and one woman!

8.4. What information about the illumination of individual receptors must be determined for you to derive the description that you recorded? Have you obtained enough information to identify all the details in your description of one event and to be able to make comparisons between successive tests? Using combinations like those described in chapter 6, attempt to define an arrangement of interacting neurons that could accomplish a significant part of the necessary processing to make those determinations that you did accomplish. Are there identified defects remaining in your model?

8.5. A 200-msec lag in making a response to visual information would be a preliminary guess. Problems such as those presented here are the subject of research in sports medicine.

8.6. Do not restrict your schemes to those known to exist in neural pathways. On consideration of cost vs. benefit, design complexity, and so on, do you find any of the existing biological schemes to be unusual?

8.7. Extend your considerations to figures 8.5 and 8.6. Give arguments to defend each of the following (conflicting) theses: (1) Object recognition is not based on initial recognition of features that are then combined. (2) Objects must be recognized by examination of a global pattern. (3) Different objects are recognized by different basic approaches of the same neural system.

8.8. This is not a trivial problem! Pattern recognition is an area in which large amounts of research effort are currently being invested.

8.9. Although we do not recognize any "correct answer" to this problem, your exploration of tentative and partial answers should be a rewarding exercise.

8.10. If you are not comfortable with matrix manipulation, a less elegant approach can be made with elementary algebra of simultaneous equations.

Noise that is large with respect to the signal size can cause the signal be unresolvable. The relative size of the signal and noise where this occurs depends on the retrieval method that is used. It is reasonable to assume that the nervous system does not use a retrieval method that could reliably extract a signal if the noise is equal to the signal size. When a signal is generated through the summation of several components, noise in one component can obscure the signal in that component.

8.12. There is no one-to-one relationship between locations in world space and its mapping into the nervous system. Likewise, world time relationships do not necessarily map onto corresponding time relationships within the nervous system.

8.13. Drawing a simple lens diagram can be useful in this problem. It may be helpful to use two colors to represent the changes resulting from adding an external lens. For your first solution to the bifocal problem, assume that one of the lenses is equivalent to the eye with no lens and the other corresponds to the single lens previously diagrammed.

8.15. During the manual exploration of an object, spatial, temporal, and magnitude information all contribute to the recognition of characteristics of the object. How can different combinations of these inputs be combined to produce the same correct interpretations of the shape when different explorations follow different patterns?

8.16. If you used a deck of playing cards, your knowledge of the shape and colors of the symbols might be used in combination with a limited observation to give a description that is more detailed than the actual observation. How might you alter your experimental design to test this possibility?

8.17. These calculations are greatly simplified by a relative approach. Base the reference frame on either the viewer or on the object location and replace the absolute movements with the convergent paths resulting from the two movements.

8.19. What other independent methods of identifying "cat" do you use? Use your examples to discuss redundancy and underdetermined identifications in perceptual function. Relate your selected examples to a multidimensional basin representation.

Chapter 9

9.1. Try to analyze the means by which you retrieved these memories. For instance, did you make use of associated or partial memories and then fill in the missing details?

9.2. An extensive literature can be found in psychology journals that describes experimental studies of learning. An important part of this literature is the identification of experimental artifacts and interpretation traps.

Chapter 10

10.1. It might be of interest to note that the resistivity of mammalian saline is about 60 Ω-cm and that of oil may be roughly 10^{15} Ω-cm.

10.2. You could, for example, make a table of I, t, and $I \times t$ using $I_0 = 1$, $k = 10$, and $0.1 < I > 100$. By all means, though, feel free to use other values if you would prefer!

10.4. If you would like to be more specific about your circuit design, microelectrodes typically have resistances between 1 and 10 MΩ, and the differential input impedance of a typical FET operational amplifier may be about 10^{10} Ω.

10.7. The pathological data given here are from W.F. Brown, *The Physiological and Technical Basis of Electromyography* (1984, p. 138).

10.8. An equivalent current density through an 18-gauge lamp cord would be produced by a current of about 60 A. What effect would such a current have on this copper wire (R = 2 $\times$ $10^{-4}\Omega$/cm)? What effect might this current density have at the fine tip of a microelectrode?

10.9. There has been almost a half century of attempts to automate EEG reading but, until the advent of fast and moderately priced computers, practiced human readers have been faster and better than any machine-aided analysis. Current machine-aided analysis has reached the point where it reveals significant details that are not obvious on normal inspection (see, for example, Jansen, 1991). Machine-aided analysis allows subtraction of defined parts, comparison of activity in different parts, and the generation of false color maps for selected properties. This latter, enhanced toposcopy often shows activity that flows over the surface in distinctive patterns involving large parts of the cortex.

Chapter 11

11.1. $q = C_m V_m = (1 \times 10^{-6} \text{ F/cm}^2) \times (100 \times 10^{-3} \text{ V}) = 1 \times 10^{-7} \text{ C/}cm^2$

(We have approximated Faraday's constant as 10^5 C/mol):

$$\frac{1 \times 10^{-7} \text{ C/cm}^2}{10^5 \text{ C/mol}} = 1 \times 10^{-12} \text{ mol/cm}^2$$

Of interest is the fact that this is only about 1 part in 10^5 of the concentrations adjacent to the membrane.

11.4. If you need a clue to answering this question read again the conditions necessary to establish potentials across membranes.

11.5. For K^+ alone we use the Nernst equation:

$$E_m = E_K = 62 \text{ mV} \log \frac{4}{155} = -98.5 \text{ mV}$$

For K^+ and Na^+ we now use the Goldman-Hodgkin-Katz equation:

$$E_m = 62 \text{ mV} \log \frac{1 \times 4 + 0.01 \times 145}{1 \times 155 + 0.01 \times 12} = -90.2 \text{ mV}$$

Thus this small Na permeability displaces the membrane potential by 8.3 mV away from the potassium equilibrium potential toward the sodium equilibrium potential.

11.6. As we have seen already, the Goldman-Hodgkin-Katz equation predicts a membrane potential of -90.2 mV with these permeabilities and $[K]_o = 4$ mM. Resolving the equation with $[K]_o = 6.5$ mM, we get

$$E_m = 62 \text{ mV} \log \frac{1 \times 6.5 + 0.01 \times 145}{1 \times 155 + 0.01 \times 12} = -80 \text{ mV}$$

Thus this degree of hyperkalemia would cause nearly 10 mV of depolarization in muscle cells.

11.7. $E_{Ca} = \dfrac{RT}{2F} \ln \dfrac{[Ca]_o}{[Ca]_i} = \dfrac{62 \text{ mV}}{2} \log \dfrac{10^{-5}}{10^{-8}} = 186 \text{ mV}$

The driving force, $E_m - E_{Ca}$, is then $(-90) - (+186) = -276$ mV, quite a substantial electrochemical gradient to move Ca^{2+} into the cell!

Chapter 12

12.1. Use figure 11.3 as a reference. What types of information must be retained with either local or long-distance signaling?

12.2. The following values, measured in mammalian motoneurons, are given in Eccles (1964), *The Physiology of Synapses* (table 1, p. 42). Time to peak of the postsynaptic response = 1.2 msec, time constant of decay of postsynaptic response = 4.9 msec, and time constant of postsynaptic membrane = 3.2 msec.

12.4. You might be wondering about the values given in problem 12.2 with regard to your answer to this question. Eccles explains that the decay of the postsynaptic response is delayed by the presence of residual transmitter.

12.5. Hint: do your calculations in terms of numbers of space constants.

12.6. $\dfrac{100 \times 10^{-3} \text{ V}}{100 \times 10^{-10} \text{ m}} = 10^7 \text{ V/m}$

It is not surprising that protein configuration changes can occur in such a field when one considers that the dielectric of air breaks down and sparks occur at about this field strength.

12.7. If you would like to answer this question quantitatively, you might use the Goldman-Hodgkin-Katz equation for your calculations.

12.8. In using a voltage clamp, usually one begins with low gain in the feedback circuit and then turns up the gain until just before ringing is observed.

12.9. Of course, if the stimulus strength is not sufficient to overcome the relative refractoriness of the membrane, the firing rate will be less than this maximum.

12.10. Hint:

$$I_c = C_m \frac{dV}{dt} \qquad C_m = 1 \text{ } \mu\text{F/cm}^2 = 10^{-14} \text{ F/}\mu\text{m}^2$$

solution:

$$I = (1 \times 10^{-14} \text{ F/}\mu\text{m}^2) \times \left(\frac{100 \times 10^{-3} \text{ V}}{1 \times 10^{-3} \text{ sec}} \right) = 10^{-12} \text{ A/}\mu\text{m}^2 = 1 \text{ pA/}\mu\text{m}^2$$

Thus, 1 Na channel per square micrometer is all that is necessary to discharge the membrane capacitance this rapidly. As we have noted in chapter 11, Na channel density is hundreds of times this great! What would be the evolutionary advantage of an excess of Na channels? If there are 300 channels per square micrometer and each channel protein molecule has a diameter of 50 Å, what percentage of the membrane is actually taken up with channels?

12.11. The shielding effect of external Ca^{2+} on fixed membrane changes is complicated but may cause almost 20 mV shift in the field sensed by channel gating sensors per 10-fold change in external Ca^{2+} concentration. For a more extensive discussion of this effect read chapter 17 in Hille (1992), *Ionic Channels of Excitable Membranes*.

12.12. These calculations can be made as a continuous function and plotted on a computer screen, or at discrete points, and simply calculated with a calculator.

12.14. Warming an axon by 10°C speeds the channel gating processes by 2- to 4-fold and will have approximately the same effect on action potential duration.

Chapter 13

13.1. Current supplied by the presynaptic nerve:

$$I = (1 \times 10^{-3} \text{ A/cm}^2) \times (2 \times 10^{-5} \text{ cm}^2) = 2 \times 10^{-8} \text{ A}$$

Necessary postsynaptic current:

$$I = \frac{E}{R} = \frac{40 \times 10^{-3} \text{ V}}{40 \times 10^{3} \text{ } \Omega} = 10^{-6} \text{ A}$$

Under what conditions of pre- and postsynaptic morphology might the presynaptic nerve be able to supply sufficient current to bring the postsynaptic cell to threshold? What factors would affect the resistance of the postsynaptic cell?

13.2. See Vincent et al. (1989).

13.3. Remember that Avogadro's number is 6.02×10^{23} molecules per mole. Would you anticipate any osmotic effects of such a concentration of ACh within the vesicle? (You might be interested to know that synaptic vesicles contain storage proteins that can bind a large number of transmitter molecules.)

13.4. Remember that Faraday's constant is 96,500 C/mol and do not forget Avogadro's number.

13.5. $E_{\text{EPP}} = 62 \text{ mV} \log \dfrac{1 \times 145 + 1 \times 4}{1 \times 12 + 1 \times 155}$

Just to be certain that you are getting sufficient calculator practice, we will not carry this solution any further!

13.7. The partial solution given for problem 13.5 should be sufficient to point you in the correct direction to solve this problem.

13.8. For two variables to be derived from two unidimensional signals, it is necessary that the signals are at least partially independent.

Chapter 14

14.3. There is an intuitive basis for distinguishing the activity of muscle fibers that are excited as a motor unit and the activity of muscle fibers that are self-excited.

14.4. Calcium is found in millimolar concentrations outside the cell and in tens or hundreds of nanomolar concentration inside the cell, thus its electrochemical gradient will cause an influx through open channels. Will this depolarize or hyperpolarize the cell? Calcium is an important transducer of nonelectrical events in cells. Here muscle contraction is initiated by an increase in intracellular calcium.

14.5. As it happens these two distances bracket the T-tubule to sarcoplasmic reticulum distance. The distances are given in problem 12.12 and at the beginning of chapter 13.

14.6. One extensive starting reference is the *Handbook of Physiology,* Section 10: *Skeletal Muscle*. Since this book was published in 1983, it will be necessary to do forward searching from references given in the book.

14.7. This question can be dealt with on as quantitative a level as you desire. You might consider such topics as conduction velocity, ion diffusion rates, and actin-myosin interaction kinetics. Some suggestions for a quantitative answer to this question can be found in chapter 8 of *Nerve and Muscle Membranes, Cells, and Systems* by Richard Stein.

14.9. Hooke's law states that $F = kx$ where F is the force exerted by an elastic element, x is the length of that element, and k is the "spring constant" for that elastic element. Stiffness is the force necessary to produce a given change in length. The elastic components of muscle do not obey Hooke's law.

Chapter 15

15.1. If you are at all stymied here, begin by going back and reading the section on conduction in chapter 2.

15.4. The acceleration of gravity on earth is about 9.8 m/sec or 9.8 mm/msec. If you are really having difficulty remembering your physics, $v = at$, and $x = 1/2at^2$.

15.5. If, after designing the experiment, you are unable to carry it out, look up the results as published by Gilson et al. (1944). Can you explain these results?

15.6. Other factors that should be considered in a more complete model are chemical reaction dynamics, diffusion to the removal site, enzyme saturation, and multiple dissipation pathways. An interesting example of successive chemical signals occurs when a neurotransmitter's action is followed by the action of a second messenger.

15.7. If the muscle response amplitude falls by about 1.5 log at a signal frequency of 4 Hz, at what frequency would the summation of EPSPs driving a motoneuron have fallen by a similar amount?

15.8. A comparison of the time courses of two subjective experiences is difficult. If you did not find this difficult, perhaps you have not considered all aspects of the problem.

15.10. The proposed model includes several simplifying assumptions, but the principles shown by this first approximation are of primary importance. A classic study that dealt with some of these questions was published by B.H.C. Matthews in 1931.

15.11. Did you consider the information that is available from comparing a single signal after it has been subjected to two different conduction delays?

15.12. Programming suggestions: A pulse rate that is proportional to the generator potential is one in which the time integral of the generator potential in each interpulse interval is equal to a constant. Thus, starting at zero after each pulse, the generator potential is integrated over time until it reaches some criterion value at which time the next pulse is generated and the cycle is repeated. You might want to refer to the comments in chapter 2 about pulse coding in general, and about this specific integrate and fire model in particular. If you have not previously modeled dynamic systems, this problem should be both instructive and, in spite of the suggestions, challenging.

15.14. After completing this experiment, you might want to redo experiments 3.4 and 4.2 considering what you have learned from this experiment.

Chapter 16

16.1. An indication of the anatomical relationships of the interacting neuronal circuits is shown in *The Synaptic Organization of the Brain* by Shepherd (1979).

16.2. Are there any differences between biological parallelism and "back-up systems" that are commonly used in engineering?

16.4. In answering this question, one might wish for more understanding of how such diverse signals are actually handled in the cortex. For an introduction to the current knowledge and its limitations see the *Handbook of Physiology,* Section 1, Volume 3, and especially chapters 5 and 18. The article "Brain maps and parallel computers" by Nelson and Bower (1990), provides some additional insight into this question.

16.5. At a given moment, different fibers may represent different modalities, conditions at different locations, the same signal with different delays, or different receptor dynamics. Other fibers may carry essentially the same information or may carry the same information about one factor that has been combined with different information about other factors.

16.7. Some block diagram reductions are valid for one use but not for another.

16.8. Figure 15.1 shows the anatomical basis for the stretch reflex. In considering this problem, it is advisable to dimension the variables described in the verbal description of the reflex.

16.9. For some readers, this problem may be best solved by taking various partial derivatives in order to describe the sensitivity of each output to changes in the operating characteristics of components or in the input signals.

16.10. Low-frequency sounds pass around a solid object with less sound shadow than do high-frequency sounds. It is important to consider the wavelength of a particular sound and the width of the human head.

16.11. In stating this problem it is assumed that any sign change in the loop is represented in either the sign of G or H.

16.13. One convenient way to treat this problem is as a graphic representation with approximate scale identification.

16.14. For more accuracy, use a video camera and frame-by-frame measurements. There is both a feedback component and an elastic-inertial interaction involved (Feldman, 1974). Identify other oscillations that involve neuronal function in their generation.

16.15. This exercise is most useful if you predict each effect before confirming your prediction experimentally.

16.16. Remember that a pendulum is described by second-order differential equations that become significantly nonlinear when the movement amplitude is large.

Chapter 17

17.1. Sometimes an adaptive control for one condition is simultaneously maladaptive for another.

17.4. Heart rate and blood pressure can be conveniently monitored with readily available digital devices. However, periodic "analog" measurements should suffice. Would you expect different results from a naive subject than from yourself?

17.5. Consumption rate:

sedentary = 2500 Cal/day

8 hours heavy work = 5000 Cal/day

body mass = 70 kg

thermal capacity = that of H_2O

17.9. *Suggestions:* The matrix can be started by inserting rows and columns representing just the controllers of blood O_2, blood CO_2, and body temperature, and then adding one controller and one set of table descriptions at a time. The rows and columns correspond to the outputs and inputs of individual blocks in the expanded version of the block diagram suggested earlier in this chapter. Other combinations also can be added individually in a similar manner but care should be taken to avoid duplicating either a row or a column. Ideally, only direct effects should be shown in a single intersection with indirect effects broken down into intermediate parts where they are known. Sometimes the addition of a new input column will show a variable that acts on an already identified effect. Likewise, a previously described input may act on a newly added response row. Do not forget to add all the indicated details to the interaction table. If you use a color code in labeling the rows and columns, it will be easier to distinguish among internal and input neural signals, endocrine signals, physical quantities, and memory information. Depending on your orientation and time limitation, you may choose to emphasize the expansion of the matrix with a limited table or refinement of the table of interactions with a less complete matrix. For long-term usage, it is advisable to include an identification of the source of information in the accompanying table.

Glossary

Absolute refractory period [12]   Time period immediately after an action potential during which a second action potential cannot be initiated. This results from inactivation of sodium channels.

Accommodation [2, 10, 12, 15]   (1) An increased threshold for excitable tissue with sustained or slowly applied stimuli that results from a gradual inactivation of sodium channels. (2) [5] The adjustments of the optical system of the eye for near objects. This response includes convergence of the eyes by extraocular muscles and contraction of the internal muscles that allow the lens to thicken so that the focal length shortens.

Acetylcholine (ACh) [13]   A neurotransmitter of the biogenic amine group that acts peripherally at skeletal neuromuscular junctions, in junctions of the autonomic nervous system, and extensively within the central nervous system.

Acetylcholinesterase (AChE) [13]   An enzyme that hydrolyzes acetylcholine into acetate and choline.

Actin [14]   The primary protein molecule of the thin filaments of muscle.

Action potential [2, 12]   The stereotypic, all-or-nothing voltage pulses produced by the ion channels of the membranes of excitable cells; the basis of signaling over a distance in the nervous system and along muscle fibers. *See Impulses.*

Activating systems [16]   Neuronal systems that increase the general level of excitation of other parts of the CNS.

Activation [12]   Characteristic of certain ion channels in which gates are opened in response to depolarization.

Activation heat [14]   Heat, measured early in a muscle twitch, that is probably associated with Ca^{2+} movement and the initial interaction of actin and myosin.

Active state [14]   The increase in stiffness that follows the rise in sarcoplasmic Ca^{2+} at the beginning of a twitch in a muscle fiber.

Numbers in brackets indicate chapters where further discussion can be found.

Active zone [13]   Regions of a presynaptic nerve terminal adjacent to folds of the postsynaptic membrane where large concentrations of neurotransmitter vesicles are located.

Adaptation [4, 15]   A declining response with time to a constant stimulus. *See Dark adaptation.*

Adrenergic [13]   Synaptic transmission that utilizes adrenaline (epinephrine) or noradrenaline (norepinephrine).

Affector [2]   An input, or sensory, receptor of the nervous system.

Afferent fibers [2]   Fibers that originate peripherally in sensory receptors and pass in to terminate at various locations within the central nervous system.

Afterdischarge [6]   A response that continues for longer than the conduction delay following termination of a stimulus.

Afterhyperpolarization [12]   That late portion of an action potential during which the intracellular potential is more negative than the resting potential.

Agnosia [4]   Loss of ability to recognize or correctly interpret a familiar sensory stimulus.

Akinesia [7]   Failure to execute normal movement.

All-or-nothing [2, 12]   A description of the stereotypic nature and stimulus independence of action potentials.

Amnesia [7]   Neurological classification of many types of pathologic memory loss including some of psychiatric origin. *See Anterograde amnesia; Infantile amnesia; Retrograde amnesia.*

Anions [10]   Negatively charged ions that migrate toward an anode.

Anisotropic bands (A bands) [14]   Transverse dark bands that are prominent in striated muscle under a light microscope. *See Isotropic bands.*

Anodal block [10]   Block of a transmitted impulse that occurs as a result of the hyperpolarization at the anode of a stimulator.

Anode [10]   A positive electrode.

Anode break excitation [10]   Excitation, occurring on ending a long period of hyperpolarizing stimulus current, that results from the removal of inactivation from the sodium channels in the excitable membrane.

Antagonistic muscles [7]   Muscles that, during a given motor action, oppose each other's torque. *See Synergistic muscles.*

Anterograde amnesia [9]   A loss of memory of events subsequent to a trauma or seizure.

Antidromic [2, 10]   Propagation of a nerve impulse in the direction opposite to that of normal conduction. *See Orthodromic.*

Associative learning [9]   Learning conditions in which the subject learns a relationship between simultaneously or successively occurring stimuli or between a stimulus and a behavior.

Associative memory [9]   Memory in which the recall of each item of information is derived from its content.

Astigmatism [5]   A condition in which the refraction along different meridians of the eye is different. Generally astigmatism results from a nonspherical surface of the cornea as a result of asymmetric elasticity.

Attractor [16]   A point, line, or region on a phase plane to which successive trajectories converge.

Autonomic nervous system [7]   The division of the nervous system that innervates smooth and cardiac muscle and glands. The motoneurons of this system are located outside of the central nervous system. *See Parasympathetic nervous system; Sympathetic nervous system.*

Auxotonic [7, 14]   Normal contractile activity of muscle in which length, velocity, and force all change.

Axon [2]   A long neurite that conducts impulses away from the cell body. (Sometimes used more generally to indicate any long neurite.)

Axon hillock [13]   The junction of the neuronal cell body with the axon, a region that generally has the lowest threshold for action potential initiation.

Axoplasmic flow [14]   The subcellular movement of substances from the cell body to axon terminals and from the periphery back to the cell body.

Basilar membrane [5]   The membrane found in the cochlea of the inner ear that is vibrated by traveling sound pressure waves. The specific auditory receptor cells distributed along this membrane are excited in a pitch-dependent manner related to their location.

Basin [8]   The whole range of inputs that separately evokes a particular perception.

Basin of an attractor [16]   Region within which all trajectories converge on the particular attractor.

Block diagrams [16]   A formal algebra that defines acceptable manipulations of operations within a group of functionally connected elements.

Buffering [3]   An action that opposes a change, usually in the concentration of some chemical substance; also applied to analogous effects in mechanical displacement.

Cable conductor [2]   A passive circuit with resistive and capacitive elements that produces the decremental spread of electrical current. Membranes of nerve and muscle cells typically have these properties.

Cable theory [12]   The theory derived originally for submarine telegraph cables, which also has been shown to account for the electrical spread of subthreshold potentials along a nerve fiber. *See Space constant.*

Calcium hypothesis [13]   A well established hypothesis that Ca^{2+} is responsible for excitation-secretion coupling.

Capacitive current [10, 11]   Current that flows across a capacitor as a result of the addition of charges on one plate and removal of similar charges from the other plate. *See Resistive current.*

Capacitor [11]   A device that separates and stores electrical charges of opposite sign. *See Membrane capacitance.*

Cardiac muscle [1]   Muscle of the heart, which is structurally and functionally distinct from skeletal and smooth muscle.

Cathode [10]   A negative electrode.

Cations [10]   Positively charged ions that migrate toward a cathode.

Channel [11]   Intrinsic membrane protein molecules that permit the transit of charged ions through hydrophobic biological membranes. *See Ligand-gated channel.*

Channel conductance (γ) [12]   The electrical measurement of the ease with which the selected ion flows through an open channel.

Channel gating [12]   The property of ion channels that allows them to either conduct or not conduct specific ions.

Channel selectivity [12]   The property of ion channels that allows passage of specific ions and excludes other ions.

Channel sensor [12]   The portion of an ion channel that regulates gating in response to a voltage or ligand signal.

Chaos [16]   Deterministic and limited but nonpredictable behavior of certain nonlinear dynamic systems.

Cholinergic [13]   Synaptic transmission that utilizes acetylcholine.

Chronaxie [10]   The stimulus duration necessary to stimulate an excitable tissue when applied at twice rheobase strength. *See Strength-duration relationship; Rheobase.*

Cisternae [14]   Specialized regions of close juxtaposition of the sarcolemma with the sarcoplasmic reticulum.

Classical conditioning [9]   The association of two stimuli such that one develops a response that initially would have occurred only in response to the other stimulus (e.g., Pavlov's experiments in which salivation was conditioned to occur in response to a bell).

Clonus [16]   A cyclic movement of reflex origin most often elicited in response to a quick stretch in conditions of exaggerated reflex action.

Cochlear microphonic [10]   Extracellular potential that can be recorded with an active electrode on the skin near the cochlea of the inner ear that gives a faithful representation of auditory stimuli.

Cognitive learning [9]   Learning that requires an involvement of the intellect (e.g., understanding the concept of a derivative).

Compliance [3]   The displacement of an object produced by a unit force with a purely elastic load; equivalent to the inverse of stiffness.

Compound action potential [10]   A conducted impulse recorded extracellularly on a nerve trunk. This potential waveform results from the summation of unitary action potentials propagated at different velocities along the individual nerve fibers.

Conditioning   *See Classical conditioning; Operant conditioning.*

Conductance (G) [12]   The ratio of the current in a conductor to the potential difference between its ends; equivalent to the inverse of resistance.

Conduction [1]   Transmission of impulses between locations in an excitable cell.

Conduction delay [15]   Time delay resulting from the finite conduction velocity of action potentials along a nerve fiber.

Conduction velocity [2]   The speed with which an action potential is propagated along a muscle or nerve fiber.

Conductivity [12]   The ratio of current density to the voltage field driving that current, characteristic of a particular conducting medium.

Convergence [6, 16]   Coming together of multiple signals from different sources onto a single neuron or group of neurons.

Current sink [10]   The point at which current flows into a tissue or a nerve or muscle cell.

Cybernetics [16]   The study of control and communication in complex biological and technical systems.

Cyclic nucleotides (cAMP, cGMP) [13]   Molecules derived from ATP or GTP that carry out important second messenger functions in cells.

Dale's principle [13]   States (incorrectly) that a neuron can secrete only one type of neurotransmitter.

Dark adaptation [15]   Increase in sensitivity of the retina as a result of continual exposure to low light levels.

Decibel (dB) [3]   One tenth of a Bel. A measure of the ratio of two powers. Frequently used in studies of sound. *See SPL.*

Dendrite [2]   Neurites that conduct impulses toward their cell body.

Depolarized [11]   Condition in which the membrane potential is less negative than at rest. *See Hyperpolarized.*

Discharge zone [6]   Those neurons that are always fired by a given input.

Disinhibition [9]   Restoration or enhancement by the action of a novel stimulus in a conditioned reflex that has been partly or completely extinguished.

Distributed memory [9]   Memory in which particular details are represented by a characteristic combination of conditions at multiple sites.

Dorsal root potential [10]   Electrotonically spread extracellular potential recorded near the sensory roots of the spinal cord following certain sensory stimuli.

EEG spike [10]   A sharp electrical spike that occurs in focal seizures, roughly 100 times longer in duration than a nerve action potential.

Effector [1, 2]   An output element, often a muscle, controlled by the nervous system.

Electrical potential (E) [11]   The work required to bring two unit charges together. *See Potential.*

Electrocardiogram (ECG or EKG) [14]   Externally recorded potentials from the contracting muscle of the heart. ECGs are used for clinical diagnosis of many cardiac conditions.

Electrochemical gradient [11]   A difference in concentration and charge between two points (usually across a membrane).

Electrocorticogram (ECoG) [10]   Electrical activity recorded directly from the surface of the cortex representing the summed effect of local potentials in the large numbers of nearby neurons.

Electroencephalogram (EEG) [10]   Electrical activity recorded on the scalp representing the summed effect of local potentials in the large numbers of nearby neurons.

Electrogenic [11]   A characteristic of some membrane pumps whereby the total charge moved in one direction is different from that moved in the other direction. A net current is thus generated.

Electromyogram (EMG) [14]   Extracellularly recorded potentials from contracting muscle fibers. EMGs have many important uses in clinical diagnosis.

Electromyography [10]   The technique of recording extracellular potentials from muscle fibers.

Electrophoretic equation [11]   Equation that relates the flux of a charged ion to a potential gradient.

Electroretinogram (ERG) [10]   Extracellular potential, recorded with electrodes on the cornea, that results from the summed local potentials in the retina in response to a bright light flash.

Emergent properties [16]   Properties of a system that are not identifiable in the properties of the constituent parts of that system.

Endplate potential (epp) [13]   The postsynaptic electrical response in a muscle following the release of neurotransmitter from a presynaptic nerve terminal.

Engram [9]   Changes in the nervous system by which memory is stored (memory trace).

Enkephalins [13]   Neuropeptides that bind to receptors to which opiate drugs can also bind.

Equilibrium potential [11]   Electrical potential difference at which the tendency of ions to move in one direction as a result of the electrical force on them is balanced by the tendency for them to move in the other direction as a result of diffusion down their concentration gradient.

Evoked potentials [10]   Electrical potentials in the central nervous system following a stimulus to some sensory system. Their measurement usually requires the averaging of multiple episodes following each of a series of synchronized stimulations.

Excitability [1]   The property, characteristic of nerve, muscle, and secretory cells, by which the cell actively responds, usually by a change in electrical potential, to an appropriate stimulus.

Excitation-contraction coupling [11, 14]   The coupling, by means of Ca^{2+} ions, of the electrical event at the muscle cell membrane with the mechanochemical process of contraction.

Excitation-gating coupling [11, 13]   The coupling, through second messengers, of a membrane potential change with the gating of ion channels that are not primarily voltage sensitive.

Excitation-secretion coupling [11, 13]   Coupling through Ca^{2+} ions, of the depolarization of a secretory cell (including a presynaptic terminal) to the release of that cell's secretory product (including neurotransmitters).

Excitatory postsynaptic potential (EPSP) [13]   Potential changes in a postsynaptic neuron that result when neurotransmitters open gated channels for ions whose reversal potential is more depolarized than the resting potential.

Exocytosis [13]   The secretion of a material by a cell as a result of fusion of internal vesicles with the cell membrane followed by release of the vesicles' contents outside of the cell.

Exteroceptors [4]   Sensory receptors that transduce signals that originate outside the organism.

Facilitation [6]   An increased neuronal response due to a previous stimulus on the same or a converging pathway.

Fasciculations [10]   Spontaneous discharges of whole motor units resulting from disease of motoneurons or peripheral motor axons.

Fast muscle fibers [12]   Muscle fibers (usually in "white" muscle) that have short duration twitches and thus require a high rate of stimulation to produce fusion. These fibers are particularly sensitive to fatigue.

Feedback [6, 16]   A closed-loop pathway in which the output of an operation determines in part the input to that same operation, thus altering that pathway's output.

Feedback, negative [9]   A closed-loop pathway in which a static returned signal is of the opposite sign from the original input. This tends to decrease the overall response to an input and the effect of certain internal characteristics but can cause oscillations.

Feedback, positive [9]   A closed-loop pathway in which a static signal is returned to the input in such a way as to increase the overall response of the loop. This tends to accentuate effects of properties of components of the loop.

Fibrillations [10, 14]   Spontaneous discharges of single muscle fibers following loss of innervation.

Fick's equation [11]   Equation that relates the flux of a substance to the gradient of concentration of that substance.

Final common pathway [6, 8]   A single motor unit that, on different occasions, can be used in different functions. A term first introduced by Sherrington.

Flicker fusion frequency [15]   Frequency at which light flashes are perceived as a continuous light.

Flow field [8]   The visual sensory experience associated with movement toward or away from an array of identifiable points.

Focal stimulation [10]   Stimulation in which the stimulating electrode is placed near the excitable cells, and an indifferent electrode is located remotely.

Force velocity effect [14]   The dependence of force generated by an excited muscle on the rate of change of muscle length.

Formant [8]   An individual frequency component of a phoneme of spoken sound.

Functional electrical stimulation (FES) [10]   Electrical stimulation of muscles or nerves to produce useful function in the absence of normal neural action.

Fusion [14, 15]   Summation of individual twitches into a smooth response without observable variations of tension.

Gamma fibers [5]   The principal group of efferent fusimotor nerves composed of small fibers with conduction velocities in the gamma range. This term is often used improperly to refer to all fusimotor nerve fibers.

γ-Aminobutyric acid (GABA) [13]   Amino acid that serves as a neurotransmitter whose effect is usually inhibitory.

Gate theory of pain [13]   A theoretical basis, assuming presynaptic inhibition, for the observation that certain sensory inputs can depress the central response to painful stimuli.

Goldman-Hodgkin-Katz equation [11]   The equation that describes the electrochemical potential across a membrane with multiple ion permeabilities.

Habituation [9]   Learning conditions in which the subject decreases the level of response to a repeated, nonnoxious stimulus.

Half center [16]   One of two reciprocally acting actions of the control center for an oscillatory action such as walking or breathing (e.g., within the respiratory center there are inspiratory and expiratory half centers).

Heat   *See Activation heat; Maintenance heat; Recovery heat.*

Helicotrema [5]   A small passage joining the two chambers of the cochlea through which low-frequency oscillations of pressure are equilibrated without producing a displacement of the basilar membrane.

Hodgkin cycle [12]   Positive feedback cycle in which depolarization increases sodium permeability, which, in turn, causes more depolarization.

Homeostasis [7]   A tendency to uniformity or stability in internal conditions in living organism.

Homunculus [8]   A point-to-point mapping of somatotopic afferent information onto the surface of the brain.

Hooke's law [14]   The change of length of an elastic structure is proportional to the applied force.

Hormones [2]   Chemical communication agents of the endocrine system that are broadly distributed to one or more sites of action within the body.

Hyperalgesia [15]   Excessive sensitivity to pain often associated with recent tissue damage.

Hyperopia [5]   Farsightedness. A condition that results when the focal length of the optics of the eye is too long for the length of the eyeball and near objects are only focused behind the retina. *See Myopia.*

Hyperpolarized [11]   Condition in which the membrane potential is more negative (more polarized) than at rest. *See Depolarized.*

Hyperreflexia [6]   Reflex response that is greater than would normally be expected for a given stimulus.

Hysteresis [9]   Dependence of the state of a system on its previous history.

Iconic memory [9]   A transient (visual) response that remains briefly after removal of the stimulus.

Impedance [5]   A measurement of the total resistance seen by time-varying signals. *See Impedance matching; Mechanical impedance.*

Impedance matching [5]   Adjustment of the load and source impedances such that maximum power is transferred from source to load.

Imprinting [8]   A narrowing of the stimuli effective for filial responses to those first encountered during a short period after birth.

Impulses [2]   Synonym for action potential, especially to emphasize the discontinuous nature of the signal.

Inactivation [12]   Channel process that results in closure of gates as a result of depolarization.

Indifferent electrode [10]   An electrode, often large, placed at a distance from an active electrode to complete the circuit for stimulating or recording.

Inertia [3]   The property of a body that opposes change in its rotational and translational motion.

Infantile amnesia [9]   The lack of recall by adults of early childhood events.

Inhibition [6]   An active process by which one neural input decreases the response of another neuron or effector. Distinguished from a response to reduced excitation.

Inhibitory postsynaptic potential (IPSP) [13]   Potential changes in a postsynaptic neuron that result when neurotransmitters open gated channels for ions whose reversal potential is near to or more hyperpolarized than the resting potential.

Initial segment   *See Axon hillock.*

Inner ear [5]   The cochlea of the auditory system and the structures of the vestibular apparatus. These specialized structures are fluid-filled compartments surrounding mechanosensitive hair cells.

Instantaneous frequency [2]   The inverse of an interval between two successive pulses.

Integration [6]   In the general context of nervous system function, this refers to the bringing together of inputs to produce an output.

Interference record [10]   The record obtained from a group of asynchronously activated impulses interacting to produce sequences of added and subtracted electrical record that depend on the relative timing of different unit activities.

Interneuron [2]   Neurons that carry internal information between various locations entirely within the central nervous system.

Interoceptors [4]   Sensory receptors that transduce information that originates within the viscera.

Intrafusal fibers [5]   A specialized type of muscle fiber that produces minimal force but acts to modify the response of spindle stretch receptors. The motor nerves driving these fibers are called fusimotor nerves.

Ion channel   *See Channel.*

Ionotropic neurotransmitter receptor [13]   A neurotransmitter receptor in which the ion channel is an intrinsic part of the receptor molecule.

Iris [5]   The circular pigmented membrane behind the cornea of the eye that is perforated by the pupil. The iris is supplied with circular and radial muscle fibers that adjust the size of the pupil.

Isometric [7, 14]   Condition of constant length during muscle contraction.

Isotonic [7, 14]   Condition of constant force during muscle contraction.

Isotropic bands (I bands) [14]   Transverse light bands that are prominent in striated muscle fibers as seen under a light microscope. *See Anisotropic bands.*

Kinematics [7]   Study of the changing geometric configurations that occur during a movement without reference to the forces involved.

Kinesiology [7]   Study of the details of the involvement of various muscles in specific motor functions.

Kinetics [7]   Study of mechanical movement and the forces involved.

Labeled lines [4, 8]   Nerve fibers committed to specific types of sensory information.

Ladder network [12]   An electrical circuit containing series and parallel resistors.

Lag [15]   A dynamic delaying of the output of a system with respect to the input. Lag alters the wave shape of a signal in contrast to signal delay, which produces an equal time shift of all components of the signal.

Lateral inhibition [4]   Depression of the activity of neurons by parallel adjacent neurons.

Lead [15]   The signal modification by an adapting receptor in which rate of change of stimulus provides a prediction of the future course of a continuously changing input.

Learning [9]   An increase of memory content, resulting from processing of sensory information often in combination with motor information. *See Associative learning; Cognitive learning; Habituation; Motor learning; Nonassociative learning; Operant conditioning; Sensitization.*

Length tension effect [14]   The dependence on muscle length of contractile and passive force.

Lens diagram [5]   A geometric construction, appropriate for thin lenses, that provides a graphic determination of an image location given the object location and the focal length of the lens.

Ligand-gated channels [13]   Gated ion channels whose sensors are receptors for specific chemical substances (ligands).

Limit cycle [16]   The constant amplitude oscillatory response of a system that is the limit approached by expanding smaller oscillations or damping larger oscillations.

Local circuit currents [12]   Decrementally spread currents that flow between nearby unexcited regions of the membrane and a region of excitation.

Local memory [9]   Memory in which each particular detail is represented by the condition at a single location.

Local sign [6]   The specialization of a response to represent the specific location of a stimulus (i.e., reflex scratching at the point of irritation).

Long-term memory [9]   A memory that develops slowly and is resistant to disruption by periods of unconsciousness and, in spite of gradual degradation, can last for years.

Long-term potentiation (LTP) [9]   An increased synaptic efficacy that can last for hours after the end of the excitatory input. Commonly studied in the hippocampal formation of the brain.

Loudness [3]   A perceived characteristic of sound that changes nonlinearly with the amplitude of the sound pressure waves.

Low-pass filter [15]   A component that allows low-frequency signals to pass while attenuating high-frequency signals.

Maintenance heat [14]   Heat, measured during a continued isometric muscle contraction, that is generated by the continued turnover of cross-bridges between thin and thick filaments.

Mean quantal content [13]   The average number of quanta of neurotransmitter released by a given presynaptic excitation.

Mechanical impedance [7]   The ratio of a dynamically changing force and the resulting movement of an object. Includes elastic, inertial, and viscous components.

Membrane capacitance [2]   The electrical property of cell membranes by which they are capable of maintaining a separation of charges with a voltage gradient.

Membrane potential [11]   Voltage differences found across the membranes of many cells.

Membrane receptors [9]   Specialized protein molecules in the cell membrane of most cells that bind specific messenger molecules and subsequently initiate a cellular response.

Memory [5, 9]   The maintenance of learned knowledge over time in a form that alters some future action. *See Associative memory; Distributed memory; Iconic memory; Local memory; Long-term memory; Memory consolidation; Short-term memory.*

Memory consolidation [9]   The conversion of short-term memories to long-term memories.

Metabotropic neurotransmitter receptor [13]   A neurotransmitter receptor whose intracellular signaling is accomplished through G proteins and does not necessarily involve the action of ion channels.

Meta control [7, 8]   The adjustment of the rules of the controller.

Middle ear [5]   An air-filled chamber located between the tympanic membrane (eardrum) and the entry to the cochlea. The bony levers and the different areas of the two membranes serve to match the impedance between external air and the fluid-filled cochlea. Pressure in this chamber is equilibrated with that of external air by intermittent opening of the eustachian tube.

Miniature endplate potential (mepp) [13]   Subthreshold, spontaneous postsynaptic responses to the release of quanta of neurotransmitter by the unexcited motor nerve terminal.

Modality [3, 4, 5]   (1) The specific form of energy to which a type of receptor best responds. (2) A category of sensation (e.g., touch, sight, or hearing).

Monosynaptic reflex [6]   A reflex involving a single or parallel afferent neurons, a single level of synaptic junctions, and parallel efferent neurons, the shortest possible reflex pathway.

Motoneuron pool [6]   The group of motoneurons that innervates a particular muscle.

Motor learning [9]   Subconscious learning of motor skills (e.g., becoming proficient at riding a bicycle or typing).

Motor unit [7, 10, 14]   The motor neuron, its axon, and all of the muscle fibers innervated by its terminal branches.

Motor unit spike [10]   The action potentials generated by the nearly synchronous activity muscle fibers of a motor unit, larger in voltage and slightly longer in time than the action potential of a single muscle fiber.

Muscarinic acetylcholine-gated channels [13]   Ligand-gated ion channels whose receptors bind acetylcholine but also can be activated by muscarine and blocked by atropine. *See Nicotinic acetylcholine-gated channels.*

Muscle   *See Cardiac muscle; Fast muscle fibers; Intrafusal fibers; Skeletal muscle; Slow muscle fibers; Smooth muscle; Striated muscle.*

Muscle spindle [5]   An encapsulated group of specialized, intrafusal muscle fibers and associated stretch receptors.

Myelin [2, 12]   An electrically insulating, fatty covering around many nerve fibers.

Myopia [5]   Nearsightedness. A condition that results when the focal length of the optics is too short for the length of the eyeball and distant objects are focused in front of the retina. *See Hyperopia.*

Myosin [14]   The primary protein molecule of the thick filaments of muscle.

Myotatic reflex [16]   Monosynaptic reflex involving stretch receptors, α-motoneurons, and extrafusal muscle fibers.

Myotonic potentials [10]   High-frequency repetitive discharges in EMGs originating in the muscles of patients with muscle disease such as dystrophy.

NMDA receptors [13]   A specific class of receptors for the amino acid transmitter glutamic acid that are also activated by *N*-methyl-D-aspartate. These are an important category of excitatory receptors that play a role in learning, long-term potentiation, the regulation of neuronal growth, response to ischemia, and epilepsy.

Na-K pump (Na-K-ATPase) [11]   Carrier molecules in the membranes of most cells that move Na out of the cell in exchange for moving K into the cell. These movements against the ionic concentration gradients require that the pump utilize energy in the form of ATP.

Negative feedback   *See Feedback, negative.*

Negentropy [17]   Increases in structural organization occurring within the nervous system. This can occur because the nervous system is open and acquires organizing energy from outside sources. The organization of these sources is degraded; however, energy and organization are provided to the neural system with an overall increase of entropy.

Nernst equation [11]   The equation that describes the electrochemical equilibrium potential of a species of ions across a semipermeable membrane as a function of concentration difference.

Nerve fiber [2]   Any long neurite.

Neurite [2]   Any extended process of a nerve cell. *See Axon; Dendrite; Nerve fiber.*

Neuromuscular junction [13]   The structurally complex synapse between a motor nerve and the muscle fiber that it innervates.

Neuron pool [6]   A contiguous group of neurons that acts in common on a particular target.

Neuropeptides [13]   Small protein molecules that act as neurotransmitters and neuromodulators in the nervous system.

Neurotransmitter [9]   Specific chemical substances released by terminals of one neuron that cause excitation or inhibition of an adjacent second neuron. *See Acetylcholine; enkephalins; γ-aminobutyric acid; neuropeptides; norepinephrine; putative neurotransmitter.*

Nicotinic acetylcholine-gated channels [13]   Ligand-gated ion channels whose receptors bind acetylcholine but also can be activated by nicotine and blocked by curare. *See Muscarinic acetylcholine-gated channels.*

Nociceptors [4]   Receptors that respond across a wide range of physical dimensions but only to stimulus levels approaching or exceeding that sufficient to cause tissue damage.

Nodal cells [14]   Specialized muscle cells of the heart that produce pacemaker potentials and determine the rhythm of cardiac muscle contraction.

Node of Ranvier [2, 12]   Periodic (roughly 1 mm apart) interruptions in the insulating myelin around a nerve fiber through which local currents can easily flow.

Nonassociative learning [9]   Learning conditions in which the subject learns specific properties of a stimulus.

Norepinephrine [13]   A neurotransmitter of the biogenic amine group that is involved, among other things, in the response to emergency situations.

Obligatory synapse [13]   A synapse in which each presynaptic action potential produces a postsynaptic action potential.

Occlusion [6]   A nonlinear response of a reflex in which the response to combined inputs is appreciably less than the sum of the responses to the inputs when tested separately.

Operant conditioning [9]   The development of a reflex response to a particular stimulus condition as a result of association of reward with those occasions in which the subject's behavior approached the desired response.

Orthodromic [10]   Propagation of a nerve impulse in the direction of normal conduction of the fiber. *See Antidromic.*

Outer ear [5]   The external ear (pinna) with the external auditory canal.

Overshoot [12]   That portion of an action potential during which the intracellular potential exceeds zero (as contrasted to simple depolarization).

Overtone [3]   A complex tone made up of components above the fundamental frequency.

Pacemaker potentials [14]   Repetitive, self-generated potentials of nerve or muscle cells.

Pacinian corpuscle [5]   A mechanically sensitive receptor found in the skin, joints, and periosteum that is formed by a mechanoreceptive nerve ending encapsulated in fluid-filled layers of connective tissue. Responds to continuous vibration but only to the beginning of a steady displacement.

Parallel elastic elements [14]   Elastic structures that occur in parallel with the contractile elements of muscle.

Parallel operation [16]   The same or related signals carried simultaneously on multiple pathways.

Parasympathetic nervous system [7]   That portion of the autonomic nervous system that originates in the brainstem and sacral portion of spinal cord.

Passive spread [2]   Decremental spread of current or voltage along a cable conductor.

Pattern code [4]   Representation of neural information by means of a unique neural firing pattern.

Perception [3]   The conscious impression of events and objects based on sensory information.

Phase plane graph [16]   A graph in which the horizontal axis represents the magnitude of some function and the vertical axis represents the rate of change of that function. Slope of the line describing a trajectory on this plane is determined by a relationship between acceleration and velocity.

Phoneme [3, 8]   Specific speech sounds, composed of multiple frequency components, and, in some consonants, transitions in frequency and loudness.

Pitch [3]   A characteristic of sound that is closely related to the frequency of the sound pressure waves.

Poisson distribution [13]   The probability distribution of the number of rare events occurring in a particular time period.

Polarized [11]   With reference to neuron electrical properties, indicates a (negative) potential difference across the cell's membrane.

Polysynaptic pathways [6]   Neural pathways, usually involved in reflex action, that involve a sequence of more than two neurons, thus passing through two or more synapses.

Positive feedback   *See Feedback, positive.*

Postganglionic fibers [2]   Fibers that originate in (autonomic) peripheral ganglia and carry signals to glands, blood vessels, the heart, and other visceral structures.

Postsynaptic [13]   The neuron that receives information at its synapses. At a chemical synapse, this neuron has receptor sites for neurotransmitter.

Posttetanic potentiation [9]   An increase in response to an individual stimulus that occurs following a train of rapidly repeated stimuli.

Posttranslational modification [9]   Modification of a protein molecule (for example by addition of a phosphate molecule) after the basic molecule has been synthesized.

Potential   *See Action potential; Compound action potential; Dorsal root potential; Electrical potential; Endplate potential; Equilibrium potential; Evoked potentials; Excitatory postsynaptic potential; Inhibitory postsynaptic potential;*

Membrane potential; Miniature endplate potential; Myotonic potentials; Pacemaker potentials; Receptor potentials; Resting potential; Reversal potential; Ventral root potential.

Presbyopia [5]   A condition that develops with age as the lens becomes less elastic, observed as a reduced range of accommodation.

Presynaptic [13]   The neuron or part of the neuron that delivers information to a synapse. At a chemical synapse, the terminal that releases neurotransmitter.

Presynaptic facilitation [9]   Neuromodulation in which one neuron, through an axoaxonal synaptic contact onto a second neuron, increases the amount of an excitatory transmitter that this second neuron releases at its synapse onto a third neuron.

Presynaptic inhibition [6, 13]   Neuromodulation in which one neuron, through an axoaxonal synaptic contact onto a second neuron, decreases the amount of excitatory transmitter that this second neuron releases at its synapse onto a third neuron.

Primary efferent fibers [2]   Fibers that originate in the central nervous system (brainstem or spinal cord) and pass out to terminate on muscles or peripheral ganglia.

Proprioceptors [4]   Receptors that transduce information regarding the location of body parts with respect to each other.

Pulse-encoded signals [2, 8]   Information transmitted in the intervals between a time-varying series of constant sized pulses.

Putative neurotransmitter [13]   Chemical compounds that have met some, but not all, of the requirements for identification as a specific neurotransmitters.

Quantum [13]   An event of fixed amplitude. In synaptic transmission, the effect of a single vesicle of neurotransmitter.

Receptive field [5]   That fraction of the total energy of a particular modality that initiates a response in an individual receptor or sensory responsive neuron.

Receptor [1]   An element that responds in a specific way to a particular type of input. (1) **Sensory receptor** The transducer of characteristic stimuli into neural activity. (2) **Membrane receptor** A molecule in a membrane that reacts with a specific chemical entity to initiate some local response. (Often used without modifier and differentiated by context.) *See Exteroceptors; Interoceptors; Nociceptors; Proprioceptors; Somatoceptors; Stretch receptors; Teloceptors.*

Receptor potentials [4, 12]   Nonpropagated, graded potentials produced in sensory receptors in response to a stimulus; a first step in the transduction process.

Recovery heat [14]   Heat, measured over a period of minutes following muscle contraction, that represents the cost of the chemical work of replenishing stored energy.

Recruitment [6, 14]   The increase of activity in a particular neural pathway that is accomplished by bringing into action previously silent units in that pathway.

Recruitment order [14]   The order in which new muscle fibers are activated with increasing neuronal signals, generally first slow, fatigue-resistant fibers and then progressing to large, fast fibers.

Referred pain [17]   The sensation of pain that is perceived at a different location than its (usually visceral) source.

Reflex [6]   Stereotypic motor responses involving a specific sensory stimulation, conduction over a neural path with only simple central processing, and an effector response. *See Monosynaptic reflex; Reflex arc; Stretch reflex.*

Reflex arc [2]   Pathway over which impulses are transmitted from sensory receptors in the periphery to the central nervous system and then, after processing, are transmitted back to effectors in the periphery.

Refractory period [2]   A period following an action potential during which an excitable cell is either unexcitable or has reduced excitability. *See Absolute refractory period; Relative refractory period.*

Relative refractory period [12]   Time period following the absolute refractory period during which a second action potential can be initiated but requiring a higher threshold.

Renshaw pathway [16]   A feedback pathway from a motoneuron back onto that same motoneuron.

Resistance (R) [12]   The ratio of the potential difference between the ends of a conductor to the current through it; inverse of conductance.

Resistive current [12]   Electrical current that flows through a conductor and represents the continuous movement of electrons or charged ions from one end of the conductor to the other end. *See Capacitive current.*

Resting potential [10, 11]   A constant potential across the membrane of an unstimulated excitable cell.

Retrograde amnesia [9]   A loss of memory of events before a causative insult, abolishing especially short-term memory.

Reversal potential [13]   The membrane potential at which an electrical response (e.g., postsynaptic current) reverses direction. Term originated in the experimental method used to determine the equilibrium potential under different conditions in intact cells.

Rheobase [10]   The minimum current that, with prolonged application, can cause stimulation of a nerve or muscle.

Safety factor [2, 12]   An amount by which a functional capability exceeds that necessary to maintaining basal activity for that function. Can be expressed quantitatively as the dimensional excess of the available function beyond that necessary or as the dimensionless ratio of the excess to the basal need. Examples: (1) The current resulting from a local action potential related to that needed to propagate the action potential. (2) The endplate potential at a nerve muscle junction related to that necessary to excite a muscle action potential. (3) The vector redundancy of information transduced by multiple receptor types and units.

Saltatory conduction [12]   Conduction in myelinated axons in which the action potential occurs only at the nodes of Ranvier. Although the word saltatory derives from the Latin word for jumping, it is the potential change that occurs only at the nodes; local currents flow continuously between nodes.

Sarcolemma [14]   The cell membrane of a muscle cell.

Sarcomere [14]   The basic contractile unit of a muscle cell delimited by Z-lines.

Sarcoplasm [14]   The cytoplasm of a muscle cell.

Sarcoplasmic reticulum [14]   An intracellular organelle in muscle fibers (most prominently in skeletal muscle) that concentrates Ca^{2+} and releases it during excitation-contraction coupling.

Saturation [16]   Maximum level of response of a system occurring at full activation of all elements that produce unit responses.

Second messengers [4, 12, 13]   Chemical agents released within a cell that have their effects at other locations within that same cell.

Second order system [16]   A system whose function is entirely defined by a second-order differential equation.

Semicircular canals [5, 8]   A set of three fluid-filled, semicircular tubes joined into closed paths by a common chamber. These parts of the inner ear are called the vestibular apparatus. The planes of the three canals form the basis of a Cartesian coordinate system that senses rotational movement. Mechanically sensitive hair cells embedded in the *cupulae* that occlude each canal are the sensory receptors.

Sensitization [9]   Learning conditions in which a novel stimulus increases the response to a second or continuously repeated nonnoxious stimulus.

Sensory fiber [2]   Any afferent neurite.

Separatrix [8]   The divisions between basins.

Serial sequence [16]   The output of one operation used as the input to the next operation in a series of connected neurons or even within a single anatomical element.

Series elastic elements [14]   Elastic structures that occur in series with the contractile elements of muscle including both elements of the tendons and parts of the contractile system itself. *See Parallel elastic elements.*

Short-term memory [9]   A memory trace that is easily disrupted persisting over a period of minutes to hours of maintained attention.

Signal [1, 2]   Anything that conveys changing information from one site to another.

Skeletal muscle (voluntary, striated) [1, 7]   Muscle fibers, innervated by the somatic nervous system that have microscopic cross-striations. These muscles are usually under voluntary control and are most often attached to the skeleton.

Slow muscle fibers [14]   Skeletal muscle fibers (dominant in "red" muscle) that have long duration twitches and will exhibit fusion with a relatively low rate of stimulation. These fibers are relatively fatigue resistant.

Smooth muscle [1]   Nonstriated muscle, not usually under voluntary control, often associated with blood vessels and hollow organs of the viscera.

Somatoceptors [4, 6]   Receptors that transduce information that is presented at the body surface.

Somatotopic [8]   Representation of touch and pressure information mapped onto the central nervous system in a pattern related to the different body locations.

Sonogram [8]   A three-dimensional representation of a vocal sound, the coordinates being frequency (y axes), time (x axes), and intensity (represented by shading intensity or color).

Space constant [12]   The distance along a cable conductor from a point of applied potential to where the potential falls to $1/e$ ($\approx 1/3$) of its original value.

Spatial summation [6]   The cumulative effect of inputs from different sources acting on a neuron or neuron pool. *See Temporal summation.*

Spinal shock [6]   A period of abolished spinal reflexes followed by reduced reflex action after transection of the spinal cord.

SPL (sound pressure level) [3]   Decibel notation used in acoustics in which the reference pressure is taken to be 20 μPa, approximately the minimal threshold for hearing.

Starling's law [14]   With more filling of the heart, the contraction force is greater and can compensate with increased blood output.

Stevens' law [4]   Statement that there exists a power relationship between stimulus strength and perceived sensation. *See Weber–Fechner law.*

Stiffness [14]   The ratio of force applied to resulting change in length.

Strength-duration relationship [10]   The approximately inverse relationship between duration and intensity of stimulus current necessary to produce a threshold response. *See Chronaxie; Rheobase.*

Stretch receptors [5]   Two major classes of displacement-sensitive receptors located on the surface of intrafusal fibers within muscle spindles.

Stretch reflex [6]   Myotatic reflex, tendon reflex, tendon jerk. A reflex that produces contraction of a muscle in response to stretch of the spindle receptors in that muscle acting by way of a monosynaptic path.

Striated muscle [14]   Muscle fibers with microscopic transverse bands that generally move the skeleton, and are usually under voluntary control. *See Skeletal muscle.*

Subliminal fringe [6]   Neurons that are brought closer to, but still not to their threshold, by a given input.

Subthreshold [2]   A stimulus of insufficient intensity to initiate a response.

Summation [15]   Addition of inputs to a neuron, usually in the form of synaptic potentials, with either (+) or (−) signs of action.

Supranormal period [2]   A period following an action potential in some nerves during which threshold is below that of a resting nerve.

Suprathreshold [2]   Any stimulus that exceeds the minimum amplitude needed to initiate a response.

Sympathetic nervous system [7]   That portion of the autonomic nervous system that passes through the chain of autonomic ganglia and originates in the thoracic or lumbar portions of the spinal cord.

Synapse [13]   The junction between two neurons at which information is transferred. *See Adrenergic; Cholinergic.*

Synaptic cleft [13]   The space immediately between the presynaptic terminal and the adjacent surface of the postsynaptic neuron.

Synaptic vesicle [13]   Small structures that contain neurotransmitter and are found abundantly in presynaptic terminals.

Synergistic muscles [7]   Muscles that act together in accomplishing a particular motor action. *See Antagonistic muscles.*

Synthetic senses [8]   Perceptions that arise only as an interpretation of the relative activation of more than one type of receptor (e.g., smell and color senses).

Teloceptors [4]   Receptors that transduce information that originates with remote sources (e.g., vision).

Temporal summation [6, 15]   The cumulative effect of successive inputs by way of the same input path, acting on a single neuron or neuron pool. *See Spatial summation.*

Tetanic fusion [14, 15]   Summation of individual muscle twitches at a sufficiently high frequency to produce a smooth contraction.

Tetanus [14]   Smooth, maintained tension resulting from fusion of a train of rapidly repeated twitches.

Thick filament [14]   A complex of myosin molecules that constitutes one part of the interdigitated structure within a sarcomere.

Thin filament [14]   A macromolecular complex that constitutes one part of the interdigitating structure of muscle.

Threshold [2, 12, 16]   The demarcation between those stimulus intensities that generate a response and those that do not.

Time constant [12]   The time required for a system to change to within $1/e$ ($\approx 1/3$) of its final value after the occurrence of a step change of a driving voltage or other quantity.

Tonotopic [8]   Representation of auditory information in the central nervous system with different pitches mapped at different locations.

Tonus [14]   A low level of contractile activity commonly found in both skeletal and smooth muscle. In skeletal muscle this is based on a low level of activity of motor nerves.

Tracts [2]   Bundles of related fibers coursing together in the central nervous system.

Trajectory [16]   The trace of sequential states of a system as it changes over time.

Transduction [2, 4]   A process that transforms a signal in one physical form into a representation of the same signal in a different physical form.

Transverse tubules (T-tubules) [14]   Periodic invaginations of the sarcolemma into the interior of a muscle fiber.

Tropism [1]   Movement that orients an organism to achieve a certain relationship to a particular stimulus such as light or gravity.

Tropomyosin [14]   A long filamentous molecule associated with actin that regulates the availability of myosin binding sites on the actin filament.

Troponin [14]   A molecule associated with tropomyosin that binds Ca^{2+} and sterically regulates the tropomyosin molecule.

Twitch [14]   The single rapid contraction of a muscle followed by a relaxation back to its resting condition occurring in response to a single adequate stimulus to the muscle nerve or directly to the muscle.

Valsalva maneuver [5]   Inflation of the eustachian tube by closing the nose and mouth and attempting forcible expiration.

Ventral root potential [10]   Extracellular potential recorded on the motor roots of the spinal cord following volley stimulations to sensory nerves that represents the sum of electrotonically spread effects of motoneuron postsynaptic potentials.

Vestibulo-ocular reflex [6, 8]   Reflex eye movements resulting from rotational stimulation of the semicircular canals.

Volley [6]   Nerve impulses on multiple fibers that arrive at a neuron or in a neuron pool nearly synchronously, usually as a result of an artificial stimulus.

Voltage clamping [10]   A technique using negative feedback by which the voltage within an excitable cell is held at a controlled value while the related current is measured.

Wave summation [15]   Summation of muscle contraction with successive stimulus pulses.

Weber-Fechner law [4]   States that there exists a logarithmic relationship between stimulus strength and perceived sensation. *See Stevens' law*

White matter [2]   Aggregates of nerve fibers within the central nervous system that appear white in an unstained sample because of their myelin sheaths.

Z-line [14]   Structure to which the ends of the thin filaments are attached in muscle. Forms the bounds of a sarcomere.

Bibliography

Preface

Aristotle *De Partibus Animulium*. In *The Works of Aristotle,* Vols. 8 and 9. R.M. Hutchins (ed). Encyclopedia Britannica, William Benton, 1952.
Bacon, F. (1620) *Novum Organum.* In *Francis Bacon,* Vol. 30. R.M. Hutchins (ed.). Encyclopedia Britannica, William Benton, 1952.
Galvani, L. (1791) *De Viribus Electricitatis in Motu Musculari Commentarius.* Published in *Scientiarum et Artium Instituto atque Academia Commentarii,* Vol. VII pp. 363–418. (English translation by R.M. Green. Elizabeth Licht, Cambridge, Mass., 1953.)

Chapter 1

References

Brookhart, J.M., and Mountcastle, V.B. (eds.) (1981) The Nervous System. *Handbook of Physiology.* Williams & Wilkins, Baltimore.
Helmholtz, H. (1850) Messungen über den zeitlichen Verlauf der Zuckung anamalischen Muskeln und die Fortpflanzungegeschwindigkeit der Reizung in den Nerven. *Arch. Anat. Physiol.* 276–364.

Additional Reading

Kirk, T.G. (1978) *Library Research Guide to Biology.* Pierian Press, Ann Arbor.

Searle, J.R. (1990) Is the brain's mind a computer program? *Sci. Am.* 262:26–31.

Swinscow, T.D.V. (1978) *Statistics at Square One.* Reprinted from *British Medical Journal,* British Medical Association, London.

Chapter 2

References

Adrian, E.D. (1928) *The Basis of Sensation.* Norton, New York.

Helmholtz, H. (1850) Messungen über den zeitlichen Verlauf der Zuckung anamalischen Muskeln und die Fortpflanzungegeschwindigkeit der Reizung in den Nerven. *Arch. Anat. Physiol.* 276–364.

Matthews, B.H.C. (1931) The response of a single end organ. *J. Physiol.* 71:64–110.

Netter, F.H. (1986) *The CIBA Collection of Medical Illustrations, Vol 1. The Nervous System.* Ciba Pharmaceutical Co., Summit, N.J.

Sargent, P. (1989) What distinguishes axons from dendrites? *Trends Neurosci.* 12:203–206.

Weber, E. (1846) Muskelbewegnung, pp. 1–122. In *Handwörterbuch der Physiologie,* Vol. III, Abt. 2. R. Wagner (ed.). Bieweg, Braunschweig.

Addtional Reading

Eckert, R., Naitoh Y., and Machemer, M. (1976) Calcium in the bioelectric and motor functions of *Paramecium.* In *Calcium in Biological Systems.* Symposium 30, Society of Experimental Biology. C.J. Duncan (ed.). Cambridge University Press, London.

Galvani, L. (1791) *De Viribus Electricitatis in Motu Musculari Commentarius.* Published in *Scientiarum et Artium Instituto atque Academia Commentarii,* Vol. VII, pp. 363–418. (English translation by R.M. Green. Elizabeth Licht, Cambridge, Mass., 1953.)

Hedge, G.A., Colby, H.D., and Goodman, R.L. (1987) *Clinical Endocrine Physiology.* Saunders, Philadelphia.

Korn, G.A., and Korn, T.M. (1961) Shannon's sampling theorem. In *Mathematical Handbook for Scientists and Engineers.* G.A. Korn and T.M. Korn (eds.). McGraw-Hill, New York.

Leader, R.W., and Stark, D. (1987) The importance of animals in biomedical research. *Perspect. Biol. Med.* 30:470–485.

Schmidt-Nielsen, K. (1975) Temperature effects. In *Animal Physiology.* Cambridge University Press, London.

Tufte, E.R. (1983) *The Visual Display of Quantitative Information.* Graphics Press, Cheshire, Ct.

West, J.B. (ed.) (1991) Endocrine Systems. In *Physiological Basis of Medical Practice,* 12th edition. Williams & Wilkins, Baltimore.

Williams, P.L., Warwick, R., Dyson, M., and Bannister, L.H. (1989) *Gray's Anatomy.* Churchill Livingstone, Edinburgh.

Chapter 3

References

Bernard, C. (1865) *Introduction a l'étude de la Médecine expérimentale.* Baillière, Paris. (English translation by H.C. Green, Dover, New York, 1957.)

Pierce, J.R. (1983) *The Science of Musical Sound.* Freeman, San Francisco.

Williamson, S.J., and Cummins, H.Z. (1983) *Light and Color in Nature and Art.* Wiley, New York.

Additional Reading

Gelfand, S.A. (1990) *Hearing: An Introduction to Psychological and Physiological Acoustics.* Marcel Dekker, New York.

Handbook of Chemistry and Physics, 71st edition. (1991) CRC Press, Boca Raton, Fla.

Withers, P.C. (1992) *Comparative Animal Physiology.* Saunders, Philadelphia.

Chapter 4

References

Art, J.J., and Fettiplace, R. (1987) Variation of membrane properties in hair cells isolated from the turtle cochlea. *J. Physiol.* 385:207–242.

Bernstein, J. (1876) *The Five Senses of Man.* Henry S. King, London.

Fechner, G. (1860) In *Elements of Psychophysics.* D.H. Howes and E.G. Boring (eds.). (English translation by H.E. Adler. Holt, Rinehart & Winston, New York, 1966.)

Matthews, B.H.C. (1931) The response of a single end organ. *J. Physiol.* 71:64–110.

Newton, I. (1687) *Philosophiae Naturalis Principia Mathematica,* London. A. Koyré, and I.B. Cohen (eds.). Cambridge University Press, Cambridge, 1972.

Stevens, S.S. (1953) On the brightness of lights and the loudness of sounds. *Science* 118:576.

Weber, E.H. (1846) Der Tastsinn und das Gemeingefühl. In *Handwörterbuch der Physiologie,* Vol. III, Abt. 2. R. Wagner (ed.). Bieweg, Braunschweig.

Withers, P.C. (1992) *Comparative Animal Physiology.* Saunders, Philadelphia.

Additional Reading

Daw, N.W., Jensen, R.J., and Brunken, W.J. (1990) Rod pathways in mammalian retinae. *Trends Neurosci.* 13:110–115.

Dennett, D.C. (1991) *Consciousness Explained.* Little, Brown, Boston.

Dionne, V.E. (1988) How do you smell? Principle in question. *Trends Neurosci.* 11:188–189.

Kandel, E.R., Schwartz, J.H., and Jessell, T.M. (1991) Sensory systems of the brain. In *Principles of Neural Science,* 3rd edition. Elsevier, New York.

The Merck Manual, 15th edition (1987) R. Berkow (ed.). Merck & Co., Rahway, N.J. (Use figure 254-1 chart for estimating extent of burns.)

Partridge, L.D. (1978) Methods in the study of proprioception. In *Handbook of Engineering in Medicine and Biology.* CRC Press, Boca Raton, Fla.

Schmidt, R.F. (1978) *Fundamentals of Sensory Physiology.* Springer-Verlag, New York.

Sherrington, C.S. (1906) *The Integrative Action of the Nervous System,* Yale University Press, New Haven.

Chapter 5

References

Brookhart, J.M., and Mountcastle, V.B. (eds.) (1981) *Handbook of Physiology,* Section I, *Neurophysiology,* Vol. III. Williams & Wilkins, Baltimore.

Helmholtz, H. (1856) *Handbuch der physiologischen Optik.* Voss, Leipzig. (English translation by P.C. Southall, Optical Society of America, Menasha, Wisc., 1909–1911.)

Helmholtz, H. (1877) *The Sensation of Tone as a Physiological Basis for the Theory of Music.* (Translation Dover, New York, 1954.)

Kandel, E.R., and Schwartz, J.H. (1985) *Principles of Neural Science,* 2nd edition. Elsevier, New York.

Loewenstein, W.R., and Mendelson, M. (1965) Components of receptor adaptation in a pacinian corpuscle. *J. Physiol.* 177:377–397.

Additional Reading

Bracewell, R.N. (1989) The Fourier transform. *Sci. Am.* 260:86–95.

Kandel, E.R., Schwartz, J.H. and Jessell, T.M. (1991) *Principles of Neural Science,* 3rd edition. Elsevier, New York.

Mendelson, M., and Lowenstein, W.R. (1964) Mechanisms of receptor action. *Science* 144:554–555.

Chapter 6

References

Gesell, R. (1940) A neurophysiological interpretation of the respiratory act. *Eugebn Physiol.* 43:477–639.

Gesell, R. (1951) An electrical study of manifestations of paired motor half-centers. *Am. J. Physiol.* 170:702–716.

Gesell, R., Hansen, E.T., and Siskel, J. (1947) On the electrotonic nature of stimulation, inhibition, summation, and afterdischarge of nerve centers. *Am. J. Physiol.* 148:515–529.

Graham-Brown, T. (1912) The intrinsic factors of progression in the mammal. *Proc. Roy. Soc. London* 84:308–319.

Kim, J.H., and Partridge, L.D. (1969) Observations on types of response to combinations of neck, vestibular, and muscle stretch signals. *J. Neurophysiol.* 32:239–250.

Ling, G., and Girard, R.W. (1949) The normal membrane potential of frog sartorius fibers. *J. Cell. Comp. Physiol.* 34:383–396.

Lloyd, D.P.C. (1946) Facilitation and inhibition of spinal motoneurons. *J. Neurophysiol.* 9:421–438.

Melzack, R., and Wall, P.D. (1965) Pain mechanisms: A new theory. *Science* 150:971–979.

McKendrick, J.G. (1899) *Hermann Ludwig Ferdinand von Helmholtz.* Longman, London.

Rall, W. (1967) Distinguishing theoretical synaptic potentials computed for different soma-dendritic distributions of synaptic input. *J. Neurophysiol.* 30:1138–1168.

Sherrington, C.S. (1898) Decerebrate rigidity, and reflex co-ordination of movements. *J. Physiol.* 22:319–332.

Sherrington, C.S. (1906) *The Integrative Action of the Nervous System.* Yale University Press, New Haven.

Sherrington, C.S., and Leddell, E.G.T. (1925) Further observations on myotatic reflexes. *Proc. Roy. Soc. London.* 97B:267–283.

Shik, M.L., Orlouowski, G.N., and Severin, F.V. (1968) Locomotion of the mesencephalic cat elicited by stimulation of the pyramids. *Biofizika* 13:127–135.

Additional Reading

Kalman, B. (1970) *Elementary Linear Algebra.* Macmillan, London.

Pavlov, I.P. (1928) *Lectures on Conditioned Reflexes.* (English translation by W.H. Gantt, International Pub., New York.)

Chapter 7

References

Berkinblit, M.B., Feldman, A.G., and Fukson, O. (1986) Adaptability of innate motor patterns and motor control mechanisms. *Brain Behav. Sci.* 9:585–638.

Bernstein, N.A. (1967) *The Coordination and Regulation of Movement.* Pergamon, New York.

Bizzi, E., Accorneio, N., Chapple, W., and Hogan, N. (1982) Arm trajectory formation in monkeys. *Exp. Brain Res.* 46:139–143.

Braun, C.W., and Fisher O. (1895) Der Gang des Menschen I. Versuche unbelasten und belasten Menschen. *Abh. Math. Phys. Kl. Koenigl. Saeschs. Ges. Wiss.* 21:153–322.

Cannon, W. (1929) Organization for physiological homeostasis. *Physiol. Rev.* 9:399–431.

Dempster, W.T. (1961) Freebody diagrams as an approach to the mechanics of posture and motion. In *Studies of the Musculoskeletal Systems.* F.C. Evans (ed.). Charles C Thomas, Springfield.

Duchenne, G.B. (1867) *Physiologie des Mouvements.* Paris. (English translation by E.B. Kaplan, *Physiology of Motion.* Saunders, Philadelphia, 1959.)

Feldman, A.G. (1966) Functional tuning of the nervous system with control of movement or maintenance of a steady posture, II: Controllable parameters of the muscle. *Biophysics* 11:565–578.

Goldstein, H. (1950) *Classical Mechanics.* Addison-Wesley, Reading, Mass.

Henneman, E., Solmjen, G., and Carpenter, D.O. (1965) Functional significance of cell size in spinal motoneurons. *J. Neurophysiol.* 28:581–598.

Lombard, W.P., and Abbott, F.M. (1907) The mechanical effects produced by the contraction of individual muscles of the thigh of the frog. *Am. J. Physiol.* 20:1–60.

Partridge, L.D. (1967) Intrinsic feedback factors producing inertial compensation in muscle. *Biophys. J.* 7:853–863.

Pavlov, I.P. *Conditioned Reflexes.* G.V. Anrep, (trans.) Reprinted 1960, Dover, New York.

Sherrington, C.S. (1941) *Man on His Nature.* Macmillan, New York.

Winters, J.M., and Woo, S.L.-Y. (eds.) (1990) *Multiple Muscle Systems: Biomechanics and Movement Organization.* Springer-Verlag, New York.

Additional Reading

Gowitzke, B.A., and Miller, M. (1988) *Scientific Basis of Human Movement,* 3rd edition. Williams & Wilkins, Baltimore.

Hedge, G.A., Colby, H.D., and Goodman, R.L. (1987) *Clinical Endocrine Physiology.* Saunders, Philadelphia.

Leeuwenhoek, A. van (1688) Letters to Royal Society of London, 7 September. In *Collected Letters,* Vol. 8(110), pp. 2–57. J.J. Swart (ed.). Swets & Zeitlinger, Amsterdam, 1967.

O'Malley, C.D., and Saunders, J.B. de C.M. (1952) *Leonardo da Vinci on the Human Body.* Schuman, New York.

Patton, H.D., Fuchs, A.F., Hille, B., Scher, A.M., and Steiner, R. (1989) The autonomic nervous system. In *Textbook of Physiology.* Saunders, Philadelphia.

Plagenhoef, S. (1971) *Patterns of Human Motion.* Prentice-Hall, Englewood Cliffs, N.J.

Sarton, G. (1954) *Galen of Pergamon*. Lawrence University Press, Lawrence, Kan.

Schmidt, R.A., (1982) *Motor Control and Learning: A Behavioral Emphasis*. Human Kinetics, Champaign, Ill.

Wells, P.N.T. (ed.) (1982) Thermographic imaging. In *Scientific Basis of Medical Imaging*. Churchill Livingstone, Edinburgh.

Chapter 8

References

Barlow, H.B., and Levick, W.R. (1965) The mechanism of directionally selective units in rabbit's retina. *J. Physiol.* 178:477–504.

Cowey, A., and Stoerig, P. (1991) The neurobiology of blindsight. *Trends Neurosci.* 14:140–145.

Creed, R.S., Denny-Brown, D., Eccles, J.C., Liddell, E.G.T., and Sherrington, C.S. (1932) *Reflex Activity of the Spinal Cord*. Oxford University Press, London.

Fields, H.L., Partridge, L.D., and Winter, D.L. (1970) Somatic and visceral receptive field properties of fibers in ventral quadrant white matter of the cat spinal cord. *J. Neurophysiol.* 33:827–837.

Gesell, R., and Dontas, A.S. (1952) An electrical study of manifestations of paired motor half centers (excitation, inhibition, precedence of stimulation, adaptation and rebound). *Am. J. Physiol.* 170:702–716.

Granit, R. (1955) *Receptors and Sensory Perception*. Yale University Press, New Haven.

Grojski, K.A., and Freeman, W.J. (1989) Spatial EEG correlates of nonassociative and associative olfactory learning in rabbits. *Behav. Neurosci.* 103:790–804.

Harmon, L.D. (1971) Some aspects of recognition of human faces. *Zeichenerkennung durch biologische und technische Systeme,* pp. 196–219. Springer-Verlag, Berlin.

Harmon, L.D. (1973) The recognition of faces. *Sci. Am.* 229: 70–82.

Hartline, H.K., and Ratliff, F. (1957) Inhibitory interaction of receptor units in the eye of *Limulus. J. Gen. Physiol.* 40:357–376.

Hsu, F., Anantharaman, T., Campbell, M., and Nowatzyk, A. (1990) A grandmaster chess machine. *Sci. Am.* 263:44–50.

Hubel, D.H., and Weisel, T.N. (1962) Receptive fields, binocular interaction and functional architecture in the cat's visual cortex. *J. Physiol.* 160:106–154.

James, W. (1890) *The Principles of Psychology*. Holt, New York.

Kim, J.H., and Partridge, L.D. (1969) Observations on types of responses to combinations of neck, vestibular, and muscle spindle signals. *J. Neurophysiol.* 32:239–250.

Magnus, R. (1924) *Körperstellung*. Springer-Verlag, Berlin.

Maturana, H.R., Lettvin, J.Y., McCulloch, W.S., and Pitts, W.H. (1960) Anatomy and physiology of vision in the frog (*Rana pipiens*). *J. Gen. Physiol.* 43:129–175.

McCulloch, W.S., and Pitts, W. (1943) A logical calculus of the ideas immanent in nervous activity. *Bull. Math. Biophys.* 5:115–133.

Pellionisz, A.J. (1988) Tensor geometry: A language of brain and neural computers. In *Neural Computers*. R. Eckmiller (ed.). Springer-Verlag, Berlin.

Peterson, G.E., and Barney, H.L. (1952) Control methods used in a study of vowels. *J. Acoust. Soc. Am.* 24:175–184.

Sherrington, C.S. (1906) *The Integrative Action of the Nervous System.* Yale University Press, New Haven.

Shik, M.L., Orlouowski, G.N., and Severin, F.V. (1968) Locomotion of the mesencephalic cat elicited by stimulation of the pyramids. *Biofizika* 13:127–135.

Yates, F.E. (ed.) (1987) *Self Organizing Systems: The Emergence of Order.* Plenum, New York.

Additional Reading

Dennett, D.C. (1991) *Consciousness Explained.* Little, Brown, Boston.

Mahowald, M.A., and Mead, C. (1991) The silicon retina. *Sci. Am.* 264:76–83.

Miller, G.A. (1991) *The Science of Words.* Scientific American Library, Freeman, New York.

Peterhaus, E., and van der Heydt, R. (1991) Subjective contours—bridging the gap between psychophysics and physiology. *Trends Neurosci.* 14:112–119.

Schmidt, R.F. (1978) *Fundamentals of Sensory Physiology.* Springer-Verlag, New York.

Skinner, B.F. (1972) *Cumulative Record: A Selection of Papers by B.F. Skinner.* Appleton-Century-Crofts, New York.

Chapter 9

References

Adrian, E.D. (1947) *Physical Background of Perception.* Clarendon Press, Oxford.

Cajal, S.R. (1911) *Histologie du Système nerveux de l'Homme et des Vertébrés.* Maloine, Paris.

Descartes, R. (1637) *Discourse on Method.* (English translation by E.S. Haldane and G.R.T. Ross, Cambridge University Press, Cambridge, 1904.)

Ebbinghaus, H. (1885) *Memory: A Contribution to Experimental Psychology.* (Reprint: Dover, New York, 1963.)

Eccles, J.C. (1953) *Neurophysiological Basis of Mind: The Principles of Neurophysiology.* Clarendon Press, Oxford.

Hebb, D.O. (1949) *The Organization of Behavior: A Neuropsychological Theory.* (Reprint, Science Editions, New York, 1961.)

Laduron, P.M. (1987) Axonal transport of neuroreceptors: Possible involvement in long-term memory. *Neuroscience* 22:767–779.

Lorente de Nó (1933) Studies on the structure of the cerebral cortex. *J. Psych. Neurol.* 45:381–438.

Luria, S.A. (1987) *The Mind of a Mnemonist.* Harvard University Press, Cambridge, Mass.

McCulloch, W.S. (1945) A heterarchy of values determined by the topology of nervous nets. *Bull. Math. Biophys.* 7:89–93.

Milner, B., Corkin, S., and Teuber, H.-L. (1968) Further analysis of the hippocampal amnesic syndrome: 14-year follow-up study of H.M. *Neuropsychologia* 6:215–234.

Sherrington, C.S. (1906) *Integrative Action of the Nervous System.* Yale University Press, New Haven.

Tizard, J. (1974) Early malnutrition, growth and mental development in man. *Br. Med. Bull.* 30:169–174.

Additional Reading

Alkon, D.L. (1987) *Memory Traces in the Brain.* Cambridge University Press, Cambridge.

Goelet, P., and Kandel, E.R. (1986) Tracking the flow of learned information from membrane receptors to genome, *Trends Neurosci.* 9:492–499.

Kaczmareck, L.K., and Levitan, I.B. (1987) *Neuromodulation, the Biochemical Control of Neuron Excitability.* Oxford University Press, New York.

Kandel, E.R. (1976) *Cellular Basis of Behavior.* Freeman, San Francisco.

Kandel, E.R. (1979) *Behavioral Biology of Aplysia.* Freeman, San Francisco.

McNaughton, B.L., and Morris, R.G.M. (1987) Hippocampal synaptic enhancement and information storage within a distributed memory system. *Trends Neurosci.* 10:408–415.

Penfield, W. (1958) *The Excitable Cortex in Consious Man.* Charles C Thomas, Springfield, Ill.

Restak, R. (1984) *The Brain.* Bantam Books, Toronto.

Tank, D.W., and Hopfield, J.J. (1987) Collective computation in neuronlike circuits. *Sci. Am.* 257:104–114.

Chapter 10

References

Adrian, E.D., and Zotterman, Y. (1926) The impulses produced by sensory nerve endings. *J. Physiol.* 61:151–171.

Berger, H. (1929) Über das Elektrenkephalogramm des Menschen. *Arch. Psychiat.* 27:179–183.

Blair, H.A. (1932) On the intensity-time relations for stimulation by electric currents. *J. Gen. Physiol.* 15:709–729.

Brown, W.F. (1984) *The Physiological and Technical Basis of Electromyography.* Butterworth, Boston.

DuBois-Reymond, E. (1848) *Untersuchungen über thierische Elektricität,* Vol. 1. Reimer, Berlin.

Erlanger, J. and Gasser, H.S. (1924) The compound nature of the action current of nerve as disclosed by the cathode ray oscillograph. *Am. J. Physiol.* 70: 624–666.

Erlanger, J., and Gasser, H. (1937) *Electrical Signs of Nervous Activity.* University of Pennsylvania Press, Philadelphia.

Fritsch, G., and Hitzig, E. (1870) Über die elektrische Erregbarkeit des Grosshirns. *Arch. Anat. Physiol. Wiss. Med.* 37:300–332.

Galvani, L. (1791) *De Viribus Electricitatis in Motu Musculari Commentarius.* Published in *Scientiarum et Artium Instituto atque Academia Commentarii,* Vol. VII, pp. 363–418. (English translation by R.M. Green. Elizabeth Licht, Cambridge, Mass., 1953.)

Gasser, H.S., and Erlanger, J. (1922) A study of the action currents of nerve with a cathode ray oscillograph. *Am. J. Physiol.* 62:496–524.

Hamill, O.P., Marty, A., Neher, E., Sakmann, B., and Sigworth, F.J. (1981) Improved patch-clamp techniques for high-resolution current recording from cells and cell-free membrane patches. *Pflügers Arch.* 391:85–100.

Hodgkin, A.L., and Huxley, A.F. (1939) Action potentials recorded from inside a nerve fibre. *Nature (London)* 144:710–711.

Hodgkin, A.L., Huxley, A.F., and Katz, B. (1952) Measurement of current-voltage relations in the membrane of the giant axon of *Loligo*. *J. Physiol.* 116:424–448.

Jansen, B.H. (1991) Quantitative analysis of electroencephalograms: Is there chaos in the future? *Int. J. Biomed. Comput.* 27:95–123.

Lapique, L. (1926) *L'Excitabilitie en fonction du temps: La Chronaxis, sa signification et sa mesure*. University of France Press, Paris.

Loeb, G.E. (1989) Neural prosthetic interfaces with the nervous system. *Trends Neurosci.* 12:195–201.

Pflüger, E.F.W. (1859) *Untersuchungen über die Physiologie des Electrotonus*. A. Hirshwald, Berlin.

Ritchie, A.E. (1944) The electrical diagnosis of peripheral nerve injury. *Brain* 67:314–330.

Additional Reading

Basmajian, J.V., and DeLuca, C. (1985) *Muscles Alive and Their Functions Revealed by Electromyography*. Williams & Wilkins, Baltimore.

Conn, P.M. (1991) *Electrophysiology and Microinjection*. Academic Press, San Diego.

Halliday, D., and Resnick, R. (1981) *Fundamentals of Physics*. John Wiley, New York.

Kondo, H. (1953) Michael Faraday. *Sci. Am.* 189:91–98.

Ling, G., and Girard, R.W. (1949) The normal membrane potential of frog sartorius fibers. *J. Cell. Comp. Physiol.* 34:383–396.

Neher, E., and Sakmann, B. (1992) The patch clamp technique. *Sci. Am.* 266:44–51.

Smith, T.G., Lecar, H., Redman, S.J., and Gage, P.W. (1985) *Voltage and Patch Clamping with Microelectrodes*. American Physiological Society, Bethesda, Md.

Somjen, G. (1972) *Sensory Coding In Mammalian Nervous Systems*. Appleton-Century-Crofts, New York.

Chapter 11

References

Galvani, L. (1791) *De Viribus Electricitatis in Motu Musculari Commentarius*. Published in *Scientiarum et Artium Instituto atque Academia Commentarii*, Vol. VII (pp. 363–418). (English translation by R.M. Green. Elizabeth Licht, Cambridge, Mass., 1953.)

Goldman, D. (1943) Potential, impedance, and rectification in membranes. *J. Gen. Physiol.* 27:37–60.

Hodgkin, A.L., and Katz, B. (1949) The effect of sodium ions on the electrical activity of the giant axon of the squid. *J. Physiol.* 108:37–77.

Additional Reading

Coulomb, C.A. (1785–1789) *Sur l'electricité et le magnétisme* (7 Vols.).

Ferreira, H.G., and Marshall, M.W. (1985) *The Biophysical Basis of Excitability*. Cambridge University Press, Cambridge.

Hille, B. (1992) *Ionic Channels of Excitable Membranes*. Sinauer Associates, Sunderland, Mass.

Nernst, W. (1888) Zur Kinetik der Lösung befindlichen Körper: Theorie der Diffusion. *Z. phys. Chem.* 2:613–637.

Chapter 12

References

Adrian, E.D. (1914) The all-or-nothing principle in nerve. *J. Physiol.* 47:460–474.

Adrian, E.D., and Zotterman, Y. (1926) The impulses produced by sensory nerve endings. *J. Physiol.* 61:151–171.

Bernstein, J. (1902) Untersuchungen zur Thermodynamik der bioelektrischen Ströme. Erster Theil. *Pflügers Arch.* 82:521–562.

Catterall, W.A. (1991) Structure and function of voltage-gated sodium and calcium channels. *Curr. Opin. Neurobiol.* 1:5–13.

Eccles, J.C. (1964) *The Physiology of Synapses*. Springer-Verlag, New York.

Hodgkin, A.L., and Huxley, A.F. (1952) Currents carried by sodium and potassium ions through the membrane of the giant axon of *Loligo*. *J. Physiol.* 116:449–472.

Hodgkin, A.L., and Huxley, A.F. (1952) The components of membrane conductance in the giant axon of *Loligo*. *J. Physiol.* 116:473–496.

Hodgkin, A.L., and Huxley, A.F. (1952) The dual effect of membrane potential on sodium conductance in the giant axon of *Loligo*. *J. Physiol.* 116:497–506.

Hodgkin, A.L., and Huxley, A.F. (1952) A quantitative description of membrane current and its application to conduction and excitation in nerve. *J. Physiol.* 117:500–544.

Hodgkin, A.L., and Katz, B. (1949) The effect of sodium ions on the electrical activity of the giant axon of the squid. *J. Physiol.* 108:37–77.

Rall, W. (1977) Core conductor theory and cable properties of neurons. In *Handbook of Physiology,* Vol. 1. Williams & Wilkins, Baltimore.

Rall, W., and Rinzel, J. (1973) Branch input resistance and steady attenuation for input to one branch of a dendritic neurone model. *Biophys. J. Biophys. J.* 13:648–688.

Additional Reading

Hille, B. (1992) *Ionic Channels of Excitable Membranes*. Sinauer Associates, Sunderland, Mass.

Hodgkin, A.L. (1977) Chance and design in electrophysiology. In *The Pursuit of Nature*. Cambridge University Press, Cambridge.

Jack, J.J.B., Noble, D., and Tsien, R.W. (1983) *Electric Current Flow in Excitable Cells*. Oxford University Press, Oxford.

Chapter 13

References

Bormann, J., Hamill, O.P., and Sakmann, B. (1987) Mechanism of anion permeation through channels gated by glycine and γ-aminobutyric acid in mouse cultured spinal neurons. *J. Physiol.* 385:243–286.

Cajal, S.R. (1908) *Neuron Theory or Reticular Theory? Objective Evidence of the Anatomical Unity of Nerve Cells.* (English translation by M.U. Purkiss and C.A. Fox, Consejo Superior de Investigaciones Científicas Instituto Ramón y Cajal, Madrid, 1954.)

del Castillo, J., and Katz, B. (1954) Statistical factors involved in neuromuscular facilitation and depression. *J. Physiol.* 124:574–585.

Du Bois Reymond, E. (1875) *Gesammelte Abhandlungen der allgemeinen Muskel und Nervenphysic.* Veit, Leipzig.

Eccles, J.C., Fatt, P., and Landgren, S. (1956) Control pathway for direct inhibitory action of impulses in largest afferent nerve fibers to muscles. *J. Neurophysiol.* 19:75–98.

Elliot, T.R. (1904) On the action of adrenalin. *J. Physiol.* 31:20–21.

Fatt, P., and Katz, B. (1951) An analysis of the end-plate potential recorded with an intracellular electrode. *J. Physiol.* 115:320–370.

Fatt, P., and Katz, B. (1952) Spontaneous subthreshold activity at motor nerve endings. *J. Physiol.* 117:109–128.

Hamill, O.P., Marty, A., Neher, E., Sakmann, B., and Sigworth, F.J. (1981) Improved patch-clamp techniques for high-resolution current recording from cells and cell-free membrane patches. *Pflügers Arch.* 391:85–100.

Kodahl, I. (1966) *Nerve as a Tissue.* Harper & Row, New York.

Liley, A.W. (1956) The quantal components of the mammalian end-plate potential. *J. Physiol.* 133:571–587.

Loewi, O. (1921) Über humorale Übertragbarkeit der Herznervenwirkung. *Pflügers Arch.* 189:239–242.

Loewi, O. (1960) An autobiographical sketch. In *Perspectives in Biology and Medicine,* Vol. 4, pp. 3–25. University of Chicago Press, Chicago.

Melzack, R., and Wall, P.D. (1965) Pain mechanisms: A new theory. *Science* 150:971–979.

Sherrington C.S. (1897) Foster's *Textbook of Physiology,* 7th edition. Macmillan, London.

Snyder, S.H., and Bredt, D.S. (1991) Nitric oxide as a neuronal messenger. *Trends Pharmacol. Sci.* 12:125–128.

Vincent, A., Lang, B., and Newsom-Davis, J. (1989) Autoimmunity to the voltage-gated calcium channel underlies the Lambert-Eaton myasthenic syndrome, a paraneoplastic disorder. *Trends Neurosci.* 12:496–502.

Additional Reading

Bacq, Z.M. (1974) *Chemical Transmission of Nerve Impulses.* Pergamon, Oxford.

Eccles, J.C. (1964) *The Physiology of Synapses.* Springer-Verlag, New York.

Heuser, J.E., Reese, T.S., Dennis, M.J., Jan, Y., Jan, L., and Evans, L. (1979) Synaptic vesicle exocytosis captured by quick freezing and correlated with quantal release. *J. Cell Biol.* 81:275–300.

Korn, H., and Faber, D.S. (1991) Quantal analysis and synaptic efficacy in the CNS. *Trends Neurosci.* 14:439–445.

Sudarsky, L. (1990) *Pathophysiology of the Nervous System.* Little, Brown, Boston.

Chapter 14

References

Bizzi, E., Accorneio, N., Chapple, W., and Hogan, N. (1982) Arm trajectory formation in monkeys. *Exp. Brain Res.* 46:139–143.

Blix, M. (1893) Die Länge und Spannung des Muskels. *Skand. Arch. Physiol.* 4:399–409.

Ernst, E. (1963) *Biophysics of the Striated Muscle*. Hungarian Academy of Science, Budapest.

Feldman, A.G. (1966) Functional tuning of the nervous system with control of movement or maintenance of a steady posture. II: Controllable parameters of the muscle. *Biophysics* 11:565–578.

Fenn, W.O. (1945) Contractility. In *Physical Chemistry of Cells and Tissues*, p. 475 ff. R. Höber (ed.). Blackiston, Philadelphia.

Galvani, L. (1791) *De Viribus Electricitatis in Motu Musculari Commentarius*. Published in *Scientiarum et Artium Instituto atque Academia Commentarii*, Vol. VII, pp. 363–418. (English translation by R.M. Green. Elizabeth Licht, Cambridge, Mass., 1953.)

Gordon, A.M., Huxley, A.F., and Julian, F.J. (1966) The variation of isometric tension with sarcomere length in vertebrate muscle fibers. *J. Physiol.* 184:170–192.

Hill, A.V. (1965) *Trails and Trials in Physiology*. Williams & Wilkins, Baltimore.

Huxley, A.F., and Simmons, R.M. (1971) Proposed mechanism of force generation in striated muscle. *Nature (London)* 233:533–538.

Huxley, H.E. (1956) The ultra-structure of striated muscle. *Br. Med. Bull.* 12:171–173

Levin, A., and Wyman, J. (1927) The viscous elastic properties of muscle. *Proc. Roy. Soc. London* 101B:218–243.

Loewy, A.G. (1952) An actinomyosin-like substance from the plasmodium of a *myxomycete*. *J. Cell. Comp. Physiol.* 40:127–156.

Partridge, L.D. (1966) Signal-handling characteristics of load-moving skeletal muscle. *Am. J. Physiol.* 210:1178–1191.

Partridge, L.D. (1967) Intrinsic feedback factors producing inertial compensation in muscle. *Biophys. J.* 7:853–863.

Partridge, L.D., and Benton, L.A. (1981) Muscle, the motor. *Handbook of Physiology, The Nervous System*, Vol. II, Ch. 3. Williams & Wilkins, Baltimore.

Squire, J.M. (ed.)(1990) *Molecular Mechanisms in Muscular Contraction*. CRC Press, Boca Raton, Fla.

Starling, E.H. (1918) *Linacre Lecture on the Law of the Heart*. Longmans Green, New York.

Stein, R.B. (1980) *Nerve and Muscle Membranes, Cells, and Systems*. Plenum, New York.

Weber, E. (1846) Muskelbewegnung. In *Handwörterbuch der Physiologie*. R. Wagner (ed.). Bieweg, Brunswick.

Additional Reading

Basmajian, J.V., and DeLuca, C. (1985) *Muscles Alive and their Functions Revealed by Electromyography*. Williams & Wilkins, Baltimore.

Best, P.M., Kwok, W., and Xu, X. (1991) Calcium channels in excitation-contraction coupling. In *Calcium Channels: Their Properties, Functions, Regulation, and Clinical Relevance*. L. Hurwitz, L.D. Partridge, and J. Leach (eds.). CRC Press, Boca Raton, Fla.

Huxley, A.F. (1977) Looking back on muscle. In *The Pursuit of Nature*. Cambridge University Press, Cambridge.

Johnston, F.D. (1961) The electrocardiogram. In *Pathologic Physiology,* pp. 449–471. Sodeman, W.A. (ed.). Saunders, Philadelphia.

Chapter 15

References

Gilson, A.S., Walker, S.M., and Schoepfle, G.M. (1944) The forms of the isometric twitch and isometric tetanus curves recorded from the frog's sartorius muscle. *J. Cell. Comp. Physiol.* 24:185–199.

Matthews, B.H.C. (1931) The response of a single end organ. *J. Physiol.* 71:64–110.

Nelson, M.E., and Bower, J.M. (1990) Brain maps and parallel computers. *Trends Neurosci.* 13:403–408.

Additional Reading

Adrian, E.D., and Zotterman, Y. (1926) The impulses produced by sensory nerve endings. *J. Physiol.* 61:151–171.

Schmidt, R.F. (1978) *Fundamentals of Sensory Physiology*. Springer-Verlag, New York.

Chapter 16

References

Abraham, R.H., and Shaw, C.D. (1987) Dynamics, a visual introduction. In *Self Organizing Systems,* pp. 543–597. F.E. Yates (ed.). Plenum, New York.

Chua, L.O. (cd.) (1987) Special issue on chaotic systems. *IEEE Trans. Biomed. Eng.* 75:979–1120.

Cotterill, R.M.J. (1988) *Computer Simulation in Brain Science.* Cambridge University Press, Cambridge.

DeFelipe, J., and Jones, E.G. (1988) *Translation of the Writings of Cajal on the Cerebral Cortex*. Oxford University Press, New York.

Devaney, R.L. (1989) *An Introduction to Chaotic Dynamical Systems*. Addison-Wesley, Reading, Mass.

Feldman, A. (1974) Change of muscle length as a consequence of a shift in an equilibrium of muscle load system. *Biofizika* 19:534–538.

Gesell, R. (1939) An electrical study of manifestations of paired motor half centers (excitation, inhibition, precedence of stimulation, adaptation and rebound). *Am. J. Physiol.* 170:702–716.

Getting, P.A. (1989) Emerging principles governing operation of neural networks. *Annu. Rev. Neurosci.* 12:185–204.

Gleick, J. (1987) *Chaos: Making a New Science*. Viking, New York.

Graham, D., and McRuer, D. (1961) *Analysis of Nonlinear Control Systems*. Wiley, New York.

Graham-Brown, T. (1911) Studies in the physiology of the nervous system. IX: Reflex terminal phenomena-rebound-rhythmic rebound and movements of progression. *Q. J. Exp. Physiol.* 4:331–397.

Grillner, S. (1975) On the generation of locomotion in the spinal dogfish. *Exp. Brain Res.* 20:459–470.

Handbook of Physiology, Section 1, Vol. 3 (19xx). Williams & Wilkins, Baltimore.

Heymans, J.F., and Heymans, C. (1927) Sur le tonus respiratoire pneumogastrique et le réflexe de la respiration. *Soc. Biol. C.R.* 94:399–402.

Kandel, E.R., Schwartz, J.H., and Jessell, T.M. (1991) *Principles of Neural Science,* 3rd edition. Elsevier, New York.

Liddell, E.G.T., and Sherrington, C.S. (1924) Reflexes in response to stretch (myotatic reflexes). *Proc. Roy. Soc. London* 96B:212–242.

Lorente de Nó (1933) Vestibulo-ocular reflex arc. *Arch. Neural Psychiat.* 30:245–291.

Marmarales, P.Z., and Marmarales, V.Z. (1978) *Analysis of Physiological Systems, the White Noise Approach.* Plenum, New York.

Merton, P.A. (1953) Speculation on the servo control of movement. In *The Spinal Cord,* pp. 247–260. J.A.B. Grey and G.E.W. Wolstenholme (eds.). Little, Brown, Boston.

Merzenich, M.M., Nelson, R.J., Stryker, M.P., Cynader, M.S., Scheppmann, A., and Zook, J.M. (1984) Somatosensory cortical map change following digit amputation in adult monkeys. *J. Comp. Neurol.* 224:591–605.

Nelson, M.E., and Bower, J.M. (1990) Brain maps and parallel computers. *Trends Neurosci.* 13:403–409.

Netter, F.H. (1986) *The CIBA Collection of Medical Illustrations, Vol 1. The Nervous System.* Ciba Pharmaceutical Co., Summit, N.J.

Pellionisz, A. (1985) The tensorial brain theory in cerebellar modelling. In *Cerebellar Functions.* J. Bloedel, and J. Dichyans (eds.). Springer, Heidelberg.

Shepherd, G.M. (1979) *The Synaptic Organization of the Brain.* Oxford University Press, New York.

Shepherd, G.M. (1988) Locomotion. In *Neurobiology,* 2nd edition. Oxford University Press, New York.

Sherrington, C.S. (1941) *Man on His Nature.* Macmillan, New York.

Shik, M.L., Orlouowski, G.N., and Severin, F.V. (1968) Locomotion of the mesencephalic cat elicited by stimulation of the pyramids. *Biofizika* 13:127–135.

Smith, B. (1988) *New Directions in Dynamic Systems.* London Mathematical Society Lecture Notes Series 127. Cambridge University Press, Cambridge.

Smith, J. (1987) Hind limb locomotion of the spinal cat: Synergistic paths, limb dynamics and novel blends. In *Neurobiology of Vertebrate Locomotion.* S. Grillner, P.S.G. Stein, A. Fossberg, D.G. Stuart, and R.N. Herman (eds.). MacMillan, London.

Wiener, N. (1948) *Cybernetics.* John Wiley, New York.

Suggested Reading

Anderson, J.A., and Rosenfeld, E. (1989) *Neurocomputing: Foundations of Research,* MIT Press, Cambridge, Mass.

Galileo (1632) *Dialogo di Galileo Galilei Linceo.* (English translation, *Dialogue Concerning the Two Chief World Systems.* S. Drake, trans. University of California Press, Berkeley, 1953.)

Korn, G. (1991) *Neural Network Experiments on Personal Computers and Workstations*. MIT Press, Cambridge, Mass.

Livingstone, M.S. (1988) Art, illusion and the visual system. *Sci. Am.* 258:30–37.

Penrose, R. (1989) *The Emperor's New Mind*. Oxford University Press, Oxford.

Poincaré, H. (1899) *Les Méthodes Nouvelles de la Méchanique Céleste*. (Reprint Dover, New York, 1957.)

Chapter 17

References

Barcroft, J. (1928) *Features in the Architecture of Physiological Function*. Cambridge University Press, Cambridge.

Bayliss, W.M., and Starling, E.H. (1899) The movement and innervation of the small intestine. *J. Physiol.* 24:99–143.

Bernard, C. (1878) *Leçons sur les phénomènes de la vie communes aux végétaux*. B. Baillière et Fils, Paris

Cannon, W. (1929) Organization for physiological homeostasis. *Physiol. Rev.* 9:399–431.

Frédéricq, L. (1884) Influence des variations de la composition centésimade l'air sur l'intestite des echanges respiratoires. *Acad. Sci. C.R.* 94: 1124–1125.

Herring, P.T. (1927) *Die Karotissinus reflexe auf Herz und Gefässe*. Steinkopff, Leipzig.

Heymans, J.F., and Heymans, C. (1927) Sur le tonus respiratoire pneumogastrique et le réflexe de la respiration. *Soc. Biol. C.R.* 94:399–402.

Pflüger, E.F.W. (1877) *Der teleologische Mechanik der lebendigen Natur*. M. Cohen, Bonn.

Wiener, N. (1948) *Cybernetics*. Wiley, New York.

Additional Reading

Dörr, F., Schuster, P., and Renger, G. (1983) Energetics and statistical relations. In *Biophysics*. W. Hoppe, W. Lohmann, I.H. Mark, and H. Ziegler (eds.). Springer-Verlag, Berlin.

Fuchs, A.F., Hille, B., Scher, A.M., and Steiner, R. (1989) *Textbook of Physiology*. (Section IX, Circulation; Section XV, Digestion; Section XVI, Metabolism and Energy Regulation) Saunders, Philadelphia.

Gershorn, M.D. (1981) The nervous system of the gut. *Gasteroenterology* 85:929–937.

Gershorn, M.D. (1986) Insights into neural development provided by the bowel. *Fidia Research Foundation Neuroscience Award Lectures*. Liviana Press, Padua.

Gesell, R. (1939) Respiration and its adjustments. *Annu. Rev. Physiol.* 1:185–216.

Gould, J.L., and Gould, C.G. (1988) *The Honey Bee*. Freeman, New York.

Trendelenburg, P. (1917) Physiologische und pharmakolische Versuche über die Dunndarm peristaltik. *Naumyn-Schneedenbergs Arch. Exp. Pathol. Pharmacol.* 81:55–129.

West, J.B. (1991) *Best and Taylor's Physiological Basis of Medical Practice*. (Section 2, Cardiovascular System; Section 6, Gastrointestinal System; Chapter 69, Visceral Control Mechanisms). Williams & Wilkins, Baltimore.

Wiener, N. (1948) *Cybernetics or Control and Communication in the Animal and the Machine*. MIT Press, Cambridge, Mass.

Index

Note: Starred terms are defined in the glossary; figures are indicated by italic *f,* tables by *t,* and appendixes by *a.*

Memory (cont.)
  short-term, 210
  synthetic mechanisms, 219
mepp. *See* Miniature endplate potential*
Merkel's disk response, 95*f*
Meromyosin, 260*f*, 341*f*–342
Metabotropic neurotransmitter receptor,*
  323
Meta control
  empty box, 149
  load change, 141
  rule adjustment, 168
Metazoan, multistage control, 428
Microelectrode, 245*f*
  intracellular, 106
  resistance, 244
Middle ear,* 87*f*, 91
Milner, H.H., 217
Mind, evolution, 137
Miniature endplate potential (mepp), 301*f*, *
Mitochondria, muscle, 340
Mnemonist, 205
Mobility, ionic, 245
Modality,* 63, 83–84*f*
Model
  computer, 13
  defects, 113
  distributed memory, 454*a*–455*f*
  Hodgkin and Huxley, 286
  incomplete representation, 378
  junctional function, 113
  learning, 218
  matrix, 178
  muscle, 135
  network, 222, 389, 394
  omissions defined, 378
  role, 179
  semicircular canals, 384
  serial processing, 179
  state, 395
  tensor, 178
  vector, 178
Modulation, 319, 441
Molecular receptor, 307
Moment of inertia vs. body configuration,
  146
Momentum conservation, 157
Monosynaptic pathway, 105, 363*f*

Monosynaptic reflex,* 114
Morphological memory, 219
Motion, visual stimulus, 81
Motoneuron pool,* 109
Motor
  learning,* 205
  map, 182
  prosthesis, 359
  pulse rate signals, 31*f*
  response, sensory dependence, 124
  unit,* 105, 328, 333
Motor control, 1, 160
  anticipatory adjustments, 149
  autonomic, 129
  centrifugal forces, 157
  complex coordination, 149
  coordinates, 156
  coordination: body, head, eye, 99
  crude globally, refined locally, 141
  defects, 246
  distributed spatially, temporally, 176
  dynamic equilibrium, 153
  excess muscles, 156
  exchange of energy, 139
  feedback insufficient, 142
  force, 132
  frequency range, voluntary, 102
  genetic basis, 156
  good enough, 156
  gravity, 143
  heat, 131
  imperfect, 157
  joint stabilization, 142
  kinematic, 135
  kinetic, 136
  learned patterns, 156
  load, 136–137
  low-level contraction, 134
  mechanical limits, 144
  meta control, 141
  multiple joint, 156
  nonlinearities, 160
  phoneme, 134
  posture basis, 142
  prosthetic, 235
  relative, 159
  robotics study, 154
  sensory, 76*f*, 187